THE HISTORY AND GEOGRAPHY OF DISEASES

THE HISTORY AND GEOGRAPHY OF DISEASES

BY FOLKE HENSCHEN

TRANSLATED BY
JOAN TATE

A SEYMOUR LAWRENCE BOOK
DELACORTE PRESS/NEW YORK

Originally published in Swedish
by Albert Bonniers Förlag
under the title *Sjukdomarnas Historia och
geografi*

© Folke Henschen 1962

English translation copyright © 1966
by Longmans, Green and Co. Ltd.

Library of Congress catalog card number: 67-13149

Manufactured in the United States of America

First American edition

Contents

Illustrations

Preface to the Swedish edition

One of the many branches of pathology, historico-geographical pathology has for more than thirty years been the object of my special interest—the study of the origins, historical development, geographical boundaries and demography of diseases, in times past as well as in our own day. I was present when the International Society for Geographical Pathology was formed in Geneva in 1931 and am probably the only surviving founder-member. Several years later in 1934 I gave in *Några blad ur sjukdomarnas historia och geografi* ('Some pages from the history and geography of diseases') a brief account of what was then known. This book has now been out of print for twenty-five years and much has changed since then. The Second World War enormously advanced the knowledge of the distribution of diseases, especially in tropical and sub-tropical parts of the world where warfare made the investigation and prevention of many diseases a matter of imperative necessity. At the same time our knowledge of the causes of diseases and other contributory conditions which favour or counteract their outbreak and continued existence, has both broadened and deepened. The account I gave in 1934 must now, therefore, be said to be quite obsolete; a new modern account of the causes, origins and historical development of diseases, their geographical distribution and frequency within different population groups, whether distinguished by race, religion, occupation or social and hygienic standards, can be said to be most timely. This book is much more than a revised edition of the earlier one. It is essentially a new book. Some of the illustrations have been retained from the 1934 edition, but most are new.

I have tried to make this account sufficiently up-to-date and abundant in scientific facts for it to be profitably read by doctors, but at the same time simple and full enough of cultural and historical information also to interest a wider readership.

FOLKE HENSCHEN

THE HISTORY AND GEOGRAPHY OF DISEASES

Introduction

Diseases are not unchanging phenomena. Their appearance and character are subject to historical development and varying geographical and demographical conditions of population. Some diseases seem able to disappear; other new ones to appear. Infectious diseases, which only one or two generations ago formed the largest group in our statistics on morbidity and mortality, have been driven back by the advance of medicine. Instead two other groups of diseases, cardio-vascular diseases and tumours, have taken the first place, a development which is partly connected with a rising average expectation of life. However, this revolution affects, above all, North America and many of the countries of Europe. But even in those countries whose populations form the great majority of the world's inhabitants, a development in the same direction has occurred. The overall picture of diseases within one country or community, which one can call the 'disease-panorama', varies then from time to time, from country to country, and from town to town.

Pathology is the study of diseases, their causes and forms, both morbid changes in organs as well as functional disturbances in the diseased organism, whether in a human being or an animal. The word pathology comes from the Greek word *pathos* which means both passion and suffering.

The object of historico-geographical pathology is to investigate the origins of diseases, their occurrence in the past and their geographical distribution among people and animals at the present. This branch of pathology also investigates the demography of diseases, i.e. their appearance and frequency within different population groups, separated from one another by race, religion or culture, by social, economic or hygienic standards, by profession or occupation, or in any other respect. Historical and geographical pathology sheds considerable light on the problem of the conditional causes of diseases, and likewise illuminates the significance of preventive, prophylactic measures and different methods of medical treatment. This branch of pathology is consequently not a specialist branch, but a method, a way of approaching the innumerable problems within pathology which have yet to be solved.

Geographical pathology has an ancient ancestry. In the classics there is the famous chapter in Hippocrates, 'περὶ ἀέρων ὑδάτων τόπων', 'on air, water and place of residence', in which 'the father of medicine' shows how environment makes its impression on human beings and their diseases. The texts which bear Hippocrates' name have long been the subject of critical examination, with the result that not one of the many works named after him can with complete certainty be attributed personally to Hippocrates. The above-mentioned chapter is said to have been written about 425 B.C. and there is reason to believe that the author of it had visited both South Russia and the Nile Valley. These writings, *Corpus Hippocraticum*, will always stand as a monument to the period of human civilisation when medicine was freed from religion and became a science.

But documents which are much older than the *Hippocratic Collection*, Egyptian papyri, the Bible, India's holy scripts and the annals of China, contain short accounts of the occurrence of diseases, as do Herodotus and Plutarch. To Thucydides and Procopius we owe a debt of gratitude for the description of some of the epidemics of the ancient world. Mediaeval travellers like Marco Polo and Ibn Batuta occasionally recorded observations on diseases in the countries they visited. But the beginnings of historico-geographical pathology are first found in the eighteenth century with, for example, Linnaeus, who at his inaugural lecture as Professor of Medicine at Uppsala University in 1741 emphasised the importance of travel in Sweden to anyone who wished to find the causes of disease. I shall return to this remarkable lecture later. Among northern scientists who later studied similar problems must here be named the Finn Ilmoni, who in his *A History of Diseases of the North* (1846–53) gave an account of the knowledge of that time. A number of German and French works of the eighteenth and nineteenth centuries—by Finke, Schnurrer, Mühry, Boudin and Lombard—must be mentioned in passing. They are all predecessors to the great and justly praised standard work in this field, A. Hirsch's *Handbook of geographical and historical pathology* (3 vols, London 1883–86). As a result of the rapid development of medicine since the 1880s, this is now naturally in many respects out of date, but its abundance of valuable detail is imposing.

A modern scientific work of geographical pathology, however, has not been possible until this century. The last white patches on the map have vanished, great distances no longer matter, and all parts of the world have become more closely linked, commercially, politically and culturally. Both world wars spurred on an intensive investigation of social, hygienic and medical conditions in countries that had been largely unknown. As a result a huge amount of previously little-known material became available and has been made use of in the rapidly expanding micro-biological and medical field of research. Many countries have become sanitated and therefore the disease-panorama has undergone fundamental changes. All this must be regarded as a happy consequence of the international complications of the last decades and a reward for labours in research in the different fields of medicine.

It should perhaps be stated that the objectives of historico-geographical pathology are quite different from those mentioned when one talks of the history of man, the geographical distribution of animals or plants, or the appearance of a certain mineral. Diseases are not living entities as man occasionally imagined in earlier times, nor concrete phenomena which can be thought to exist freely without relation to human beings. A disease is in itself an abstraction; in fact, there are only diseased people. One can only establish the elements and species of disease by vigilant observation and experience, through the study of a number of cases. Not even in those cases where one can directly indicate the cause of the disease, for instance a parasite which can perhaps even be seen by the naked eye, is one entitled to put an equals sign between the distribution of the disease and the appearance of the parasite, for the latter is only *one* of the factors entering into the pathogenesis of the actual disease.

Historico-geographical pathology is a border region between pathology on the one hand and history, geography and demography on the other. Often doctors, hygienists, zoologists and botanists, historians, geographers, geologists, anthropologists, ethnographers, sociologists and statisticians must co-operate to bring in a good harvest from this large and fruitful field, to utilise every possibility and to avoid mistakes. In this field of research with its world-wide programme, international co-operation is more than ever necessary; this necessity has found expression in the 'International Society for Geographical Pathology' (Geneva, 1931). The World Health Organisation (WHO) gives information on many diseases in its *Annual Epidemiological and Vital Statistics* and monthly *Epidemiological and Vital Statistics Reports*. Maps are needed clearly to demonstrate geographical-pathological conditions and the best of these are found in the great work *Global Epidemiology* and in Jusatz's fine atlas.

3

Historical pathology has many points of contact with the history of medicine but should not be confused with it. The history of medicine considers the development of the art of healing from ancient times and also gives an account of the lives of great doctors. The theme of historical pathology is the appearance of diseases in ancient and modern times.

The history of disease stretches very far back in time, for as long as man has existed he has been tormented by disease. If one also includes animal diseases, then one must take the history of disease back to early pre-history, measured in geological periods of time. This branch of pathology is called palaeopathology. How late one should talk of palaeopathology is perhaps a matter of taste; many people use the expression for changes in disease of a relatively recent period, for instance in referring to the diseases of the Indians during the pre-Columbian period in the New World. Historical pathology is not, however, interested only in diseases of eras long since vanished, but also in the nutritional disturbances and the new disease-panorama which during and after both world wars appeared in the many belligerent countries as well as in various neutral countries afflicted with food-supply crises.

The records of historical pathology fall into three different categories of somewhat different scientific value: written records, representations and nature's own records.

1. Written records, whether accounts of variations in diseases or descriptions of epidemics, are often extremely subjective and more or less coloured by prevailing medical trends of thought or by lay prejudice and beliefs. Not infrequently the descriptions are obscure or ambiguous, and in some cases the meanings of the symbols are obscure and incomprehensible, as in some of the Egyptian papyri which otherwise give us accurate information on diseases in Pharaonic times. Accounts of epidemics, such as the famous plague in Athens during the Peloponnesian War, are often so generalised and hard to interpret that they give rise to endless disputes. Even when one comes to the diseases of the late Middle Ages and the Renaissance, the descriptions are often so summary, obscure and lacking in clarity that one cannot interpret them. The best example is the early history of syphilis.

2. Representations of diseased conditions, whether drawings, paintings or models, can be very valuable. In the art of ancient Egypt a great many representations of diseases and deformities have

4

been found, and also in the realistic pottery of ancient Peru which often portrays diseases, deformities and mutilations. But even these must be used critically. They are not infrequently diagrammatical, subjective and founded on misapprehensions which make possible strongly divergent interpretations.

3. In contrast to the above, the lesions created by nature itself are absolutely reliable but unfortunately not always easy to interpret and often of uncertain origin. So it mostly comes down to the pathology of hard tissues, morbid changes in bones and teeth, which often do not allow any more than general conclusions about the nature of the disease. Occasionally stone formations in the bladder and gall bladder are found and also calcified foci of pus, tuberculous soft tissue or tumours. The pathology of soft tissues is really only possible in the case of the mummies of ancient Egypt and pre-Hispanic Peru. There, with suitable methods, one can disclose a great deal of disease changes in the internal organs—arteriosclerosis, lung and pleural sac changes, calcified lymph nodes, enlarged spleens, growths in the abdominal cavity, parasite eggs and even bacteria. Research into blood groups too can produce results from archaeological material, as has been recently shown by one of the representatives of palaeoserology, Madeleine Smith. At the larger and scientific excavations of human remains, as in the great Egyptian necropolises or Europe's many churchyards and burial grounds, statistical and genealogical calculations can also be carried out—of hereditary skeletal types and deviations from the norm, of the occurrence of joint and spinal lesions of degenerative type, of the frequency of dental diseases, of child mortality and of the then composition of the population (Gejvall).

Geographical pathology, which is closely allied to historical pathology, during the last thirty years has developed to an incredible extent. However, one must here emphasise the importance of criticism and sufficient statistical foundations for general opinions on the distribution of a disease and its frequency in a certain country. Unfortunately in some recent publications a number of accounts of the occurrence of diseases have been published without due attention to statistics and exact methods of investigation. A clinical and pathological-anatomical terminology must be formed in accordance with international regulations. Every report on the incidence of a certain disease should always be accompanied by the number of observations on which it is founded, further reports on the division

5

of age-groups, on the relative number of men to women, on the division of those cases between rural and urban districts, on different races and religions should these apply, on occupations and social groups and finally definite figures on morbidity and mortality rates. In certain cases it is also necessary to have adequate information about the number and quality of hospitals, on the extent of the population's willingness to co-operate (hospital-phobia) and on the possibilities of receiving hospital treatment as well as the availability of doctors in general. In certain countries, for different reasons, many more men than women go into hospital. When it finally comes to the diagnosis, the degree of reliability should always be given, i.e. whether the diagnosis is from a post-mortem (autopsy), from a microscopic investigation of samples from a living person (biopsy), purely clinical, at a hospital, by a private practitioner or wherever it may be given.

The demands one should make on statistics and other information in relation to the occurrence of a disease are thus substantial, and unfortunately they are seldom fulfilled. Often the real differences between two periods of time or two towns in different countries are not so great as one is perhaps inclined to think if one just reads what is stated as fact. As evidence of how lively the interest is in geographical pathology, it can be mentioned that under the auspices of the World Health Organisation there has been issued a special handbook (by Doll) on the methods to be used, in which the importance of the necessary criticism is fittingly emphasised.

The pathogenic factors to be considered in historico-geographical pathology are of course generally the same as in pathology. It should be stressed, though, that certain conditions are perhaps not understood or appreciated to the full if one is not sufficiently aware of the predominating endogenous (internal) or exogenous (external) factors, at that point in time or in that place, and therefore does not understand their significance. For this reason there follows here a brief account of pathogenic matters which are especially important in historico-geographical pathology.

Hereditary, constitutional factors in some ways occupy a special position in geographical pathology. Morbid hereditary factors and their eventual consequences, hereditary diseases, are mainly independent of outward influences or dependent on them only to a limited extent. Hereditary tendencies follow the carrier and his descendants wherever they go; for instance if they move from Sweden to America.

In most of Europe and especially in the United States the mingling
of different hereditary tendencies has now advanced so far that it is
hardly possible to carry out a study of the geography of hereditary
diseases. However, in Scandinavia, in certain parts of Switzerland
and Italy and in the Balkans—not to mention many of the remoter
parts of the world—the population until the last generation has
in many places remained so stable, living in, geographically speaking,
more or less isolated areas, where they have been limited in marriage
to a small circle, that a geographical survey of hereditary diseases has
been and still is possible. (And even isolation of a religious and
social nature is sometimes of great significance.) For such family
investigations, however, something else is required which is available
only in exceptional cases—namely good archives which go far back
in time. These irreplaceable documents have unfortunately been
destroyed in many countries, the Scandinavian countries generally
constituting an exception in this matter. In primitive communities
there is usually little possibility of acquiring reliable information
about family circumstances and diseases of earlier generations.

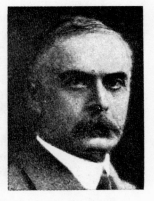

Karl Landsteiner, the dis-
coverer of human blood
groups, b. in Austria 1868,
Professor in Vienna and
later in USA, awarded
Nobel Prize for Medicine
in 1930, d. in USA 1943.
His discovery of blood
groups (Menschliche Blut-
gruppen, *1900*) *opened*
an immense and valuable
field of research.

Hereditary characteristics include, as we know, the blood groups,
as well as a number of little-known anthropological-genetic conditions such as the ability to sense the smell of prussic acid in a
weak solution or the bitter taste of phenolthiocarbamide. The
significance to pathology of research into blood groups is still in its
early stages; what is known will be set out under the respective
diseases. About the significance of the other hereditary characteristics we know extremely little.

Among the exogenous, environmental pathogenic factors are

several which occupy little space in current text-books on pathology and internal medicine and perhaps in the public eye, but which are of considerable significance to geographical pathology. These are factors of environment which change violently from time to time, from place to place, from country to country, and occasionally can even be of decisive significance. Among them are the geology and chemical composition of the soil and the surface of the earth and the composition of water, especially the quality of drinking water. Of these factors, whose importance in the pre-bacteriological era was considerably overrated, very little factual knowledge exists. We still know all too little of the significance of micro- or trace-elements in our food and drink. There has been a renewed interest in water with the research into the effect of fluoride on the teeth; the cause of goitre is still even today only partly realised and perhaps the solution lies in conditions which are now understood.

With geography and geology one must consider the altitude conditions of the surface of the earth. Human beings who permanently work at great heights are exposed to strong rays from the sun and to other rays. The temperature there is often low, the air pressure constantly low, and most important of all, the inhabitants live in a perpetual shortage of oxygen. The most complete example of these conditions and their significance is found in the South American Andes; we shall return to them later.

It is an ancient conclusion that climatic conditions influence the state of health of more sensitive people, but only in latter years has it been possible to investigate more deeply the complex nature of the weather and its influence on the human organism. Medical meteorology, which studies the climate's influence on biological reactions, sensitivity to climatic conditions and the climate and its fluctuations as a cause of disease, has grown into a special branch of research. A survey of these and related problems can be found in Hellpach's book *Geopsyche* amongst others.

Some elementary medical concepts

When accounting for the incidence of diseases, their variations and significance, their presence in the past and today, it is necessary to explain briefly several medical concepts and anthropological questions with which we shall be concerned in what is to follow.

Pathology is the study of disease; in this context the Greek word *pathos* means suffering, disease. To explain what is meant by

8

'disease' in a few words is not so easy as one might think. Perhaps it is easier to define its opposite, health. In Hippocratic medicine, from which all later scientific medicine is descended, health is a state of equilibrium, a state in which all the organs of the body function in perfect harmony, adapting themselves to each other and to the outer world and its stresses. One would not be far wrong if one simply said that disease is a disturbance of this harmony, but the concept of disease can perhaps be best defined as a disturbance of this equilibrium, this balance, under the influence of abnormal internal and external conditions, i.e. as a failure of adaptability. A person can be ill without feeling ill, because the disease is subjectively latent, i.e. does not show any noticeable symptoms, as for instance in an early cancer, or because the person concerned finds himself in such a condition that he does not notice the disturbance. But the opposite also not infrequently occurs: one can have a strong sense of not feeling well although not even the most searching examination can detect any disturbance; it is not necessarily a case of an imaginary illness.

In general a disease is not something static, at a standstill, but rather a series of reactions within the cells, tissues and organs of the organism, which follow on each other and have an effect on each other. These reactions succeed one another with a greater or lesser degree of rapidity.

However, pathology does not only concern itself with the abnormal phenomena and manifestations of life which we usually call diseases. It is also concerned with other deviations from the normal which, in everyday speech at least, are not regarded as diseases: for example the remaining consequences of disease, like atrophy, withering and paralysis after polio, or certain deformities; a person with a hare-lip, webbed fingers or a birth-mark is not diseased in the usual meaning of the word.

The causes of diseases are of many and varied kinds. Often the cause is so self-evident that any further explanation is unnecessary, but in most cases the cause or causes, as everyone knows, are by no means so obvious or easily understood. Our present-day understanding of the causes of diseases has grown from the methods of observation used in the past. Most of us no longer believe that diseases are due to the evil eye or possession by evil spirits, as is so often stated in the Bible, but this ancient medical way of looking at diseases as demonic can be said to survive, in a modern form, in

9

today's widespread fear of bacteria, the fear of small invisible dangerous beings. Nor do we connect disease with the position of the planets, or earthquakes and other natural disasters, or regard them as punishments from God for offences against His commandments and a sinful life.

Hippocratic medicine taught that diseases were due to an incorrect mixing of the '*humores*', the four body fluids or cardinal juices. This ancient method of observation, the humoral-pathological method, which was further developed by the doctors of ancient times, notably Galen (A.D. 129–*c*. 199), dominated medicine for thousands of years. In the middle of the last century it was followed by another system, the cellular-pathological system. Disease came to be regarded as a disturbance in the life of the cell, tissue or organ. Cellular pathology, which was essentially created by Virchow, meant an incomparable step forward in medicine, but to present-day eyes it seems in many respects very one-sided.

The great bacteriological discoveries of the latter part of the nineteenth century similarly led to imbalance in the understanding of the causes of diseases; the newly discovered microbes were considered the overriding cause of nearly all diseases.

Medical research has, however, revealed that in most cases diseases are not the result of one single active harmful factor, e.g. a certain pathogenic microbe, but that usually it takes several, perhaps a whole set of contributing factors for a disease of a definite type to manifest itself. Occasionally a whole constellation of different causal momenta is present, perhaps acting in separate directions, though usually one of them is dominant.

Among all the many different factors which can influence the occurrence of a disease, one can in general distinguish two principal groups: internal or endogenous factors which lie hidden in the person's individuality, his inherited constitution and his perhaps more fortuitous condition and disposition, and the external or exogenous factors which assert themselves from the outer world, surroundings and environment. One can therefore in general distinguish between internal and external causes of diseases, between endogenous and exogenous pathogenic factors.

Internal causes of disease

Experience shows that if a number of individuals is exposed to the influence of an exogenous causal factor, for example to rapid chilling, poisoning, bacterial or virus infection, then they react in highly different ways: some are perhaps not affected at all, others insignificantly, and others react very strongly or even with such a severe illness that death follows. One can denote this as varying individual predisposition. Some individuals lack predisposition, are insusceptible or immune, others are in a greater or lesser degree predisposed. No one is exactly the same.

Predisposition can be of a varying nature. It can be the expression of an inherited characteristic which is confined to the individual, the family or the population, which the individual retains all his life and which is then called constitution. The concept of constitution is in this case closely tied to the concept of heredity and the constitution becomes the sum of all the individual physical and psychological characteristics which depend on heredity and are fixed in genetic types.

However, the individual, from the moment of the sperm's union with the ovum right up to his death, becomes exposed to an uninterrupted series of influences from his environment which to a great extent affect and certainly are capable of changing his constitutional character. Already in the womb these are in evidence: for instance, if the mother during pregnancy falls victim to German measles or syphilis, or to today's thalidomide. Diseases, even if apparently insignificant, perhaps hardly observed, such as a slight primary tuberculous infection in childhood, can have the greatest influence on the individual's reaction and powers of resistance later on. Economic, social and hygienic conditions, especially during the growing years, bad habits in food and drink, nutrition, too hard a struggle for existence, all these often become of radical importance; they can reshape both body and soul, and make their impression on the whole individual and his disposition. Individual condition, disposition, is thus not something constant but dependent on significant variations.

The old observation that individuals with a certain affinity, for instance a single race or a population, are similar to one another physically and that one can arrange at least some of them by body structure into certain categories or types, led Hippocratic medicine to the formulation of two constitutional types: *habitus phthisicus*, the tall, flat-chested, long-necked, thin type with a disposition to phthisis, consumption; and *habitus apoplecticus*, the shorter, squatter, short-necked, fatter type with a disposition to apoplexy, stroke.

Modern constitutional research has taken up the question of body structure with renewed interest and has set up new types which only in some respects coincide with the ancient Hippocratic ones.

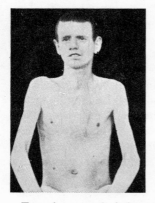

Young man with leptosome body type of asthenic build (after Kretschmer, Korperbau und Charakter, 1929).

French research defines four types, using self-explanatory terminology: *respiratorius*, *cerebralis*, *muscularis* and *digestivus*. Tandler differentiates between a hypotonic type, with low blood pressure, and a hypertonic, with high blood pressure. The types coincide on the whole with the old type *phthisicus* and *apoplecticus*. Best known is Kretschmer's division into two extreme main types, a leptosome, tall, slim type, and a pyknic, shorter, thick-set, squat type, as well as a type to one side of them, an athletic, muscular type. It should be stated here that this division is carried out in men and is more difficult to apply to women and to some young leptosome individuals who with age seem to become more of a pyknic type. Despite criticism and many weaknesses and difficulties in application, this division of types of constitution has shown itself highly convenient and valuable. Kretschmer has also carried out systematic investigations into the physical and psychical constitution of human beings under normal and pathological conditions. The psychophysical types or units which he set out in this way were in fact known in outline to Hellenic doctors and philosophers. Who is not reminded here of Shakespeare's words put into the mouth of Caesar: 'Let me have men about me that are fat; sleek-headed men and such as sleep o'nights.'

Research has gone further: there is reason to connect body types with a number of more or less obvious constitutional metabolic and organic diseases, such as arteriosclerosis, arcus senilis (literally 'old man's eye arc'), hypertension (high blood pressure), diabetes, gout, adiposity and gallstones, and diseases of the skeleton and joints. These diseases, which are important from the geographical and anthropological point of view, will be dealt with later.

A step further into constitutional research and anthropology was taken with Landsteiner's discovery of blood groups and isohaemo-agglutination, i.e. the condition in which certain people's red blood cells are agglutinated or bound together in serum from certain other people. This characteristic of blood cells and serum belongs to the individual's genotype which remains unchangeable throughout his life, and permits a classification of individuals into four main groups (by the ABO-system) according to the presence of one or both of the factors which are called A and B, or the absence of both, which is called O. By subdividing the four groups in the ABO-system the classification can be made more elaborate but this would take too long to go into further here.

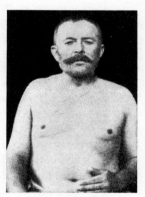

Man of about 50 with pyknic body type (after Kretschmer, 1929).

Constitutional research can hardly be said to be of great interest to historico-geographical pathology if it cannot be shown that the distinguishing characteristics of the individual constitution are present in a great number of individuals of the same race or population and within a geographical area which has been inhabited by this population for a long time, perhaps hundreds or thousands of years.

As long as we are only concerned with the three main great races —in everyday speech, black, white and yellow—who are sharply distinct from each other, who have long inhabited different parts of the world's surface where they are still present in reasonably pure conditions, then the bodily and spiritual differences are so obvious that it is unnecessary to mention them here. External dissimilarities in physique, skin and colour of the eyes correspond to internal dissimilarities, in the skeleton, muscular system and internal organs, and amongst the latter in the brain and its weight and structure. The ancient Egyptian had, in relation to size of body, a heavier brain than the modern European; the same applies to the Chinese whose brain shows certain deviations from the Westerner's. The negro brain is also of a certain type. Such comparative investigations are extremely lengthy, for the study of racial differences within the brain must be based on a very large number of investigations. Even the endocrine organs yield certain racial differences which would explain certain psychical differences and racial predispositions to diseases.

Within the white race one can without difficulty differentiate between certain relatively pure main types. In large areas of Europe, however, and even more so in North America, the mixture of these main groups is now so great that it is generally extremely hazardous to carry out a physico-anthropological classification of types. Despite all the difficulties it is still of some interest to investigate statistically how the above-mentioned different constitutional types are distributed within different populations and how the classification turns out proportionately. Certain populations seem to be tolerably unified as regards constitutional type, such as the Eskimoes who show a preponderance of the French *typus digestivus* (see p. 12). The difficulties of such research are great and much depends on the investigator's acuteness and objectivity. Here earlier research into race has left a great deal to be desired. A well-known responsible researcher in a study of the different peoples of Germany has found the following proportional values in the classification of anthropological types in the northern, central and southern parts of the country. The agreement between the constitutional types and the anthropological types is remarkable and seems even to correspond with the divisions of psychical and psychiatric types within Germany.

	Constitutional type Leptosome and muscular	Pyknic	Anthropological type 'Nordic'	'Alpine'
North Germany	88	12	96	4
Central Germany	70	30	82	15
South Germany	65	35	45	55

In research into blood groups a great many interesting results have been achieved; here exact methods of investigation and the use of modern statistics can give exact results, though these are not always easy to interpret. It has been shown that different human races, and different populations in a section of the world, even in a single country, show notable and constant differences as regards proportional classification into the four groups in the ABO-system and its sub-divisions; this Beckman has demonstrated, especially in connection with Sweden. The gypsies in Hungary are a good example of how constant is the proportional division of blood groups. Despite the fact that they have lived for many hundreds of years in what is for them an alien climate and among alien people, their blood groupings do not seem to have undergone any changes. They still show a remarkable correspondence with those of certain Indian population groups, the inhabitants of the gypsies' original country.

What do these more or less prominent constitutional differences, which one can show in different main races and populations, mean to the origin of diseases? Have race and attachment to a certain population any significance as commanding factors? These questions are naturally of considerable interest to geographical pathology.

From the study of earlier literature on this subject one easily gains the impression that race and attachment to a population would play an exceedingly large role in the appearance of diseases of very different kinds. A critical look at the facts, however, shows that it is extremely difficult to reach any clear conclusion. A great mistake has been made in the past in underrating the significance of environment in all its forms. Insufficient attention has been paid to the fact that the different races and populations have lived and are living under utterly different conditions as regards climate, food and drink, clothing, living habits, occupation, hygiene and past and present diseases. This applies too to population groups living side by side which though they live in the same geographical area, are differentiated in other respects, for instance the three groups living in South Africa, whites, Indians and negroes. Many other examples could be given in which religious, social, economic, hygienic and other differences must be of great significance to the species and frequency of diseases.

The geographical classification of certain infectious diseases and especially the absence of such diseases in distant islands and isolated land areas were often in the past taken to show a deficient constitution, to show immunity in the inhabitants. However, this is nearly always a misapprehension which has had to be corrected. The spread of infectious diseases in the world cannot generally be explained by a hereditary and greatly variable immunity or disposition in different populations; and there are other factors which are decisive. The problem of whether there exists any disposition, or immunity, in a particular race or population can only be solved when two or more races, or population groups, live side by side in contact with each other and under as similar circumstances as possible, without any mixing of blood. One might cite the examples of Europeans, Indians and Africans in South Africa, and possibly Jews and non-Jews in North Africa and North America, or whites and coloureds in America, but none of these examples entirely fulfils the above conditions.

Negroes, during the time they have lived in North America, have adapted themselves to the climate and a sizeable number of them live in the sub-arctic parts of Canada. Certain American writers maintain that as regards resistance to infectious diseases in the USA, one can make three population categories: the Jews, who are said to be the most resistant, the descendants of northern Europeans, who take a central position, and the Negroes who are the least resistant. In the white population, gastro-intestinal diseases predominate with endocrine and nervous disturbances, and in the negro population the infectious diseases, especially lung diseases. To what extent this information can be completely credited would be hazardous to say; it seems as if many of these differences in disposition and immunity would be more easily explained by differences in ways of life, occupation and profession, hygiene, caution and inclination to seek timely medical advice, as well as by other psychological reasons. The question of predisposition to cancer and the incidence of cancer within different races and population groups will be dealt with later.

The abundant information on predisposition and immunity to cosmopolitan infectious diseases like tuberculosis, leprosy, measles, rheumatic diseases, alveolar pyorrhoea (chronic infection round the roots of the teeth) and others should therefore be received with some discrimination. The same applies to the information on tropical diseases, towards which whites in certain cases are said to be more predisposed than coloureds. In general coloureds and whites live in the tropics under conditions altogether too dissimilar for a simple statistical comparison to be of any value in solving this problem. The native population is fully acclimatised and above all it has almost certainly since childhood built up an immunity against many infectious diseases with which the whites have had no contact. On the other hand the whites' more rational clothing and hygiene form a protection which the bare-footed and extremely lightly clad natives usually lack. I have reason to return to these matters later on.

In certain cases it is precisely such a difference in social and perhaps intellectual standards which explains different statistics for different groups, which may easily be taken as signs of different dispositions. Elephantiasis in North Africa, caused by guinea worm, is most common in negroes, less common among Arabs and seldom found among Jews.

The further research goes, the more likely it will be that the earlier presumed differences as regards predisposition and immunity between different races and populations in fact exist only to a very limited extent. Heine, a student of the pathology of China, maintains that with continued research into diseases there, one will find that the differences between China and the West are not due at all to race but to environmental factors. In fact the different human races are probably much more closely related, as regards disposition and immunity, than, for instance, the different groups of rodents, mice, rats, guinea-pigs and rabbits, which we use in our laboratories and in which different species show clear differences in predisposition and immunity.

External causes of disease

The understanding of environment as a factor which affects human beings and is also of significance to the incidence of disease, is again found, as was intimated before, in the writings which bear the name of Hippocrates, in the famous chapter 'On Air, Water and Place of Residence':

He who wishes to study the art of healing must first and foremost observe the seasons and the influence each and every one of them exercises. . . . And further he shall take note of the warm and cold winds. . . . So should he also consider the properties of the water. . . . The healer shall thoroughly take the situation into consideration [and also] the soil, whether it is without trees and lacks water, or is well wooded and abundant with water, whether the place lies in a suffocatingly hot valley or is high and cool. Also the way of life which most pleases the inhabitants; he should pay attention as to whether they are given to wine, good living and effeminacy, or are lovers of bodily exercises, industrious, have good appetites and are sober.

Hippocrates goes on to more specifically geographical and anthropological matters, graphically describing European and Asiatic peoples whom he had personally known or had heard spoken of, and he sums up his experience with the following words:

> One will mostly find that man's outward form and character is suited to the nature of the country. Namely where the soil is rich, soft and well watered, so that the water is warm in the summer and cold in the winter, and also the conditions of the seasons are favourable, there the people are also fleshy, not very mobile, damp, discomforted by hardship, and usually not richly endowed. Greed and drowsiness are common among them, in arts and crafts they are clumsy, without finesse and subtlety. . . . Where the soil is bare, lacking water and wild, subdued by the cold in winter or baked by the sun, there one finds dry and slim people, mobile, energetic and with a strong growth of hair. In such natures one comes across a lively desire for activity, and alertness, but also self-awareness and stubbornness in customs and inclinations; in their character lies more defiance than meekness, in arts and crafts one finds with them more subtlety and wisdom, in warfare more skill than in others. Yes, even all else that the earth produces is in accordance with the earth's own natural quality.

This Hippocratic teaching on the influence of environment on people undoubtedly contains a great deal of truth. It has certainly not lacked opponents, for example Hume, who in the eighteenth century categorically disputed the influence of environment on the national character. The influence that 'air, water and place of residence' exercises on human beings is far too obvious to be ignored and in our times a whole literature has arisen which, with the help of all the resources of natural science and medicine, seeks to penetrate into the geophysical and geopsychical phenomena surrounding nature's influence on body and soul and health's dependence on atmospheric, climatic and geological conditions.

Hellpach has closely studied the influence of weather, climate, soil and landscape on the spiritual life of man. He has compared data on the optimal air temperature for physical and mental work and has analysed different peoples' ability to acclimatise themselves to alien climates. He considers it proved that negroes become used to a sub-arctic climate much more easily than whites do to a tropical one; worst off, he says, are 'the blond races' (i.e. blond individuals), whose psychophysical habitus is violently reversed in a tropical climate. He reports what is known on 'spiritual abnormisation through climate', i.e. neuroses and psychoses provoked by climatic conditions—'*Tropenkoller*', polar depression (Lapp-disease) and highland neuroses, etc.

Even co-operation between meteorology and medicine has begun to bear fruit. It has been shown that the so-called weather diseases should not be interpreted as merely disturbances provoked by meteorological elements; for symptoms of disease to appear, complete 'accord' of meteorological factors is demanded as well as an especially receptive individual, preferably a person with a labile neuro-vascular system, who lacks the capacity for normal adaptation.

The influence of weather-changes is presumably explained by the variations which then enter into the composition of the air and which have an effect on the organism, presumably via the vegetative nervous system. Of very great interest are the investigations which have been made into the physiological effect of the transition from the dark to the light seasons in northern countries on both human beings and animals—'the biological spring' or 'the hormonal crisis of spring', the thyroid gland's maximum of iodine in March, the increase of psychoses and suicide and the high rates of mortality during the spring months. An interesting object of study recently has been the conditions of deer and their antlers and the connection between the increase of light, the growth of the antlers and the deer's rutting season.

As examples of diseases directly provoked by geographical factors one can name mountain sickness at great heights and the not uncommon eye afflictions in arctic regions provoked by the strong reflections of light from the snow.

The above are merely indications, and one can find an exhaustive investigation in Sorre's *Les fondements de la géographie humaine* (1947).

The importance of the geographical, climatic and other conditions which have been briefly mentioned as external causes of diseases must not be overrated. They fade into insignificance when compared with a whole series of other external pathogenic factors of many varying kinds: inadequate supplies of water, food, salts and vitamins, warmth and cold, electricity, rays of different kinds, changes in air pressure, mechanical factors, intoxicants, endocrine disturbances, as well as, first and last, parasites from the plant and animal kingdom.

These various factors can be active by themselves or in more or less involved combinations. In many cases, perhaps in most, and especially as regards the causes of parasitic diseases, the exogenous factors combine in one way or another with the endogenous. The individual's constitutional pattern, his permanent or fortuitous disposition, earlier contracted infectious diseases, often assert themselves in one way or another, so that the effect of the irritation, the entry of the infection, its course and its termination in actual fact are decided by the individual kind of person. There is no reason here to go further into the different possible combinations of external and internal factors which can be present.

However, a large section of these external pathogenic factors, however significant they may be in themselves, are of no particular interest from the geographic-pathological point of view. They are too alike and too constantly active over the whole of the inhabited world. Only those which are significant from a historico-geographical point of view will be duly considered in the following.

The historical role of diseases

For anyone who has studied at all the history of diseases and historical pathology, a perspective of historical events is opened of which the greater part seems to be more or less alien to the usual humanistic slant of historical research, or at least not to meet the appreciation it deserves. It is understandable that historians usually do not think medically. Their interest is first captured by the repeated growth of states in the course of history, their rise and fall, their religions and ideologies, their leaders, mild elders, noble tyrants or inhuman despots. For historians such themes as justice, the demand for freedom, the destructive instinct, productivity, social and economic conditions and the general development of civilisation have been of paramount importance. But powerful historical factors (and grim rulers) like crop failure, famine and in particular the great epidemics have in general hardly attracted interest to the degree they deserve. Infectious diseases, those *'compagnes fatales et constantes de notre vie'* (Nicolle), have probably been the most dangerous enemies of mankind, much more so than war and mass murder. When one studies the constant epidemics of the past and the deficiency diseases on land and at sea, one realises that the whole of civilisation could have succumbed, and one is constantly surprised that mankind has survived. But it has done so by the strength of a powerful capacity for regeneration which often followed on after the blood-lettings which the constant epidemics involved.

When it comes to the historical significance of chronic malnutrition, acute famines and great epidemics, our factual knowledge unfortunately is often somewhat limited, and we must, when we have to consider times long ago with discrimination, occasionally resort to what we do know with certainty about the conditions of more recent times and in primitive and backward peoples.

In the past, variations in the supply of food played an important role, which we with our international communications of all kinds can hardly imagine. The conditions which we today can study among the starving millions of India and China and the tribes of Africa were certainly earlier widespread in the West too, especially in prehistoric times. Of equal and perhaps even greater significance was the repeated occurrence of epidemics. Their ravages were terrible and perhaps it was just because they appeared during years of famine and in the wake of wars that they were so devastating. One realises that such afflictions as crop failures and famine, constant wars and the onslaught of epidemics on a population in many ways unprotected must have appeared as an outbreak of the wrath of God, as God's punishment for a sinful life, even as a sign of the approach of the end of the world. No wonder people saw the Riders of the Apocalypse in the sky. This life of epidemics, hunger and war, generation after generation, left its mark on people, their religion and their philosophy of life, and took expression in life-denying resignation and dumb fatalism. 'Death was once a focal point in life, as the churchyard was the focal point of the village' (Fourastié). Death became a reality which thrust men, women and children into life in quite another way to that of today, and, with death constantly in sight, mankind stood terrified and irresolute. No wonder that those innumerable 'dances of death' with their reapers and open graves saw the light of day.

Death goes from one village to the next
With his cracked old fiddle.
Old, old man but brisk and bright,
Dry bones but still frisky.

(Karlfeldt)

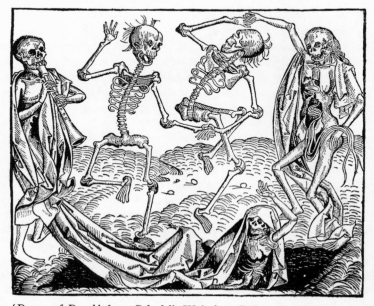

'Dance of Death' from Schedel's Weltchronik *(1493). The numerous representations of dancing skeletons date as early as the time of the Black Death in Germany in 1348 and the following years.*

Did the ancient world see death in any other way? The picture of Niobe with her seven sons and seven daughters whom the gods killed as a punishment for their pride is not all that unlike the mediaeval dances of death. Perhaps the Niobe myth is an unconscious reminiscence of an ancient epidemic. Can we believe that the Greeks in the West were inspired by the spirit expressed in Fröding's 'From Anabasis'?

But Xenophon, who remembered the great hardship
the Greeks had endured and still must expect,
and famine and frost and the dead lying,

was proud and glad to see that the Greeks could suffer
and yet could rejoice and raise themselves
to more noble things than grief over distress
and not bow as barbarians do
in madness and terror to cruel destiny.

In any case, it is of great interest that skulls and skeletons as symbols of death very seldom appeared in ancient times, but became extremely common in mediaeval times and later.

The part played by different epidemics in the past will be dealt with later. There are researchers who maintain that destroyers like malaria forced whole tribes to break away from their homelands and seek healthier places to live in, even that the great migrations of populations were not due to natural catastrophes and crop failures but in fact were occasionally set in motion by diseases. Was malaria perhaps one of the reasons why classical Greek culture wasted away? And was it malaria and smallpox which completed the break-up of the Roman Empire? Similar conditions are to be found in ancient Mexico where epidemics in the sixth and later in the twelfth centuries played a devastating role (Somolinos).

As long as communities were small and isolated from each other by poor communications, mountains, forests and water, the risk of the spread of epidemics was inconsiderable. But the concentration of huge masses of people in large cities, in field camps and armies, in concentration camps, markets and pilgrimages, was always allied to extreme risks which man neither imagined nor appreciated nor was able to remove by prophylactic or hygienic measures. Great armies and sea expeditions came to an ignominious end as a result of epidemics. That is what happened to Sennacherib when he wished to occupy Jerusalem. The plague in Athens during the Peloponnesian War, as mentioned before, is another classic example. In the First Crusade (1096–99) it was calculated that 500,000 initially took part. Of those who left the West about 300,000 are calculated to have landed at Aleppo. Antioch was besieged for a long time and when the fortress finally fell, the crusaders' army consisted of only 60,000 men. When Jerusalem was finally taken, there was only a small group of 20,000, some sick, who were able to march into the Holy City. In much the same way the great armies of the following crusades were diminished by hunger, privation and disease. And the ones who returned brought back with them smallpox, leprosy and

other infectious diseases from the Orient. The Black Death deci-
mated the peoples of mediaeval Europe and led to a mixing of
different surviving peoples, the genetic significance of which cannot
be overlooked. 'The sweating sickness' which followed after the
Wars of the Roses killed more Englishmen than all the long years of
war had done.

Let us now cross the ocean and see what the discovery and conquest of America meant. The indigenous population of America had
for thousands of years lived isolated on their double continent,
which seems to have been troubled by surprisingly few of the many
infectious diseases with which the Old World was afflicted. As a
result the Indian population had built up no resistance to them.
There is in fact a strange biological contrast between the two worlds
isolated from each other, and it is remarkable that it remained so
until 1492. But the arrival of the Europeans changed conditions with
one blow. The Spanish, Portuguese and English soldiers and colon-
isers who landed in Central, South and North America brought
with them all the infectious diseases of the Old World, measles,
smallpox, diphtheria, meningitis and so on. Cortez and the other
brave knights of the Conquistadors infected the Indians at the heart
of American civilisation and mass deaths amongst them made the
conquest easy. The same happened in North America where measles
and smallpox proved so devastating to the powerful but susceptible
Indians that whole tribes died out and their land lay waste to receive
the invaders. But in exchange the syphilis spirochaete was brought
over to the Old World.

During the Thirty Years War, Central Europe was ravaged by
famine and epidemics which cost many more human lives than the
war. The Napoleonic Wars meant a huge new blood-letting from
all the epidemics which followed on the heels of war. At the siege
of Damietta only 3,000 of the 80,000 defenders survived, the rest
of them dying of disease and scurvy. During the Peninsular Wars
of 1804–14 the French lost 100,000 men in battle but 300,000
died of infectious diseases, mainly typhus. At Torgau the French
lost 30,000 men, mostly of disease. Napoleon's advance to Moscow
cost innumerable human lives and the ones who succeeded in
returning were infected in different ways. During the Crimean
War (1853–56), 900,000 succumbed to typhus. During the American Civil War (1861–63) nearly two million, soldiers and others,
succumbed to dysentery and of these 45,000 died. During the

Franco–Prussian War of 1870–71 the number of cases of disease was between four and ten times as many as that of wounded on the battlefield, but on the other hand this war was the first with more dead in battle than of disease: 28,000 were killed in action, 15,000 died of diseases, mostly epidemics. In the Russo–Japanese War of 1904–5, the Russians lost 34,000 in battle but not more than 9,000 through disease. In both world wars the proportion of sick and dead from infectious diseases was finally reduced thanks to the advance of medicine, but even in the First World War the malarial mosquito was considered to be 'a more dangerous enemy to the British at Salonica than the Bulgarians'.

The conquest of infectious diseases has revolutionised life in many countries whose populations for thousands of years have been held down by innumerable diseases and have only been able to survive by an incredible capacity for procreation. We do not yet know what will happen when these hundreds of millions have recovered and finally shaken off the vestiges of colonialism. Will they then with their vast populations, perhaps with an unsuspected vitality, overwhelm Western civilisation which has freed them from innumerable epidemics? Where will these people find sufficient food? Have perhaps the laboratories and techniques of Europe and America disturbed nature's equilibrium, which applies to human beings as well as to rodents and insects?

There have been serious authors who have maintained that epidemics and wars have a selection value, that only the strongest and the best are left. But no one can believe that the mechanised warfare with which we are now threatened can be considered of selection value.

This short introductory survey could easily have swelled into a book, but what has been said should be sufficient to illuminate the part that undernourishment and in particular infectious diseases have played in people's lives in the past. And it applies equally to the great masses of people as it does to the personal fates of their leaders. I have good reason to repeat here the paradox which I formulated in my book in 1934:

The history of mankind is the history of its diseases.

Infectious Diseases

Introductory

Under this heading will come not only diseases caused by unicellular microbes but also those caused by multicellular parasites. When it is a matter of larger, macroscopic parasites the expressions invasion or infestation diseases are often used for convenience, the latter especially when the macroparasite attacks the surface of the body or from there penetrates into the organism.

With those diseases which occur as a result of the combination of two different—or in exceptional cases more than two—living organisms, on the one hand a microscopic organism and on the other a larger macro-organism, whether in human or animal, the pathological background and causal conditions become very complicated, whether in a single case or a number of cases, in an epidemic or epizootic (in animals), or an endemic or enzootic (more permanent diseases in humans and animals). Decisive for the origin, course and termination of different disease forms are the general biological properties of the organisms, microbes and macro-organisms, reacting with each other, but apart from this, different environmental factors partake which can hinder or favour the individual disease, be it epidemic or epizootic. Among these environmental factors, all the preventive (prophylactic) and healing (therapeutic) measures which are taken at the threat or onslaught of infectious diseases, naturally take first place. In addition many other circumstances can influence the disease and its spread. The factors which particularly favour the spread of the infective agent include, first and foremost, malnutrition, poor hygiene and the concentration of large numbers of people in confined areas such as detention camps, as well as, above all, in armies, naval expeditions and war. Even the peaceful movement of large numbers of people, in pilgrimages and emigration, has been of great importance. Chinese coolies are said to have spread leprosy to Australia and the South Sea Islands, and it is said to have come to North America partly through immigrating Norwegians and Icelanders, partly through African negro slaves. Echinococcus disease is also supposed to have been brought to North America by immigrants. The great caravans, markets and peasant movements in Asia and Russia have also contributed much to the spread of infectious diseases.

Among the great advances of recent years in the field of infectious diseases are man's knowledge and understanding of the significance of animal diseases and subclinical infections, and what their infectious diseases can mean to human beings. Infections which are common to humans and animals and the diseases that follow—anthropozoones—are of particular interest to geographical pathology.

Two questions that are of focal interest to historico-geographical pathology, as to microbiology (the study of microscopic organisms), serology and hygiene, must here be dealt with briefly and in general.

1   How, when and where did the infectious diseases of today arise? Have new infectious diseases appeared during the period of hundreds or thousands of years which we can reasonably survey? Do the pathogenic microbes stay constant for great lengths of time or are they subject to biological variations? Do infectious diseases die out spontaneously and in that case what part is played by changes in the surrounding environment?

2   Have the fundamental biological elements in the human and animal organism, which we call predisposition, resistance, immunity, changed essentially during the course of history? Do there exist essential, genetically determined constitutional differences between the different human races, or between discrete populations which cannot be called races in the modern sense?

1   The interesting question of when, where and how certain microbes become pathogenic to humans or animals may never really be answered. One can hardly go any further than hypothetical evidence of probability. In most cases it is thought that pathological micro-organisms in prehistoric times developed from the harmless saprophytic parasites of humans and animals or from the microbes living free in nature. On the capacity of bacteria to remain alive almost for ever, there has been evidence from Dombrowski's investigations into the bacterial content in old salt deposits near Bad Nauheim in Nassau. These salt deposits contained, apart from pollen and small bits of wood, about forty different bacteria of which only one corresponded to a present living form. Many of them were cultivable! As the salt deposits originate from a lake in the Permian period, the bacteria's age can be estimated at 180–200

million years. He then examined rock salt from the Devonian period in America and there too could show bacteria which could not be identified with those of the Permian period in Germany or with present-day bacteria. The Devonian period was about 300 million years ago. Nicolle, who has written a work well worth reading, *Naissance, vie et mort des maladies infectieuses*, does not doubt that inoffensive microbes can be transformed into pathogenic ones, whether through a direct, gradual adaptation to warm-blooded animal organisms or through the mediation of those insects which in many cases transfer pathogenic microbes to the vertebrate animals. He comments on Pasteur's experiments with anthrax bacteria which were artificially made avirulent (harmless) but could again be made pathogenic, and also on his own experiments with subclinical (clinically unobservable) infections in animals and humans. Even the sudden changes of harmless saprophytes which live in dead organic matter, into pathogenic microbes, were possible according

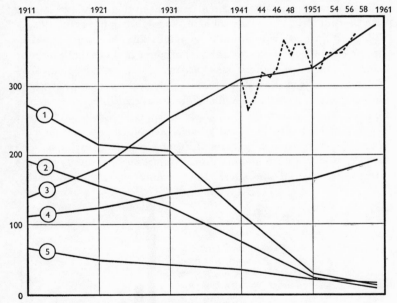

Changes in the Swedish disease-panorama during the last 50 years, from statistics on causes of death: 1. All infectious diseases. 2. Tuberculosis only. 3. Cardio-vascular diseases. (Dotted line shows rapid decline during the crisis years of 1941–42 and rapid rise in the years 1947–50.) 4. Tumours. 5. Infantile diseases.

to Nicolle, and 'what has occurred in past times or has succeeded by way of an exception in nature will always be repeated'. In the light of recent research into the genetics of microbes, these words of Nicolle's from 1930 sound almost prophetic, and the sudden change of harmless saprophytes into new pathogenic forms no longer seems as fantastic as before. The German bacteriologist Doerr in 1932 wrote, in agreement with Nicolle but with some caution: 'For the change of a saprophyte into a pathogenic parasite, reliable fixed points are lacking. We agree to this possibility only theoretically to explain the primary source of infectious diseases in prehistoric times or the appearance of previously unknown epidemics in historic times.' Manson, a famous English researcher in the field of tropical infectious diseases, goes very far back in time when his imagination leads him to the not entirely absurd hypothesis that the oldest common ancestor for the malarial mosquito and humans was the host of the malarial parasite.

Nor can one really answer the question of whether pathogenic microbes have generally remained constant in their virulence during the past hundreds and thousands of years, although a certain variability within quite wide limits is generally known and admitted, as in the case of such toxic (poisonous) bacteria as those that cause the coccus diseases, diphtheria and lockjaw. The possibility that infectious diseases can die out for purely biological reasons, i.e. without human action, also arises. Williams believes that infectious diseases can appear and then spontaneously disappear. Nicolle and others have pointed to the apparently vanished epidemic 'sweating sickness', which ravaged large parts of Europe in past centuries, as such a disease. We return to this disease later. It is naturally quite a different matter if one succeeds in eradicating a disease locally,

The most important causes of death in Sweden in 1960 per 100,000 persons: 1. Diseases of the circulation (388·13). 2. Tumours (191·11). 3. Nervous and mental disorders (149·00). 4. Diseases of the respiratory system (62·64). 5. Violent death (47·04). 6. Diseases of the digestive system (38·67). 7. Diseases of the uro-genital tract (28·84). 8. Diseases in the first year of life (15·41). 9. Infectious diseases including tuberculosis (11·30). 10. Other causes of death.

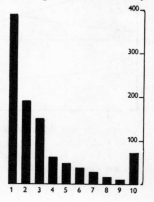

regionally or even globally by deliberate hygienic, prophylactic and therapeutic measures; this too will be dealt with later on. The graph opposite gives an idea of how rapidly the rate of mortality from infectious diseases has declined through measures taken or perhaps solely through improved economic and social standards.

2   Very little is known about man's disposition to infectious diseases and his original resistance in prehistoric and early historic times. On the other hand we have several hundred years' experience of the great risk a population can run if it is exposed to the attack of a microbe against which it lacks virtually any protection, and with this experience behind us we can have a vague idea of what it could and ought to have been like in the beginnings of history. If an infectious disease is brought into a country in which it has never before existed, or from which it has vanished for many generations, it can take on new, more severe forms because the long-spared population lacks any specific immunity. Perhaps this lack of immunity also leads to a rapid rise in virulence in the newly-arrived microbe. Later we shall return to these questions several times. It should also be stated that the conditions of immunity vary quite considerably from one infectious disease to the next. Certain infectious diseases, like common colds or gonorrhoea, give extremely little and very transitory immunity. In other cases the immunity can last a lifetime, or can even be transferred from one generation to another via the placenta or through breast-feeding.

Many infectious diseases are by nature originally cosmopolitan, but now confined to backward parts of Europe and the rest of the world, especially the great tropical and sub-tropical countries where over-population, illiteracy, malnutrition, poverty and wretched hygiene make their continued existence possible. The crowding together of so many infectious diseases in hot countries is due not only to the above failings but in many cases to the fact that the essentially cosmopolitan diseases are associated with other infectious diseases whose microbes need warmth and humidity, as do the arthropods which in the long run act as their transmitters from person to person. One sees too that occasional changes in temperature and humidity which favour the microbe and its transmitters can bring with them an unexpected expansion or a puzzling upsurge of the infectious disease. One finds more than anything else a great dependence on humid heat in the pathogenic multicellular animal parasites, worms and arthropods, which in many cases can maintain a self-sufficient existence away from the human body.

As far as the future of infectious diseases is concerned, it is precarious to prophesy. It is obvious that many epidemic and endemic infectious diseases are now in retreat all along the line, or at least in some countries. Not a few of them have been completely eradicated from country after country and have had their area of distribution considerably limited. Others have not exactly been eradicated but have apparently changed character and become milder. In many epidemics the high mortality rates of a century ago are now a thing of the past, in spite of the fact that morbidity has not tangibly decreased. It would perhaps be responsible here to issue a warning against undue optimism. Diphtheria can still occur in violent forms which are resistant to serum treatment. Gonorrhoea is still an unsolved problem, even in countries which regard themselves as most advanced like Sweden. We still have not been completely successful in eradicating nosocomial infections which manage to spread in hospitals and come from staphylococci and other microbes, but which in themselves are not usually dangerous.

Even in this century certain infectious diseases have spread outside their old-established areas. Tasmania, New Zealand and New Guinea were free of smallpox until 1905. The incidence of common colds, influenza, measles and poliomyelitis is still not under control, but vaccination against them looks promising.

So one must not forget that the disappearance of an infectious disease, whether this happens as the result of infection and natural immunisation of the whole population, or as the result of hygienic and medical measures, must bring with it a weakening or disappearance of natural resistance. Someone who has never had a primary tuberculous infection or has not been effectively vaccinated against tuberculosis, runs a greater risk of eventual exposure to the tubercle bacillus than the person who is immunised. Strict hygiene makes us in all probability more susceptible to poliomyelitis than people who live in wretched hygienic conditions. The eradication of body lice probably made Europeans more sensitive to the typhus microbe than those permanently infested with the lice.

One must therefore reckon that the human family of the future, freed from the infectious diseases which we are still fighting, will become increasingly susceptible to the impact of a virus, a microbe, from its very last stand, and might have to pay the penalty for generations of freedom from all epidemics with a sudden and violent rise in morbidity and mortality.

1 Virus Diseases

Viruses (the word *virus* essentially means poison) are parasitic microbes, usually much smaller than bacteria, which can live and increase only in living receptive cells of plants and animals. Many forms of virus can be cultivated in living hen's eggs or cultures of tissue. As the nature and biology of viruses are still incompletely understood, it is difficult to make a classification of virus diseases which would be valid in every respect. The classification in this chapter follows that given by Rivers and Horsfall in 1959. One could also advantageously classify virus diseases according to the organs which they mainly attack:

1. Predominantly neurotropic viruses, which mainly attack the nervous system (rabies, poliomyelitis, etc.).
2. Predominantly pneumotropic viruses, which attack the respiratory organs ('chills', influenza, ornithosis, etc.).
3. Dermatoepitheliotropic, which mostly attack the skin (smallpox, chickenpox, herpes, etc.).
4. Hepatotropic, which damage the liver (yellow fever, infectious hepatitis, etc.).
5. Pantropic, which attack several different organs.

Viruses transmitted by insects

Among the ten or so different viruses carried by insects which are now known, only the most important can be given here. Many of them are in any case observed only in North and South America and Japan. Several are essentially horse diseases which can easily be transmitted to humans, and one of them is worth mentioning here.

Russian spring encephalitis and the sheep disease 'louping ill'
The virus of this encephalitic form occurs in different variations, amongst others in sheep; it was first discovered by a Russian researcher. The virus is transmitted by several kinds of tick, and

35

the disease has hitherto been recorded in Siberia, Russia, Finland, the island of Åland, eastern Sweden, Austria and Poland.

Yellow fever, febris flava

Yellow fever is an endemic and epidemic disease with a high rate of mortality (20–70 per cent). It is transmitted by different species of mosquitoes, especially *Aedes aegypti* (previously called *Stegomyia fasciata*), which on account of its great sensitivity to cold and dryness has a fairly constant distribution in the world, which is also a decisive factor in its spreading potentiality. The part played by the mosquito was already realised in 1881 by Finlay in Havana. The original homeland of the disease is not known with certainty, as the nature of earlier epidemics of yellow fever is uncertain. At the arrival of Europeans in Central America an epidemic is said to have been raging amongst the Indians, thus infecting Columbus's sailors. Presumably the disease was already widespread over large parts of Central America where the first definite epidemic was described in Yukatan in 1648. In favour of an American origin is the fact that there is a forest or jungle form of yellow fever which occurs in tropical South America, and also the disease's relatively limited distribution in Africa, where it is principally confined to the west coast. It is possible that the virus could have been transmitted, even in prehistoric times, by mosquitoes carried by winds from one continent to the other.

Sorre considers that even before the first appearance of human beings yellow fever existed as an ape disease in the primaeval forest of both America and Africa. In South America this form of yellow fever is still found among apes and from them it is occasionally transmitted via mosquitoes to humans. One therefore has reason to note two variants of yellow fever: first, the one more important to human beings, called the urban, which is transmitted by 'domesticated' mosquitoes, especially *Aedes aegypti*, from person to person; secondly, the one which is of less importance to man—the theoretically and historically interesting forest or jungle form which is transmitted from apes to humans by other species of mosquitoes living in the forests. The most important species, *Aedes aegypti*, thrives best in harbour towns and on low-lying plains in a temperature preferably of 27°–32°C. In such conditions yellow fever has occasionally been endemic with epidemic outbreaks.

From Central America and the Caribbean Islands, where it

already had a wide distribution in the seventeenth century, the disease soon spread to the southernmost parts of North America and to trópical South America, principally at first to the eastern coasts and up the big river valleys, especially those of the Mississippi and the Amazon. Dirt and poverty favoured its spread and it kept a hold, especially in harbour towns. Brazil, which was relatively spared, was infected in 1849 by the brig *Brazil* which sailed from New Orleans to Bahia. On the voyage two sailors had died and soon yellow fever broke out amongst those who had been in contact with the *Brazil*. It spread round the harbour to other vessels and during the next ten years spread over the whole coastline of Brazil. Even on the west coast of South America seats of infection appeared, with particular severity in the port of Guayaquil in Ecuador. The American epidemics were widely distributed and had high rates of mortality. During the nineteenth century the mortality figures in the USA were calculated to be at least 500,000. In Rio de Janeiro, which was then a small town, more than 40,000 people died of yellow fever in the second half of the nineteenth century. A splendid example of what systematic and energetic sanitation can achieve is found in the completion of the Panama Canal. When a French company tried to carry out the construction of the canal, disease frustrated their plans, but when the Americans took over the work twenty years later, it was possible to sanitate the whole of the canal area and complete the construction.

Cuba before 1901 was one of the worst-hit areas, in some years more than half of all deaths during the summer months being ascribed to yellow fever. In 1897 nearly 2,600 people died in the military hospitals in Havana and Regla alone, and in the whole of the island over 6,000 people died out of the 30,000 who succumbed. During the Spanish-American war, yellow fever ravaged both armies. When the war was over, American army doctors immediately began to sanitate Havana. The campaign began on 15 February 1899 and every victim or suspected victim was isolated, his room was protected from mosquitoes which could transmit the parasite to others, and the mosquito was combated as extensively as possible. The result was excellent: in ninety days Havana was free of the disease and from 7 May to 1 July not a single case occurred. During the following months a few cases came in from outside but they were easily isolated and yellow fever was definitely eradicated from Havana.

37

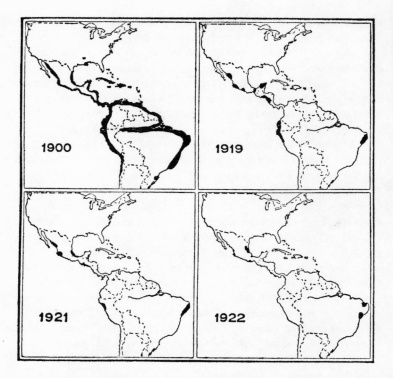

The decline of yellow fever in America 1900–22, after a Rockefeller Foundation report—the result of a consistent and energetic campaign of eradication.

Three years after the beginning of the great eradication campaign against the yellow fever mosquito, the disease flared up unexpectedly in New Orleans at the mouth of the Mississippi. It was the second outbreak, the first having come eight years previously, with resultant panic. When the epidemic broke out a second time in 1905, different, modern resources were available, and despite appalling difficulties with the open canals and water tanks where the eggs of the mosquitoes were hatched, and which often overflowed by the autumn of the same year the authorities were successful in eradicating the disease from the town.

As a result of consistent and energetic campaigns, yellow fever has since declined considerably over the whole of its western area of distribution and nowadays is of secondary importance. However, even in the 1920s and 1930s, the number of registered deaths varied from year to year. In 1928 82 cases were registered in Brazil, in 1929 444 and in 1930 only five.

The distribution of the disease in Africa has been much more limited. On the west coast it was to be found on the Gold Coast (now Ghana), in Sierra Leone, Senegal and Gambia. The famous Japanese bacteriologist, Hideyo Noguchi, who worked on solving the problem of the yellow fever microbe and believed that he had found it in a spirochaete (his assumption was false), was himself a victim of it in 1928. The age of the African seats of infection is uncertain: there are researchers who consider that the disease is in fact African, but on the other hand a great deal of the evidence points to a relatively late infection. Yellow fever, as it happens, never spread to the east coast of the continent, but Sudan had a big epidemic in 1940 with 15,000 cases and a 10 per cent mortality rate.

Remarkably enough, yellow fever has never been active in southern and eastern Asia, although the transmitting mosquito is to be found there. According to some reports, however, cases of the disease have been found in India.

During the eighteenth and nineteenth centuries yellow fever made repeated attacks on Europe, on the coasts of France, Italy and England, and especially on the ports of Spain and Portugal. The last time it was carried to Spain in 1878 by troops from Spanish Cuba.

Immunological investigations of large numbers of inhabitants of the tropics have contributed greatly to our knowledge of the true distribution of the virus and the disease. Earlier, immunity to yellow fever virus was very general, but after the eradication of the disease this immunity has largely disappeared in the Caribbean area. By contrast, large numbers of the inhabitants of tropical South America, Central America and Africa, even the children, are still immune. In Africa a wide immunity zone stretches from the west to the east coast, the northern border running along the edge of the Sahara and the southern running through Zambia.

Yellow fever is now in rapid retreat. Between 1950 and 1955 it decreased by about 50 per cent and it has lost its earlier terrifying character, but as recently as the spring of 1961 a bad epidemic broke out in south-west Ethiopia, causing several thousand deaths.

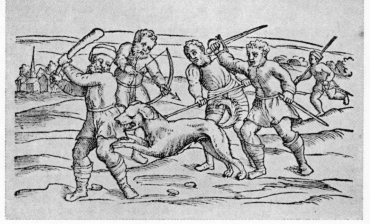

CANIS RABIOSVS.

A dog with rabies hunted by peasants. Woodcut from Commentaires de Matthioli sur Dioscoride (*Venice, 1560*).

Dengue fever

This disease, which has a relatively mild course, is characterised by pains in the joints and muscles which give the victim's movements a certain stiffness and elegance; hence the Spanish name *dengue* which means elegance. The disease is said to have been described in 1779 in Java by the Dutch doctor Bylon. It is widely distributed in the Mediterranean countries, the warmer parts of Africa and Asia, also in Japan. In the southern states of the USA epidemics occur and in 1922 between one and two million people were infected. The virus is transmitted by the same species of mosquito as yellow fever, *Aedes aegypti*. Apes can be infected too, and they probably form a host for the virus.

Papataci fever, phlebotomus fever

This non-malignant fever, which bears a certain resemblance to dengue, is thought to have been known since Napoleon's 1799 campaign and is widespread in the Mediterranean basin, South Russia, Central Asia and parts of India. Its area of distribution, between 20° and 45° N, is defined to a large extent by the temperature in which the transmitter of the virus, the sand-fly, *Phlebotomus papataci*, thrives. As with yellow fever, the insects' area of distribution is far greater than that of the disease; for example the disease is

40

supposed never to have appeared in Ceylon where the sand-fly is common. Papataci fever has never appeared in America either, but during the Second World War many American soldiers contracted the disease in different places in the Mediterranean area; 12,000 cases were reported, but probably the number of cases was much greater, as uncertain cases of fever were often reported as malaria.

Viruses transmitted from mammals

Rabies, hydrophobia

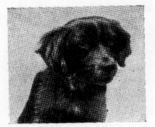

Dog with rabies, showing characteristic peering and confused expression, up-turned eyes and paralysis of the jaw muscles (after Hutyra and Marek, 1922).

This disease, which can be described as a kind of nervous or mental disease, was known long before our reckoning of time. Democritus described it in dogs and other animals *c.* 500 B.C. and Aristotle knew it too; the danger of being bitten by dogs was also observed and stressed by, amongst others, Celsus *c.* A.D. 1, Galen and other Graeco-Roman doctors. The disease was earlier very widespread and occasionally even acquired epidemic proportions as a result of stray dogs and other animals, as in the eighteenth century in Italy, France, Germany and Hungary. It occurred in the Middle Ages among the wolves of Western Europe and seems to have come to Great Britain considerably later and to North and South America in the middle of the eighteenth century. It is not known when the Scandinavian countries were infected, but it has been said that cases of rabies appeared in the spring of 1135 in the old town of 'Konghäll' (Kungälv, in Sweden), among dogs and humans. On the other hand it may have been long present in eastern Finland, to which it had been carried by wolves from Russia. In Helsinki there is the Pasteur Institute for the treatment of rabies, as there is a risk of

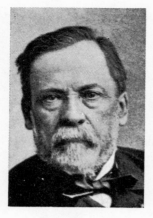

Louis Pasteur (1822–95). Pasteur, who was originally a chemist, first studied fermentation and decomposition processes and vine diseases, and later continued his pioneering investigations in the institute in Paris which bears his name. Most celebrated is perhaps his discovery of protective inoculation against rabies. Pasteur, one of the greatest names in medicine, lies in a mausoleum in the institute where he worked.

infected wolves coming in from Russia. In Sweden rabies has long since been eradicated, largely owing to the compulsory dog tax. Apart from dogs—which in 80 to 90 per cent of cases transmit the disease—in rabies-infected countries one has other animals to reckon with, such as cats (7–8 per cent), horses (cases appeared several times during the First World War) and in rare cases even cattle, sheep, pigs, geese and also, among wild animals, foxes as well as wolves. After the Second World War rabies became widespread in Central Europe where small wild animals are virus carriers. The same applies to North America where rabies is very widespread among foxes, prairie wolves and smaller furred animals, especially skunks, and is therefore very difficult to eradicate. In Florida bats also transmit the disease, and the blood-sucking bats of Brazil and Surinam, vampires, play the same part. In very rare cases one human has infected another. In the USA 10,540 cases were known up to 1944, among them:

Dog	Cattle	Cat	Pig	Sheep	Horse	Goat	Other animals	Human
9067	561	49	43	40	32	14	311	53

The disease is very widely distributed over the whole of Asia, especially in India where annually there are large epizootics among dogs and numerous deaths among humans. Hundreds of thousands of people seek treatment but many do not bother as it is known from experience that only a small number of those bitten by dogs really succumb to the disease. In China rabies has been very common, and in Japan in 1924 there was a large epizootic among dogs in which many people were bitten and 235 died. In tropical America and Africa a great number of different wild animals play an important part—wild and half-wild dogs, other carnivores, hyenas, jackals, weasels and flying foxes—and also domestic animals such as donkeys and camels.

The vaccination of those bitten by dogs, evolved by Pasteur in 1881–89, has been of outstanding therapeutic and prophylactic significance. Before his discovery, the mortality rate after dog bites was as much as 16–20 per cent and no less than 60–90 per cent after wolf bites; by vaccination it has been reduced to hardly 1 per cent.

Other virus diseases

Poliomyelitis

Sixty years ago, poliomyelitis, then normally called infantile paralysis, was considered a new disease, but it appears that it existed in ancient Egypt. A mummy of *c.* 3700 B.C. examined by Mitchell may be the oldest known case. Good evidence can be found in a stone relief in the Glyptotek in Copenhagen (page 45), which shows a priest from the eighteenth Dynasty, *c.* 1500 B.C., with an atrophied shortened leg, undoubtedly the result of polio in childhood. Pharaoh Siptah's mummy from the nineteenth Dynasty shows similar variations. In the writings of Hippocrates there is mention of an epidemic on the island of Thasos which may well have been polio, and Graeco-Roman doctors seem to have known of the disease. Ireland was smitten in A.D. 707 with an epidemic, 'that pestilence that is called lameness', which MacArthur considers to have been polio. Good clinical accounts of the disease by English and Italian doctors of the late eighteenth and early nineteenth centuries appear to consider it a new disease. Its symptomatology is described by Heine (1840) and by Medin (1887) who observed an epidemic in Stockholm of forty-four cases. An epidemic in Sweden in 1905 of previously unknown magnitude, with no fewer than 1,031 cases, is excellently described by Wickman (1905–11), who established its transmission from person to person. Already in 1909, however, the Nobel prize-winner Landsteiner had shown that the disease could be transmitted to apes from bacteria-free material from humans. One cannot entirely exclude the possibility that humans can be

43

infected by animals, such as apes and others which have shown paralysis, as well as through sores.

The poliomyelitis virus is widespread all over the world. In countries with poor standards of hygiene the disease seems to be considerably rarer than in those with high ones, presumably because in more primitive countries small children are infected early, directly or indirectly, in which case more severe symptoms need not appear and a satisfactory immunity remains. Severe limited epidemics are also known in tropical areas and in the Near East.

In Europe and the United States, the earlier more sporadic appearances of poliomyelitis have been replaced by large epidemics. In Stockholm the polio rate was lowest in 1920–24 with seven cases per year (1·7 per 100,000), then it increased in 1950–54 to 180 cases per year (23·8 per 100,000) (Ström). It is in general more common in rural areas than in towns. At the same time it has increasingly become an adult disease. Whereas in the first severe epidemics in Sweden, the USA and Australia, 90 per cent of the children affected were under five, during the last twenty years there has been a movement towards a higher age-group. Nowadays it is principally on isolated islands and in other remote places that cases among children predominate. In the severe epidemic (with 1,095 cases) on the island of Mauritius, 95 per cent of the child cases were under ten. In epidemics in the Union of South Africa, predisposition to the virus has been shown to be about ten times greater in whites than in blacks. Similar conditions were found when British and American troops came into contact with primitive peoples in North Africa; the natives seldom succumbed but there were, on the other hand, a considerable number of cases among the foreign troops. The world-wide vaccination against polio which is now being carried out appears to be having satisfactory results but it is too early yet to talk of the future.

Coxsackie virus group (among others Bornholm disease or myalgia epidemica)

This disease, which in Scandinavia is usually known as Bornholm disease, is said to have been already described in 1856 by Finsen in Iceland. Sylvest published cases from Bornholm. Coxsackie is the name of a village in the USA where the character of the virus became established in an epidemic. Virus diseases of this kind are known in all parts of the world.

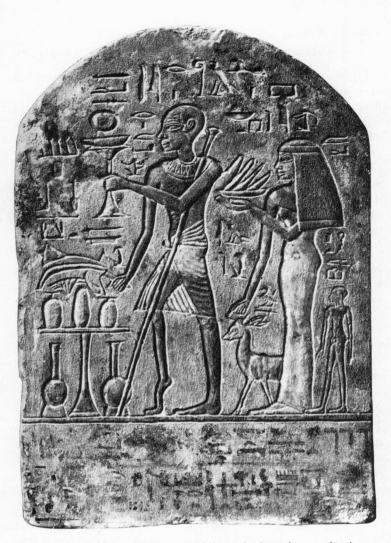

An Egyptian stone relief from the Glyptotek, Copenhagen, showing a priest from the Eighteenth Dynasty, followed by his wife, offering sacrifices to the god of health, Istar. The priest's right leg is short and thin and he has a typical 'pointed foot' and supports himself with a stick. The deformed leg is undoubtedly a result of poliomyelitis in early childhood.

Viral hepatitis

There are at least two varieties of viral hepatitis known at present.

(*a*) *Infectious hepatitis, 'catarrhal' jaundice.* This virus disease has been known for centuries, partly in isolated cases and partly in epidemics. Such an epidemic occurred in 1745 in Minorca, and later ones followed in the Mediterranean basin; Napoleon's army in Egypt was affected. In Sweden a severe epidemic occurred in 1858. Several years later jaundice raged among the Union troops in the American Civil War. During the Second World War both sides had casualties who became unfit through jaundice. A singular epidemic occurred in Sweden in 1956 as a result of virus-infected oysters and was confined to the oyster-eating upper class. The oysters had been kept in sea water too near a sewer opening.

(*b*) *Inoculation hepatitis.* The commonest virus of this form of jaundice is closely related to that of 'catarrhal' jaundice. There are accounts of epidemics in Germany in the 1880s after cowpox vaccination, and the first definite hospital epidemics after injections of different kinds are described by the Swede Flaum and others in 1926. During the Second World War inoculation hepatitis was widespread nearly all over the world. In this way 27,000 American soldiers who were vaccinated against yellow fever fell victim to a new unknown non-malignant form of jaundice.

Nasopharyngitis, common cold

This common virus disease, known since ancient times, has no special geography, but it should be mentioned that in temperate zones it is most common in autumn and spring, while in isolated arctic regions it is rare in winter.

Epidemic influenza

Epidemics, which in all probability were of influenza, are mentioned in the writings of Hippocrates; since antiquity more or less severe epidemic outbreaks have ravaged parts of the known world; and it is known that as early as the first century A.D. there were a number of severe epidemics with high mortality rates. Such an epidemic was described by St Gregory, Bishop of Tours in 591. After a long interval an epidemic broke out in 1173 and spread rapidly and violently. This, Hirsch considers to be the first absolutely definite

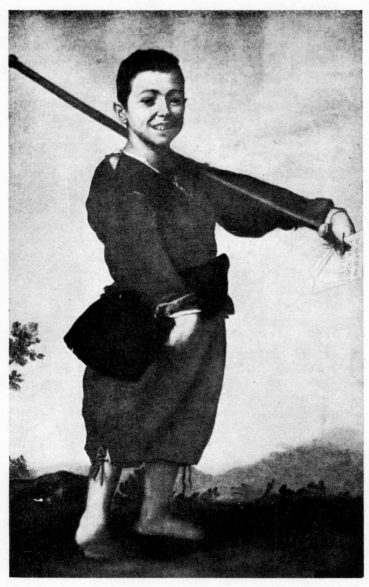

Paralysis and contraction of the right arm and leg, probably after poliomyelitis. Oil painting in the Louvre by Jusépe de Ribera (1588–1652).

one. It raged at first in Italy, Germany and England, others following in the 1300s. Since then innumerable epidemics and great global pandemics have swept over Europe, Asia, Africa and later America, and one has no hesitation in agreeing with Hirsch in naming influenza as the greatest scourge of mankind.

The name influenza is said to have been first used by an Italian writer Piero Buoninsegni about an epidemic which was raging in 1580. The German-French name for influenza, *grippe*, is said by many to derive from the French verb *agripper* (to grip or snatch).

Some pandemics have been named after the country in which they are supposed to have originated. The pandemic of 1729–33 and the outbreak in 1782 of 'Russian 'flu' were of this kind; the great pandemic of 1889–90 was similarly named when it was thought to have originated in one of the endemic seats of infection in Russia. This one was more malignant than previous pandemics and spread rapidly into European Russia and Siberia. In October 1889 it reached St Petersburg and then spread westwards over Scandinavia and Central Europe, reaching England just before Christmas, but it had already reached Quebec earlier in November and New York at the beginning of December. At the beginning of 1890 it arrived in South America. In the east, it had reached Vladivostock by May 1890; Persia had already become infected at the beginning of the year, then western India and somewhat later, in February, eastern India, followed by China in the winter and the early spring of 1890. In the south, the influenza reached South Africa in January 1890. Iceland was infected in the summer of 1890 and the Falkland Islands as late as October. Few countries escaped the infection, including the West Indies (with the exception of one group, the Ireland Islands) where an English naval squadron was infected with 'Russian 'flu' after a visit from the Swedish corvette *Saga*.

During the following years little was heard of influenza but at the beginning of this century smaller epidemics occurred in several capitals, London, Paris, Madrid and Constantinople.

In the middle of 1918, when mankind was in the throes of the greatest war the history of the world had known, a severe and at first puzzling epidemic called 'Spanish 'flu' broke out all over Europe; the outbreaks were apparently disconnected but were soon recognised as influenza. The source of the pandemic was for a long time obscure, but one thing was certain—that this pandemic, which in a few months swept round the world, did not deserve the name

'Spanish 'flu'. It was simply that the disease was first officially recognised in Spain, which did not apply the same strict censorship as the belligerent countries. Some asserted that it had first broken

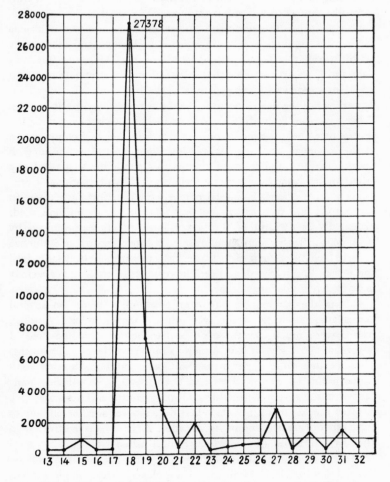

Deaths from epidemic influenza in Sweden 1913–32. After the ravages of the 'Russian 'flu' in the 1880s, influenza played an insignificant role all over Europe. Then during the First World War came the terrible 'Spanish 'flu', which in Sweden alone in 1918, 1919 and 1920 was the cause of 35,000 deaths. The diagram shows the figures from official statistics.

49

out in the trenches, and it is probable that the hardships of the war years had prepared the ground. However, it gradually appeared from reliable information that influenza had already been raging at the beginning of 1918 in America and in March in China. It spread with incredible swiftness; if influenza previously used the post-chaise, nowadays it uses the aeroplane, and when huge numbers of troops lacking any immunity were transported to Europe and other parts of the world, the disease spread like lightning. Mortality was very high and it was remarkable that it was often the strongest men and pregnant women who were victims of the infection. No fewer than 85 per cent of the deaths occurred in the strongest age-group, 17–40. What gave the 'Spanish 'flu' its most malignant character were the severe, often necrotic pneumonias which followed as a complication of the influenza itself; the expression 'lung-plague' was used with reason. In the number of its victims this pandemic surpassed any other known. According to the report of the International Commission on Hygiene, about 50 per cent of the world's population succumbed and it is calculated that at least twenty million died, principally as a result of the severe lung infections produced by streptococci. In Sweden alone over 34,000 people died of influenza in 1918–19. Since then the disease has not completely disappeared and it flared up in Sweden in certain years, as in 1922 and especially in 1927, when nearly 3,000 people died.

During the pandemic of 1918 an epizootic occurred in several places among horses, which was called horse influenza. Autopsy results were much like those on human beings who had died of influenza, and I myself had numerous opportunities to confirm this when at that time I performed autopsies on both humans and animals. Similar observations had been made earlier during pandemics in the seventeenth and eighteenth centuries (Hirsch).

After the 'Spanish 'flu' had died out, several smaller epidemics occurred during the following decades. A virus was cultivated in 1933 by Smith and others, which is now called type A. Epidemics of this virus occurred in 1936, 1943, 1947 and 1953. In 1931 Shope showed that the virus of swine fever was closely related to the A-virus but not identical. Hjärre has carried out important investigations in this field lying between human and veterinary virus research. More recent investigations by Steele and others show that horses and pigs are susceptible, naturally and artificially, to the influenza A2-virus, and that the fowl-pest virus is closely related to that of

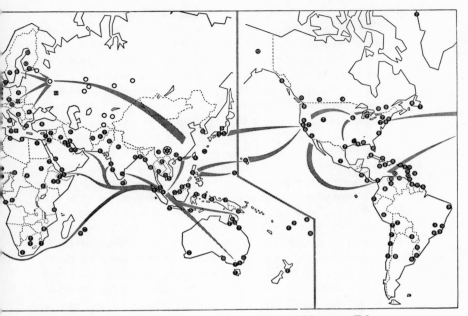

Routes by which 'Asian 'flu' spread over the world between February 1957 and January 1958. The star in southern China shows the probable source. Black dots show the first wave and the figures show the month of the first case. The white circles in Asia and Russia show the first cases from May–August 1957. (After Le Courrier, 1958.)

influenza. One might well conclude therefore that the influenza virus has its source in host animals. Another very important type of human influenza was discovered by Francis Jr. in 1940 and is now called type B. Ten years later a third type, known as type C, was isolated by Francis, and finally Kuroya and others in 1953 discovered a fourth type, D.

At the outbreak of the last great influenza epidemic, in Vladivostok in 1956, this D-type dominated. 'Asian 'flu' spread swiftly in the early spring of 1957 into northern China, in April Hong Kong was attacked and in May Japan and Singapore. The explosive flare-up of influenza in Singapore was noticed all over the world but before there was time to produce a vaccine, the influenza was in Australia. In May and June it reached the Philippines, Indonesia, India, Pakistan, Iran and the Yemen. In July it began in Iraq, Egypt, the

51

Sudan and other parts of Africa. Meanwhile it had passed rapidly across to the west coast of South America from where it quickly spread out to other parts of the continent. Finally in August and September Rumania, Greece, Central Europe and the British Isles were attacked, and then during October Scandinavia and North America. In this way, within the space of six months, the epidemic had affected practically the whole of the world; 10–35 per cent of the population sickened but mortality was low, about 0·25 per cent.

Smallpox, variola

The origins of this disease are lost in antiquity and the several hundred year old argument about its age is not yet over. It is presumed that smallpox occurred in China 1,200 years B.C. A severe epidemic is said to have raged there in 1120 B.C. and later smaller epidemics followed. In A.D. 1 smallpox was brought into China from Indo-China, and after the fifteenth century it spread extremely fast. It probably reached Japan rather later than China, and Korea in A.D. 583. Japan is said to have experienced sixty-five larger epidemics and five of her emperors are said to have died of smallpox. The earliest description of smallpox is supposed to come from a Chinese writer, Keh-Hung (281–360).

Certain reports state that smallpox occurred very early among the negro population of Central Africa. The position in ancient Egypt is obscure; according to some, the disease never reached the Nile valley, according to others a disease described in the Ebers papyrus was smallpox. A skin condition similar to smallpox in one of the mummies from the Twentieth Dynasty (1200–1100 B.C.), which was described by Ruffer and Ferguson, is, according to Unna, not smallpox but a blistering caused by gas-producing bacteria after death, which could be demonstrated. According to certain authors such as von Hagen, the plague in Athens in 430 B.C. started with an epidemic of smallpox.

The first appearance of smallpox in the Near East is a subject of sharp controversy: some authorities connect the first outbreak of the disease with the so-called Elephant War when the Christian Abyssinians laid siege to Muslim Mecca, but this is doubted by others. Egypt seems to have been infected relatively late, in A.D. 620, and Roman doctors describe an epidemic reminiscent of smallpox in the second century. There are authors who go so far as to say that the decline and fall of the Roman Empire was associated with the great epidemics of malaria, smallpox and spotted typhus. In Italy and France smallpox raged during the sixth century and the disease spread to Spain from Egypt in 714. The great Arab doctor Rhazes gives an excellent account of the disease in the tenth century.

At the beginning of the second century A.D., smallpox began to appear in Central Europe and it was not long before the whole continent was infected. It came to Denmark in the thirteenth century, from there Iceland was infected in 1306 and large and small epidemics raged there no fewer than twenty times, the infection usually being brought by Danish ships. In 1720 20,000 Icelanders are said to have died of smallpox. Greenland was also infected by Denmark, as were the Faroe Islands, but not until 1651. For many hundreds of years smallpox was one of the most common causes of death in Europe.

At this time the disease had a colossal hold on Asia too, where deaths occasionally rose to over a third of the victims. Similar conditions reigned in Africa.

The New World was infected shortly after the arrival of Europeans, the West Indies and Central America succumbing first, then in 1540 the east coast of North America and twenty years later Brazil. During the seventeenth century several terrible epidemics raged among the North American Indians, and over large areas of the east coast whole tribes of indigenous people were wiped out, people who were considered to be exceptionally strong and healthy, but who lacked immunity to a disease which was new to them. A similar fate befell the Indians in Central and South America; smallpox and other epidemic diseases from Europe contributed far more than weapons to the swift conquest of America. One might say that it was a kind of unintentional bacteriological warfare. The English Puritans thanked their God for the wonderful support He gave them when they took possession of their new country, but the Jesuits who accompanied the Spaniards and the Portuguese showed more sympathy for the Indians who were dying out.

The earliest prophylactic treatment of smallpox, variolation, which consisted of inoculating those not yet infected with the actual pox-pus, was very early used in China, where the first vaccination is said to have been done in 1022 B.C. A script of A.D. 1577 recommends the method. It is, however, possible that variolation took place even earlier in India. For a long time in Europe too, chiefly in rural areas, protection for children against smallpox had been

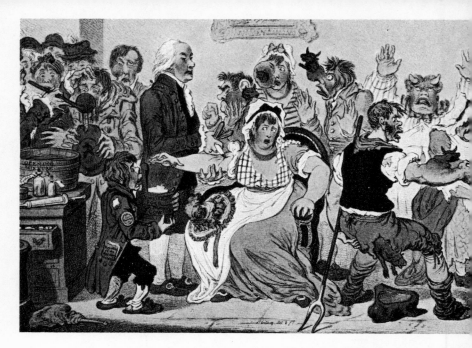

*The dangers of being vaccinated with Jenner's new serum and the
amazing consequences thereof. Cartoon by J. Gillray (1802) issued by
the British Anti-Vaccination Society.*

sought by transferring the 'infection-substance' to them locally in
different ways. The procedure was called 'buying pox' and this cost,
in what is now Polish Prussia, three to six pfennigs. Variolation was
sometimes carried out professionally by wise old women who
accompanied it with mysterious ceremonies and oaths (J. Petersen).
The great Danish anatomist Bartholin writes of variolation in 1666
and 1673. However, it was not until the beginning of the eighteenth
century that interest was taken in this folk medicine by Timoni, a
doctor in Constantinople. During the stay in Turkey of Charles XII
of Sweden, the king's surgeon, Skragge, came into contact with
Timoni and Charles arranged for Skragge's story to be sent back to
Stockholm where, however, they had more important things to
think about than variolation, and it was not until 1715 that the
method became generally known in Europe. Among those who were
treated by this not entirely safe method was Gustav III of Sweden
as Crown Prince. Jenner's discovery of vaccination in 1796 swiftly
replaced variolation. But in this too there had been precedents, for
the fact that cowpox had a protective capacity was known to milk-

maids and dairymen in various parts of Europe, including Holstein
(J. Petersen).

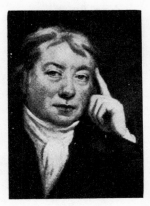

*Edward Jenner, the dis-
coverer of cowpox vaccination (1749–1823). His
discovery that cowpox
vaccination (Latin* vacca =
*cow) offered protection
against human smallpox
was first made public in
1798, more than twenty
years after he had noticed
that milk-maids were never
victims of smallpox.*

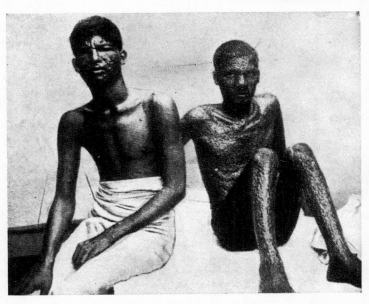

*Two Hindus with smallpox. The one on the left, with a less severe
attack, had been vaccinated seven years previously, and survived. The
one on the right, whose whole body was covered with pustules, was not
vaccinated and died four hours after this photograph was taken (after
M. Mayer,* Exotische Krankheiten, *1924).*

With the introduction of vaccination, at the beginning of the nineteenth century epidemics of smallpox rapidly decreased all over Europe and simultaneously there was a considerable decline in mortality. In all countries with strictly enforced vaccination, only isolated, usually imported cases occurred. In other countries smallpox lost its malignant character and remained as a relatively non-malignant disease called alastrim. However, in Switzerland from 1921–26 5,551 people fell victim to it, and in Great Britain from 1922–34 no less than 70,000, but mortality was very low.

Global Epidemiology gives information on the incidence of variola in Asia, Australia and Africa in the last decades. The morbidity and mortality figures stand in direct relation to how effectively vaccination has been carried out. In large parts of China, Indo-China and especially India, where vaccination extends to only 50–75 per cent of the population, smallpox is still endemic. In Africa epidemics and free periods have alternated sharply. In Egypt, where pilgrimages to Mecca constitute a great danger, 4,138 cases occurred in 1943, no fewer than 11,194 in 1944, but two years later only sixteen. In Kenya severe epidemics raged between 1943 and 1945, but when in the last epidemic mortality figures rose to 31 per cent, vaccination was introduced with very good results. Mortality rates are now slowly decreasing all over the world; in 1945–49 193,000 people died of smallpox, in 1950–54 178,000, and in China smallpox is said to have all but disappeared.

A great deal could be said about the introduction of the vaccinia-virus of cows in different parts of the world, and also about the different forms of poxes in other animals, horses, sheep, pigs and hens; one must too mention in passing the strange disease of the hands in men and women who milk cows, called *Melkerknoten*, 'milker-bumps', which is caused by a related virus, paravaccinia-virus.

Ornithosis (psittacosis), parrot disease

The virus of this disease bears the name *Miyagawanella ornithosis* (after a Japanese researcher Miyagawa). As far as one can judge, this disease has been widespread from time immemorial among birds, especially parrots and related birds in South America, and cases among humans have occurred without rousing any untoward notice. Australian parrots too are nowadays infected. A connection between parrot disease and lung infections in humans was first suspected at the end of the 1870s, and in the 1890s there was increased interest in France in this anthropozoonic, though without any further study of the conditions. Then there was a complete lull until 1929 and 1930 when it suddenly flared up in different parts of the world in the form of a strangely fulminating pneumonia, usually in owners of birds. In all, about 400 cases are supposed to have occurred and mortality was high, 35–40 per cent. All the cases seemed to be connected with a large exhibition of birds in Córdoba in Argentina at which a great many parrots died without anyone setting much store by it. At the same time a number of people died of pneumonia, but this was not connected with the death of the parrots. Not until the exhibition moved to Tucumán in northern Argentina, and both birds and people died as in Córdoba, was it realised that there was a connection between the two. However, before this was realised, parrots had been exported to North America, North Africa and Europe, and everywhere gave rise to sporadic outbreaks of a typical pneumonia and deaths in humans. Nowadays it is known that as well as parrots, other apparently healthy birds can be virus carriers, such as pheasants, hens, turkeys, pigeons, ducks, gulls, finches and canaries. The virus *Miyagawanella psittaci* was discovered simultaneously in 1930 by three Americans, Levinthal, Coles and Lillie. In several European countries epidemics have been observed from which the disease appears to involve direct infection from person to person.

In the USA and Canada, epizootics and enzootics in different kinds of birds have been described, as have major and minor epidemics among humans. In 1954 563 cases in humans were registered, of which nearly 60 per cent arose through birds other than parrots, and in 1952–59 808 cases occurred of which 55 per cent arose through parrots and 45 per cent through other birds, mostly turkeys. By the introduction of a complement-fixation test it has been possible to study further the distribution of the infection. Thus in Denmark Matthiesen found no fewer than 244 cases with positive reaction. It should be mentioned in passing that related virus forms, all called *Miyagawanella*, are known as causes of more or less malignant pneumonias in humans and animals.

Lymphogranuloma inguinale or venereum (climatic bubo, swelling or infection of the lymph nodes of the groin)

The virus of this disease, which is closely related to that of ornithosis, is called *Miyagawanella lymphogranulomatosis*. Cases, which are

57

relatively rare in northern Europe, are said to have been described by Hunter in London in 1786. By the skin test given by Frei, it has been shown that certain inflammations of the external genital organs and rectum in women, which have been known for nearly a hundred years, are caused by the same kind of virus as that of the inguinal bubos. According to Favre and Hellerström, the disease is probably ubiquitous and likely to be found in most ports, but its real distribution is not known. In the ports of the Mediterranean and the tropics with their wretchedly poor hygienic conditions, it is very common, as it is in Ethiopia. In the USA it occurs mostly east of the Mississippi.

Trachoma, 'Egyptian eye disease', and other conjunctivitis diseases (inflammation of the inner membrane of the eyelids)

Trachoma is described in the earliest Egyptian and Chinese medical works. In Hippocrates and Galen one can find notes on its incidence and treatment. Many historical characters of the past were victims, among them Roman emperors. Its distribution over Europe was aided by the Crusades and later by the Napoleonic Wars. The nature of the characteristic cell changes was shown by Halberstädter and Prowazek.

A swelling often appears in the upper eyelid, which makes it hang down. It is said that this is what gives the eye of an oriental its 'romantic' and 'melancholy' look!

Trachoma has an enormous distribution today in the great poverty-stricken and backward countries of Africa and Asia. It is calculated that at least 50 per cent of the population of the world is infected. Trachoma is one of the most significant causes of blindness. In New Guinea 53 per cent of the inhabitants were infected and in one large village 85·7 per cent of those suffering from eye disease had trachoma. Torgersruud found trachoma in 14 per cent of his eye patients in Ethiopia. Trachoma was brought to Sweden from abroad on several occasions. Huss tells of an epidemic in Östergötland at the beginning of the nineteenth century: 'From the German armies of 1814 two soldiers, Stark and Caesar, returned home to Restads village in Vånga parish, both suffering from Egyptian inflammation of the eyes which was prevalent in the Allied armies.' Many others were infected, both children and adults. Trachoma seems to have been very widespread in the parishes; a peasant woman went round treating the patients with blue vitriol and she had over 300 cases. The disease gradually disappeared. During the Second World War a number of cases came in from the Baltic to Sweden.

A form of inflammation of the conjunctiva, which cannot be distinguished from trachoma, either with the naked eye or in a microscope, called *Einschlusskonjunktivis* in German and inclusion conjunctivitis in English, occurs in many parts of the world where genuine trachoma is unknown. It was described over seventy years ago.

Morbilli, measles

This disease is undoubtedly very old indeed. Arab doctors distinguished between '*variolae*' and '*morbilli*', but whether these descriptions correspond to the medical language of today is uncertain. In the seventeenth century measles was recognised as an independent disease by Sydenham, and in 1757 Home showed that the blood of a measles patient infects healthy people. When the whole of continental Europe had long been infected, Iceland and the Faroe Islands were still free. Iceland had its first severe epidemic in 1644, the Faroes in 1781, roughly at the same time as Lapland was infected.

In Japan, measles epidemics are said to have occurred as early as 552 and 998. Despite the principally non-malignant character of the disease in Europe, it produces very high mortality when it attacks a previously un-infected population which lacks immunity. This was the case when it reached North and South America with the arrival of Europeans, and also when it came to South Africa where it was unknown before the arrival of the white man. Similarly, when it reached the Hudson Bay area, the Eskimoes were infected and died. During the American Civil War measles took many victims among the Confederate troops in 1866, as it did too in the Garde Mobile during the Siege of Paris in 1871. During the Boer War, when measles was practically an unknown disease among the Boers, a fifth of those who succumbed in English prison camps died.

German measles, rubella

This disease is also undoubtedly very old, but it was not until 1829 that Wagner recognised it as a special disease, distinct from measles and scarlet fever. Its virus was cultivated in 1954 by Anderson. To

59

the embryo, rubella in the mother involves a risk which should not be underestimated.

Chicken pox, varicella

This disease is said to have been known since the great period of Arab medicine and to have acquired its name from Rhazes; it is, however, very uncertain whether the disease he called varicella is identical with the varicella of today, a word which in general means smallpox. Chicken pox however, has nothing aetiologically to do with smallpox. It was not until the eighteenth century that a distinction was made between the two forms of pox. The virus is called *Briareus varicellae.*

Zoster (herpes zoster), shingles

Shingles, an acute inflammation in a sensory root ganglion in the spinal cord or brain, has been known since classical times; its infectious character was shown by Gruter in 1912, and the nature of its virus by Löwenstein in 1919. The virus is related to the chicken-pox virus and the description herpes should, according to Lehmann, preferably be dropped as shingles has nothing to do with lip sores, herpes simplex, a completely different virus infection. The disease has a clear socio-hygienic distribution in that it is most common in the poorer, overcrowded strata of society.

Foot and mouth disease, stomatitis aphthosa, infectious inflammation and blisters of the mucous membrane of the mouth

The first description of foot and mouth disease in domestic animals comes from Fracastorius in 1514. It is, as is well known, principally a cattle disease but also occurs in sheep, goats, camels and pigs. It has long been known, is to be found permanently in large parts of Asia and now and again spreads in large epizootics. Earlier it reached and flooded all over Europe but now its spread is much slower, thanks to effective protective measures. The epidemic has repeatedly reached Sweden, usually via Denmark, and has been the cause of huge financial losses.

Reports that human beings are infected and get blisters in the mouth exist from the past, but not much is known about the frequency of stomatitis and the formation of blisters in the foot and mouth periods. In tropical countries with poor hygiene, such as Burma and Thailand, epizootics are often said to be accompanied by epidemics in humans. Cases of 'foot and mouth disease' in humans have also been repeatedly noted in Canada, the USA and England, but in Sweden hitherto only a couple of suspected cases have occurred.

Mumps, epidemic parotitis

This disease is clearly described in the *Hippocratic Collection*, in which the usual complication in men, inflammation of the testicles or orchitis, is also mentioned. It is principally a children's disease but can be widespread in barracks and army quarters, as was the case among Confederate troops in the American Civil War.

Infectious mononucleosis, 'student angina'

This disease was first described, it is thought, in 1889 in Germany by Pfeiffer under the name *Drüsenfieber*. Since 1915 and 1920 it has been called mononucleosis. The virus is very widespread on the continent of Europe, in Great Britain and the USA. As it is often found in American students, it is occasionally called student angina. At the university of Wisconsin it is calculated that there are 4·5 cases per 1,000 students every year.

Lymphoreticulosis benigna (*in English* 'cat-scratch' *fever, in German* Katzenkratzkrankheit, KKK)

This disease was observed in the 1920s by Debré who, however, did not make his findings public. A skin test, theoretically similar to the tuberculin test, has been worked out by Hunger and Ross, by which it is shown that the disease occurs in many countries, and in Sweden too, though very seldom. The connection with scratches from cats is not always provable; the localisation of the disease varies very much according to the place of entry of the infection.

Indigenous sleeping sickness, encephalitis lethargica

Opinions differ as to the early history of this disease. Some consider it to be described in the *Hippocratic Collection* and by Graeco-Roman doctors. It is more likely, though, that the *'febris comatosa'* described by Sydenham, which raged in London in 1673–75, was sleeping sickness. During the seventeenth, eighteenth and nineteenth centuries, epidemics which may well have been sleeping sickness also occurred in Germany. General attention was directed to this form of encephalitis by von Economo's classic description of an epidemic in Vienna in 1917. Epidemics, to a great extent similar to that described by von Economo, occurred in Australia in 1917 and 1918. Epidemics with high mortality occurred in St Louis, USA, in 1933 and 1937, and in Japan epidemics have been described which at least in some respects can be said to be identical to the Vienna epidemic.

Molluscum contagiosum

This harmless skin disease, which looks like small rounded skin tumours, has been known as an especially infectious complaint since 1817. In the tropics 1 per cent of the most common skin diseases there are said to be molluscum. The virus, *Molitor hominis*, has been shown only in humans. It is supposed that wrestlers, who rub against each other, are especially susceptible.

Sudor anglicus, 'the sweating sickness'

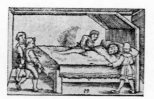

A rare picture of 'The sweating sickness'. In the patient's nightcap are openings 'damit die bösen Vapores, Dempff und Feüchtigkeit vom Houpt steigen können'.

As an appendix to this chapter on viruses, perhaps a few words should be added on the now apparently almost vanished 'sweating sickness'. Its nature as a virus disease cannot be regarded as certain. The disease, the symptoms of which are acute rash and signs of encephalitis, were observed in England in 1486 and occurred later during the fifteenth and sixteenth centuries in Great Britain in a number of epidemics with high mortality. The disease reached Hamburg in 1529 and then spread swiftly to different parts of Germany, France, Russia and Scandinavia, while southern Europe remained free. The following was written about its occurrence in Sweden: 'Anno 1529, Sweden was overcome by the so-called English Sweat from which many thousands lost their lives.'

During the eighteenth century, a similar disease appeared epidemically in Italy, France, Spain and Belgium, and everywhere mortality was high. The last severe epidemic broke out in 1844 in Italy and, somewhat earlier, epidemics had been observed in

Germany and Austria. It is said that single cases have occurred in France, southern Germany and Rumania and that the disease showed itself to be of a virus nature, but this information should be accepted with caution. Shaw has described the history and geography of 'sweating sickness'.

Malignant lymphoma in children

A disease observed in tropical Africa during the last five years. It is thought to be of a virus nature with a species of mosquito as carrier. Many hundreds of cases of this deadly disease are now known.

Leucosis in cattle

An infectious blood disease which may be caused by a virus. It should be included here as the disease has recently become very general in Sweden, especially in the south-east. It has roughly the same distribution area as 'Russian spring encephalitis' (p. 35) and piroplasmosis in cattle (p. 145) and its distribution ought perhaps to be discussed with the vaccinations which have been undertaken against piroplasmosis.

2 Rickettsial Diseases

Rickettsia is the name of a group of micro-organisms which in size generally come between viruses and bacteria. They are difficult to cultivate on artificial media, and they are parasites of arthropods —insects—which transmit them to humans. The name comes from the American pathologist H. T. Ricketts (1871–1910). Burgey's *Manual*, which I principally follow, distinguishes between nine forms, of which only the most important are dealt with here.

Typhus exanthematicus classicus, epidemic spotted fever

The microbe, *R. prowazekii*, is transmitted by the body-louse *Pediculus hominis* from person to person.

Typhus fever is an acutely infectious disease which in certain cases reminds one of ordinary measles. It is inclined to take the form of large and rapidly flaring epidemics when the population is already affected by some other disaster. During wars and famine it has spread and taken many victims, sometimes hundreds of thousands. Hence the eloquent names for this disease—camp-fever, famine-fever, ship-fever, putrid fever and jail-fever. 'The history of typhus is written in those dark pages of the world's story which tell of the grievous visitations of mankind by war, famine, and miseries of every kind.' With these words Hirsch begins his account of its history.

Typhus has been known since time immemorial. The plague which visited Athens in 430 B.C., and which Thucydides described in his history of the Peloponnesian War, has had many different diagnoses: bubonic plague, smallpox, measles, syphilis, dengue, typhus and ergotism (rye-flour-poisoning). The most likely, however, is that it was principally typhus, although one may well imagine that other epidemics raged at the same time or started each other off, for instance smallpox. Opponents of the typhus hypothesis have put forward, among other arguments, that it is hardly likely that body-lice, the transmitters of typhus, would have existed among the inhabitants of Athens who were known for the care they took of their bodies and for their cleanliness. But this probably applied mainly to the upper classes and not to the people in general or to the slaves. Keil rightly emphasises that the significance of the whole population of Attica being concentrated in Athens and the Piraeus during the war seems to have been overlooked, and that the epidemic might well have been brought in by prisoners-of-war in the fleet which was lying in the Piraeus, just where the epidemic broke out. That the lice of the poor country folk and prisoners then rapidly transferred to the inhabitants of Athens, cannot of course be proved, but it seems very likely. It can be added that Fracastoro (1483–1553) considered that the plague in Athens was identical with the typhus he himself experienced.

In ancient Rome pestilences occasionally raged, amongst which typhus was very likely one of the most malignant. Good descriptions of epidemics in Salerno and Bohemia, probably typhus, are to be found from the eleventh century. In 1501 the disease is said to have been carried from Cyprus to Italy. It became widespread at the end of the fifteenth and beginning of the sixteenth centuries in conjunction with the recurring periods of famine then prevalent in large parts of Austria, Germany, France and Spain. During the seventeenth and eighteenth centuries too, Europe suffered severely, and in the Thirty Years War epidemics, among them typhus, raged among both armies and civilians. No part of Europe was spared. In Britain typhus also broke out repeatedly and in poverty-stricken Ireland it remained for a long time. Sweden and Finland were also hard hit, especially in 1695–97.

Napoleon's retreat from Moscow brought back from Russia lice and typhus among the disintegrating armies, and with them there was in 1814 a tremendous diffusion among soldiers and civilians in western Europe. Then the disease generally retreated, only to flare up suddenly during the Crimean War in which 900,000 men sickened, and again during the Russo-Turkish War.

A fairly calm period was followed by a terrible spread of typhus during the First World War, especially in the east where the troops retreating from the Balkans and Russia brought with them lice and disease. In Serbia 150,000 people died in six months, and between 1918 and 1922 the epidemic raged in Russia, where it is calculated that 30,000,000 sickened and about 3,000,000 died.

Nicolle's discovery of the part played by lice as transmitters of the infection showed its value when the First World War could be

65

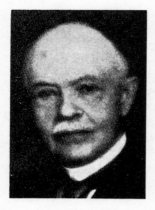

Charles-Louis Nicolle (1866–1936), the conqueror of typhus, became head of the new Pasteur Institute in Tunis. Nicolle's demonstration of the part played by lice in the spread of typhus became the basis for the measures taken in the First World War against the disease. He was awarded the Nobel Prize in 1929.

seen as a great practical experimental application of his research. The discovery of the part played by body-lice was a turning point in the history of typhus, for a once dreaded disease has become an infectious disease which has lost its importance as a devastating epidemic. But one should not therefore think that it has altogether disappeared from Europe. On the contrary, the figures below show that it still existed long after the First World War.

	Lithuania Sick	Dead	Poland Sick	Dead	Russia Sick	Dead
1927	450	214	—	—	38,566	—
1928	519	235	2,401	161	29,440	—
1929	520	151	1,988	146	30,513	—
1930	382	137	1,640	112	22,196	—

Even during the Second World War there was a fair amount of typhus, especially in North Africa and Jugoslavia, in German concentration camps and in Korea and Japan. There was typhus in Naples in 1943–44, and probably in Sicily too. Nowadays the disease is in all probability completely eradicated in Europe and North America, and elsewhere it is gradually receding. However together with three other rickettsial diseases, it is quite widespread in India, China and Korea. In Africa it occurs in many places, and in Egypt in 1943 there were 8,252 deaths from typhus, but five years later only 325.

Typhus exanthematicus endemicus (murine spotted fever), rat typhus

The microbe, *R. mooseri*, is transmitted to humans via rat-lice from rats which are hosts. This form has also undoubtedly existed for centuries and there are even researchers who consider that the murine form is historically the older of the two, probably with good grounds. Distinguishing the endemic form of typhus from the epidemic form has been the cause of considerable difficulties, and the connection between the two forms is not yet clear.

It is widely distributed over the whole of the world wherever there are rats, with the exception of western Europe. Russia, Siberia, Japan and large parts of Africa, especially the Congo, are all infected. In the USA between 1931 and 1946 there were about 42,000 cases and in some years mortality was quite high: for instance in 1945, of 5,193 cases, 214 died.

Febris tsutsugamushi, Japanese river fever, scrub typhus

The microbe, *R. tsutsugamushi*, is transmitted by a mite, *Trombicula akamushi*, and the hosts are rats and mice.

The disease was described in the sixteenth century in China and 150 years ago in Japan. It occurs in the river valleys of Japan and China, and has also been observed in Korea, Formosa, Burma and India. It is to a certain extent an occupational disease, as workers by rivers are affected. Mortality can rise to 50–68 per cent of the victims.

Rocky Mountain fever, tick typhus

The microbe, *R. rickettsii*, is transmitted by a tick, *Dermato-centroxenus*. The hosts are rodents, sheep and dogs.

The disease was discovered in 1899 in the Rocky Mountains and was first believed to be limited to that area, but it also occurs in forty-four of the states of the USA. It has also been established in Canada, Central and South America. Mortality is very high, and in certain respects it is perhaps the most severe of the typhuses. In the USA there were 4,614 cases from 1947 to 1954.

Rickettsiosis quintana, trench fever, five-day fever, Volhynia fever

In all probability this disease is described in ancient and mediaeval medical literature. During the Russo-Turkish War it was called Valakish fever, and in the First World War soldiers on both sides of the front were extensively infected (about a million cases). It occurred in the Second World War too, although on a smaller scale, especially in the Balkans and in the Ukraine.

Febris Q, Q-fever (from query (i.e. uncertain), not Queensland)

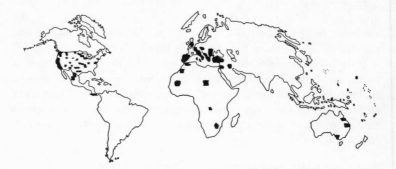

Distribution area of Q-fever.

The microbe, *Coxiella burnetii*, is transmitted to humans by ticks, *Dermacentor andersoni* and others, as well as by fleas. Its hosts are different wild and domestic animals—rats, rabbits, cattle, sheep, goats, horses, pigs and dogs.

The disease was discovered in 1935 in Queensland and in western USA, and became widespread in the Near East and the Mediterranean area in 1944–45 as a result of the Second World War. It is nowadays almost universally widespread in most parts of Europe, with the exception of Holland, Ireland and Scandinavia.

Sennetsu fever

A disease similar to infectious mononucleosis, it occurs in Japan, and has been known since 1955. It is caused by *Rickettsia sennetsu*, whose electronmicroscopic structure was established by Tanaka and Hanaoka in 1961.

As an appendix, I mention here a disease common in the forested river valleys of Peru. Its systematic position is still unclear.

Verruca peruviana, Oroya fever

From Oroya, a province of Peru; also known as Carrion's disease after a student who died after voluntarily allowing himself to be inoculated with verruca serum. The microbe *Bartonella bacilli-formis*(?) produces a peculiar skin disease with bleeding wart-like tumours. Mortality is occasionally very high.

Neorickettsiae is the name given by French researchers to a group of infectious diseases, the importance of which to humans is minimal, but which are considered significant to cattle and pigs. The microbe is said to have a position between the real Rickettsiae and the ornithosis virus. Its isolation is technically difficult.

3 Bacterial Diseases

The innumerable forms of bacteria are nowadays divided into a smaller number of large groups, of which the only two pathogenic groups are dealt with here: Spirillum and Eubacteriales.

Spirillum

Cholera asiatica, Asiatic cholera (from the Greek word cholera, alluding to the thin evacuations)

The microbe is *Spirillum (vibrio) cholerae*, the comma bacillus (Koch, 1884).

The homeland of cholera is considered to be India, especially Bengal and the Ganges delta where swamps and morasses abound. Indian writers of 400 B.C. describe epidemics with symptoms which are typical of cholera. Endemic seats of infection existed very early in eastern and western India. In China, which since records began has been affected by gastro-intestinal diseases, cholera is said to have appeared as early as the seventh century A.D. Large epidemics seem to have been first known much later, at the beginning of the fifteenth century. Vasco da Gama's expedition was probably afflicted with cholera in 1490. In Java a severe epidemic, in all probability cholera, raged in 1629. From the end of the eighteenth century the English garrisons in India lost thousands of soldiers from cholera. Pilgrims too died in tens of thousands from cholera during the eighteenth and nineteenth centuries.

1817 is a fateful year in the history of cholera. Earlier it had been believed that the disease was confined to India, but between 1817 and 1823 it spread over large parts of Asia. It came with a ship to Arabia, two years later it reached Persia; and somewhat later Turkey and Astrakhan. Simultaneously it spread eastwards to Malacca, Siam and Japan.

A larger pandemic gradually spread from India in 1826 over Persia, Arabia, Bokhara, the Volga and European Russia. In 1829–30

70

Poland, Germany, Austria and Sweden were infected, Great Britain and France somewhat later, in 1832–33 the rest of Europe; also in 1832 Quebec and New York, and then Cuba and Mexico.

There was a gap of about eight years before the next outbreak. In 1840 Malacca was affected, in the following year China. In 1844 the epidemic spread across Afghanistan and Persia, in 1846 to Mesopotamia and Arabia, and in 1847 to Asia Minor, Constantinople and south Russia; the following year the whole of the rest of Russia, Finland and Sweden were infected, and a year later the whole of Europe. North America and North Africa were also affected in 1848–49.

The Mediterranean countries were again infected in 1850, Poland and Germany in 1851, Russia again in 1853, also Scandinavia, especially Sweden, and again the whole of Europe in the next two years. Mortality was high; in France no fewer than 140,000 died, in Italy 24,000, in Great Britain 20,000. This great pandemic did not die out completely in Europe until 1856-58.

The fifth great epidemic began in China in 1860-62. In 1865 it reached Turkey, Russia and parts of the rest of Europe, which gradually became almost completely infected in 1866-68. The USA too became infected over large areas.

In 1870 a huge pandemic raged in Asia, reaching Russia the following year, the rest of Europe in 1872 and North America in 1873. In 1881-82 cholera occurred to a lesser extent in Egypt and southern Europe.

The last great pandemic began in 1891 in India, presumably among the huge crowds of pilgrims who returned home after ritual bathing in Hardivar in northern India. The disease spread to the east of the Caspian Sea, and to western Siberia and Russia, where in August it reached St Petersburg. At the end of the month cholera appeared in Hamburg which received its water from the Elbe and the whole city became infected, while its twin city, Altona, with its good drinking water, remained free. The disease reached Berlin and spread to the ports of England, France, Spain and Italy. In Russia the epidemic did not die out until 1896.

A relatively small and mild epidemic began in 1902 and confined itself to parts of Asia, Egypt and southern Europe.

The number of epidemics is questionable; here eight have been mentioned but others talk of six large epidemics. Thanks to improved hygienic measures since 1874 only in exceptional circumstances has cholera kept a hold in Europe and North America. In Asia several epidemics have again occurred more recently and Afghanistan had a serious one in 1938–39. Even in south Asia and the Far East epidemics have become somewhat rarer. China, however, had large epidemics in 1909, 1919, 1926 and 1932, 100,000 cases and 34,000 deaths being reported in this last year. India still holds a special position: between 1927 and 1930 an annual average of 313,000 people died, then the annual mortality decreased to something over 100,000 though it rose to over 236,000 in 1934. Between 1945 and 1949 824,000 deaths were reported, from 1950–54 385,000—a little progress, in fact.

In Africa, many countries have been free of cholera since the beginning of the century, and some others like Uganda, French West Africa and the Congo have generally speaking never had cholera. On the other hand, Egypt presents an exception as the

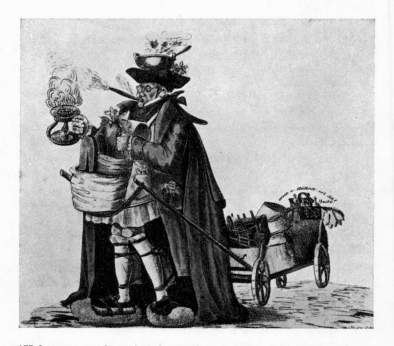

'Kolerapreservativman', colour print of 1832 with text by M. G. Saphir. It says that if one follows all the instructions, one can be certain of catching cholera.

country has suffered from the disease when returning pilgrims repeatedly brought it back with them: in one large epidemic in 1947 25,000 people died, i.e. 45–60 per cent of those who fell ill.

The name paracholera is occasionally used for epidemics with atypical spirella. In 1961 a large epidemic of this kind raged among the poor and undernourished inhabitants of Hong Kong, Formosa, the Philippines and Indonesia.

Rat-bite fever, sodoku (Japanese name)

The microbe, *Sp. minus*, was discovered in 1916 by Futaki; rats are the host animals, and scratches from cats can also transmit the infection. The disease is said to have been known in India before Christ. From there it is supposed to have gone to Japan where it seems to be quite common. It has an almost universal distribution, mostly in sporadic cases, and single cases have also occurred in Sweden.

Eubacteriales (true bacteria)

Rhinoscleroma, a tumour-like swelling of the nose

The microbe, a rod, Klebsiella, was described by Fritsch in 1882.

The disease was formerly especially common in south-east Europe among poor slaves and eastern Jews—many cases were found in the old Austro-Hungarian Empire, in Bessarabia, Rumania and south Russia. Occasional isolated cases were seen in East Prussia, Italy and Switzerland. Very few cases have been noted in Sweden. According to Dutch doctors, it is widespread in the East Indies; an especially dense seat of infection was in Sumatra, and it is also widespread in Central and South America.

Typhus abdominalis, typhoid fever, paratyphoid (earlier often called nerve fever)

The microbes, *Salmonella typhi* and *paratyphi* (Eberth, 1880) were isolated in 1885 by Pfeiffer from excreta of victims.

The history of these diseases really first began with the discovery of their microbes, for even if one can find descriptions which may be of abdominal typhus and paratyphoid in the *Hippocratic Collection* and other records of ancient times, such as Egyptian papyri, it was a long time before it was possible to distinguish them from typhus exanthematicus. From the first quarter of the seventeenth century

73

one can, thanks to Willis, Sydenham and others, see the difference more clearly. Some French clinicians gave quite good accounts, but it was Schönlein who first clearly showed the difference in 1839. Budd, in the middle of the last century, principally studied the epidemiology of the disease and its transmission via the intestinal evacuations, water and milk. Typhoid fever and paratyphoid took first place for a long time among the epidemic diseases of Europe, calmer periods alternating with great spreads of these intestinal diseases with their high mortality. Little is known about circumstances in Asia and Africa in ancient times, but these epidemics almost certainly played an important part there too. South Africa seems to have been especially affected and it is worth noting that during the Boer War mortality from these diseases among English soldiers was very high. No fewer than 31,000 soldiers had to be sent home on account of typhoid fever, while on the other hand, during the Russo-Japanese War three years later, there were only 133 cases. During the American Civil War abdominal typhus was a calamitous factor, especially for the South.

Typhoid fever and paratyphoid were still endemic in Stockholm at the beginning of this century. At the Serafimer Hospital there were nearly always patients with these intestinal diseases, which could not then be distinguished apart. In the Karolinska Institute autopsies were performed on those who died, without any special precautions being taken in the autopsy room, the contents of intestines and the rinsing water running unregarded into the Mälar channel a few hundred yards upstream from the popular Ström bathing-place. Occasionally some purifying agent would be poured into the rinsing water to do what it could.

In many places protective inoculation has had excellent results. The disease has declined or disappeared; but if people with the disease enter a country with refugees, as they did at the end of the last war, those not inoculated become extensively infected. It is not here possible to give an account of the spread of the disease, but a few figures will show what enormous numbers are involved. In India during 1938–47 the average annual number of people ill in hospital was 102,000 and mortality was as high as 82·5 per cent, which indicates that only very serious cases were hospitalised. Typhoid fever has ravaged the whole of the Far East, and an epidemic in the Philippines was especially severe, with 50 per cent mortality. In Egypt also epidemics have followed one after another, and in

Cairo and its suburbs the disease has at times been very common, occasionally with mortality as high as about 17 per cent. One can presume too that the number of registered cases of typhoid fever and paratyphoid in Asia and Africa constitutes only a fraction of the cases that in fact occur.

Bacillary dysentery

The microbe is *Shigella dysenteriae* (Shiga, 1898).

Dysentery, together with the plague, cholera and influenza, is among the severest of mankind's epidemic diseases. Dysentery-type intestinal diseases were described in Egyptian papyri and it is said that the god Horus, son of Isis and Osiris, once sickened of a form of dysentery. It played a role in Europe which now one cannot even imagine, and its spread in countries with poor hygiene is still very considerable. The difficulty in giving exact figures of morbidity and mortality is to a certain extent due to the fact that bacillary dysentery is clinically so similar to another form of intestinal disease, amoebic dysentery, caused by an amoeba, and only serological and microscopic examination can decide which form is in question.

Good accounts of dysentery are to be found in the Ebers papyrus and above all in the *Hippocratic Collection*. Graeco-Roman doctors and Avicenna also knew the disease very well. Stories of army epidemics in ancient times and in the Middle Ages give us a good picture of the part dysentery has played. Wherever large numbers of people have collected together, in barracks and on board ship, in flocks of refugees and during times of famine, outbreaks of dysentery have threatened and achieved catastrophic results. During the American Civil War of 1861–65, nearly two million people fell ill with dysentery and the number of dead was as high as 45,000.

Dysentery is supposed to have raged among the Vikings during their raids on France and also, according to Saxo, among Ragnar Lodbrok's people in Bjarmaland. In King Magnus Eriksson's common law there are two prescriptions for dysentery: 'For blood sickness' and 'This is a remedy for red sickness'. In 1452 dysentery raged in the Danish army which was in the Jönköping region, advancing towards Stockholm. A long narrative verse contains this description:

> God sent them two hard guests,
> With ills of blood-sickness and pest:

Of these much misery ensued
And great numbers of them died.

How common dysentery was in Sweden can also be learnt from
A Useful Home Doctor by Benedictus Olai (Stockholm, 1578), in
which dysentery is spoken of as 'such a sickness as is known to all'.
The severe epidemic among Swedish troops returning from the
Russian War in 1742 is also notorious.

Dysentery has played a very important role in Sweden. Bergman,
who has studied its history, says that of all the epidemics after the last
ravages of the plague, none has been responsible for so many deaths,
not even smallpox, cholera or typhoid fever. Most of its victims
were small children, more in rural areas than in the towns. To
enumerate all the epidemics which Sweden has endured would be
much too lengthy. Particularly severe were the famine years of
1695–98. The years 1736–43, 1770–73, 1808–13 and 1851–60 are
also known for their widespread dysentery epidemics with high
morbidity and mortality. During the epidemic of 1808–13 25 per
cent of the inhabitants of Älvsborg county fell ill and in certain places
it was up to 66 per cent. Occasionally over 50 per cent of those ill
died. In 1858 about a third died of all those who fell ill in the counties
of Jönköping, Östergötland, Kalmar, and Göteborg and Bohus.
During the years 1851–60 dysentery took about 25,000 lives in
Sweden, cholera about 12,000 and smallpox about 13,000. Men in
barracks were particularly affected. Among towns especially affected
was Jönköping where the flood-meadows with their canals and dykes
and the poverty of the inhabitants all presented an excellent target
for the disease.

As with so many other infectious diseases, dysentery has had its
main seat in tropical and sub-tropical areas such as India and
southern China. There it sometimes took first place among causes
of death, if one includes acute and chronic cases with cases of marasmus or wasting after prolonged illness. The possibility cannot be
excluded that in tropical and sub-tropical countries the condition
is often amoebic dysentery. About 50 per cent of the dysentery cases
in Cyprus during recent decades have been of the amoebic variety,
and in Iraq cases of amoebic dysentery were many times more
numerous than those of the bacillary type. In Lebanon a short time
ago, 50–75 per cent of the inhabitants were carriers of the amoeba,
but not all were ill.

Plague, bubonic plague, lung pest, pestis

The microbe, *Pasteurella pestis*, was discovered almost simultaneously in Hong Kong in 1884 by the Japanese Kitasato and the Swiss Yersin. In many epidemics rats and rat-fleas play a large role in the spread of the disease.

Plague has been one of the worst scourges of mankind. In past centuries it swept across huge areas of the world in giant waves and gathered victims in larger numbers than most other diseases. Before it was learnt to distinguish between epidemics, plague was the general name for all diseases with very high mortality but nowadays the name is reserved for those diseases caused by the plague bacillus.

The earliest story of the plague is to be found, as Scheuchzer showed in 1725, in 1 Samuel 5 and 6 where we read how Jehovah's hand slew the Philistines with 'emerods' (grave boils).

The Philistines had taken the ark of the Lord and placed it in the temple of Dagon. 'But the hand of the Lord was heavy upon them of Ashdod, and he . . . smote them with emerods.' Then they moved the ark to another city, but the Lord 'smote the men of the city, both small and great, and they had emerods in their secret parts'. When the ark had been in the country of the Philistines for seven months, the Philistines called for the priests and diviners and asked what they should do. They replied: 'If ye send away the ark of the God of Israel, send it not empty; but in any wise return him a trespass offering; then ye shall be healed', and when the Philistines asked what the offering should be, they received the reply: 'Five golden emerods, and five golden mice, according to the number of the lords of the Philistines: for one plague was on you all, and on your lords. Wherefore ye shall make images of your emerods and images of your mice that mar the land.'

So even then, about 1000–900 B.C., the plague was associated with rodents. There are other stories about rats and the plague in the annals of Sennacherib, in the Bible and in Herodotus. Sennacherib (705–681 B.C.) besieged Jerusalem but retreated without capturing the city. The Bible says that the angel of the Lord one night took the lives of 185,000 men in the camps of the Assyrians, while Herodotus says that countless rats broke into the camps and ate all the leather so that the siege had to be lifted. If one puts these three stories together, they show, according to von Soden, that in all probability there were so many victims of the plague caused by rats in Sennacherib's army, that he had to abandon the infected camp.

77

In the *Bhagavata Purana*, one of the most ancient and important of India's holy scripts, rats are also mentioned in association with plague. The Greek god Apollo too, in one place, is said to have sent plague through mice.

Avicenna, the great Arab doctor of the beginning of the eleventh century, mentions that when the plague drew near to the people, the rats and all the other animals that lived in the ground left their holes and reeled about like drunks. A large epidemic in China in 1643 is said to have cost 200,000 human lives. Another epidemic in the second half of the eighteenth century is described by a contemporary as follows: 'Then it happened that in Chau-chau [in Yunnan] strange rats in the middle of the day pushed their way into the houses where they lay down and died, spitting blood. Not a single man infected by the disease escaped sudden death. Tan-nan wrote a poem about it called "Death of the Rats"—it was his masterpiece. Several days later he himself died too of this strange disease of the rats.' When in 1665 the plague raged in London, every measure, as Defoe says in his classic account *A Journal of the Plague Year* (1722), was taken to get rid of the rats. His shattering realism presents a macabre picture of the suffering caused by the plague, especially among the poor.

Although rats obviously often had much to do with the spread of the plague, it is clear that not all outbreaks of plague have been followed by rats and rat-plague. There is no mention of mass deaths among rats during the Justinian plague, the Black Death or the great Moscow epidemic in 1770.

The first major historically-known plague pandemic is the so-called Justinian plague which probably began in Lower Egypt where it came via the trade routes from China. It spread in 542 along the north coast of Africa, across Palestine and Syria and then reached Europe. It affected the whole of the known world and is considered to have contributed to the decline of the East Roman Empire. It did not die out until the end of the century when it was considered that about half the population of the East Roman Empire had died of the disease or of general destitution. Contemporary eye-witnesses give us a good picture of its advance. Procopius, a prefect in Constantinople, has left a story so full of detail that there can be no doubt that it was plague, and the prefect in Antiochia, Eugarius, describes how he himself fell ill and how he lost his wife, several children, relations and friends.

During the first 1,500 years A.D., more than one hundred major outbreaks of plague are known. Best known is the pandemic which under the name of the Black Death ravaged Europe in the fourteenth century. This epidemic, which must be described as a visitation on a world-historical scale, was only to a minor extent one of bubonic plague, and rats, which are otherwise considered to be of such great significance, seem to have played a small role in the Black Death. Some authors maintain that the Black Death was a lung-pest caught through droplet-infection; others, such as Rodenwaldt, consider that this infection was spread by human fleas. It is not here possible to go into the arguments on which this is based, but they seem very convincing. Nor can one exclude the possibility that the Black Death was a combination of other simultaneous epidemics and that the black spots on the skin could have been the so-called 'black pox'. In any case certain problems still remain to be solved about this fearful pandemic, almost certainly the most terrible visitation to which mankind has ever been exposed, one which shook the foundations of the whole of Europe, bringing with it incalculable economic consequences and leaving its impression on man's whole attitude to life.

The Black Death (*La Mortalega Grande*, *La Peste Noire*, *De Groete Doet*, *Der Schwarze Tod*, *Svatur Daudi* in Icelandic, *Iso Rutto* in Finnish, *Digerdöden* in Swedish) came, like so many other epidemics, from Asia, from either China or India. In the annals of India there is mention of a lengthy epidemic between 1325 and 1351, which indicates an origin in that country. It spread across Mesopotamia, Egypt and Armenia and appeared in the spring of 1347 in Genoa and in the same year in Constantinople. John VI Cantacuzene, Byzantine Emperor when the Black Death ravaged his capital, who in 1355 became a monk and devoted the rest of his life to study and spiritual exercises, gives an excellent account of the disease. It came, he says, from the country of the Hyperborean Scythians, i.e. from the steppes north of the Black Sea. Another Byzantine writer, Nicephorus Gregoras, says the same. The Russian *Troitsky Chronicle* tells that in 1346 the plague was to be found round the Don and Volga, and in the Caucasus and Armenia. It is possible that the Tartars had got it from China, with which they then had active communications; however, the annals of China make no mention at all of the plague at that time. Another Russian document, the *Pskov Chronicle*, says that the disease came from India and this tallies with a traveller's tale of the Arab merchant

Ibn Batuta, who incidentally himself sickened of the plague in Muttra, Mohammed Tiglath's capital, probably in 1332. That the plague had raged in South Russia before it reached Europe is confirmed in the description given by the Italian Gabriele de Mussis of the epidemic in the Crimea in 1344–46. It is supposed to have been a ship from Caffa, now Feodosia, which brought the infection to the ports of the Mediterranean. Caffa was being besieged by Tartars who were themselves suffering from the plague; they hurled their dead with catapults into the city—a kind of bacteriological warfare.

Among those who had a close view of *La Mortalega Grande* in Italy were Boccaccio and Petrarch. A substantial part of the introduction of *The Decameron* is taken up by a description of the epidemic:

> In the year then of Our Lord 1348, there happened at Florence, the finest city in all Italy, a most terrible plague; which, whether owing to the influence of the planets, or that it was sent from God as a just punishment for our sins, had broken out some year before in the Levant; and after passing from place to place, and making incredible havoc all the way, had now reached the west . . .

And Petrarch wrote to the memory of his beloved Laura, who was taken by the plague on 6 April 1348, a poem called 'The Triumph of Death', in which he describes her illness and death. In his *Epistolae familiares* he gives an account of the epidemic and all the miseries that followed it. Another Italian, Agnioli di Tura, 'buried with my own hands five of my children in a single grave. Many corpses were buried so superficially that the dogs dug them up and devoured them. No bells. No tears. This is the end of the world' (Siena, 1354).

Italy seems to have suffered most. Emperors, kings and princes died of the plague and artists like Ghirlandaio, Giorgione, Perugino and Titian are supposed to have been victims.

Superstition flourished; the Jews were hounded and killed as it was believed they had caused the plague, and synagogues and ghettoes were burnt down. In a village in Savoy a doctor confessed under torture that he had poisoned the well water with a concoction of snakes, frogs, scorpions and communion wafers. The great French surgeon Ambroise Paré believed that the plague was deliberately spread by poisoners who smeared doors and walls with plague-infected matter.

Because of the ravages of the plague, Pope Clement VI advanced the Holy Year, which was to be celebrated in 1350, to 1348; at Easter 150,000 pilgrims from all over Europe visited Rome in the hope of appeasing the heavens, almost certainly contributing to the further spread of the disease. From the Mediterranean countries it slowly spread across the whole of Europe. It came by ship to Scandinavia. A plague-infected ship from London, most of the crew of which was already dead, ran aground near Bergen on the west coast of Norway and so the plague arrived.

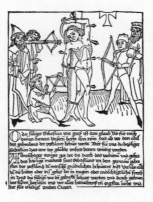

St Sebastian as the patron saint of the plague stricken (15th century German woodcut). After the Evangelist Luke, himself a doctor, more and more of the saints were regarded as patrons in sickness, especially the brothers SS. Cosmas and Damian, born in Arabia in the fourth century. In times of plague one confided especially in St Sebastian who himself had had the disease. Below is written a prayer for release from pestilence.

When it came to Sweden in 1349, King Magnus Eriksson issued a proclamation which read that God 'because of the sins of man, had had a great plague of sudden death thrown into the world, so that most of the people in the lands that lie west of our country have died of this plague; and it is now all over Norway and Halland, approaching us here'. Orders went out for the arrangement of special church services and processions, for prayers, fasts and diligent distribution of alms, but none of these helped. The disease spread and devastated the country; no Boccaccio or Petrarch has given us an account of the havoc. Trade ceased, agriculture collapsed, beasts died and famine was the result. All moral ties loosened, people fled from each other, families were dispersed, empty houses plundered and it became a matter of living well while the going was good.

The Black Death was also carried to Iceland and Greenland and was probably one of the reasons why the Nordic colony died out there; it was partly too because of the consequent lack of supplies from plague-stricken Scandinavia. Tuberculosis existed there as

81

well; it has been established in bodies in the churchyards. The western region already lay waste before 1370. Finally hostilities with the Eskimoes had their effect. They advanced on the eastern region in 1379 and the last Norsemen fell towards the end of the fifteenth century. Sea communication ceased and the country lay completely forgotten.

The most northern part of Russia and Archangel were also infected, probably by a ship from the west. Ilmoni gives an important item about the plague in Russia in 1352 which literally says that 'the disease showed itself through glands in the soft hollows of the body', clearly indicating the buboes, swellings of the lymph nodes of the armpit and groin.

It is calculated that the Black Death in Europe cost twenty-five million human lives; those terrible years have been called the black night of the Middle Ages. But after that great blood-letting, the will to live re-awoke and it is considered that the birth-rate rose rapidly. There followed the prosperity of the Renaissance.

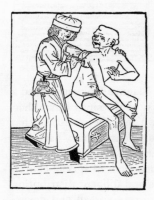

Plague doctor opening an ulcer in the lymph nodes of the armpit (German woodcut 1482). When the ulcers appeared one tried to dissolve them with different plasters and ointments and then open them. Another method 'which was highly praised by the doctors', was to bind a live plucked cockerel or a toad over the ulcer.

The plague did not loosen its grip on Europe immediately. From the end of the fourteenth century major and minor epidemics followed one another, until the pressure began to lessen at the beginning of the seventeenth century. Denmark had her last large epidemic in 1654, Sweden in 1657, England in 1666–67, but 1710 was still a bad year for Sweden, as the church registers bear witness. This epidemic, Sweden's last, did not die out until 1713, and an excellent account of it is given by the medical historian Hult (1916). In Russia and the Balkans, the plague remained for a long time.

When Peter the Great attacked Riga in 1710, thousands died of it, and from 1770–72 a terrible epidemic raged in Russia, especially in Moscow.

Our information on the plague position in south Asia and China during recent centuries is uncertain, but in general it seems to have been of a less malignant nature. This seems also to have been the case with the immensely widespread pandemic which began in the interior of China in 1893 and spread via Canton to Bombay and the rest of India during the following years, reaching Arabia, Turkey and Madagascar in 1898 and crossing to the southern hemisphere and South Africa for the first time in 1899. Then suddenly came the news that Paraguay and other South American

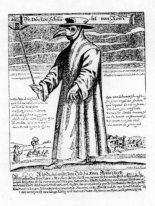

Plague doctor in protective clothing—'Doctor Schnabel von Rom' (German engraving by P. Furst after J. Colombina, 1656). The text says that the doctors of Rome were clad in this way when visiting the sick. The long beak of the face-mask is filled with 'aromatic spices', the gown is of leather or waxed cloth, and the rod is to indicate what should be done.

countries had been infected. That same year plague appeared in Oporto and Vienna, the following year in Glasgow and San Francisco's Chinatown, then somewhat later in Italy and on the east coast of Africa. Large parts of the world had thus been infected, but this time the disease was everywhere relatively mild.

Since the First World War, plague has everywhere declined, yet, for example, in 1927–30 in Argentina the average annual number of deaths from plague was 60, in Africa 5–10,000, in Dutch East Indies about 30,000 and in India 30,000–136,000. In Africa plague lingered in many places, what was then French West Africa apparently being the central seat of infection, where in 1912–46 45,000 people sickened and mortality was high, 70 per cent.

The plague-complex, an expression used by Sorre, is very elaborate. There are, according to him, many infectious forms,

83

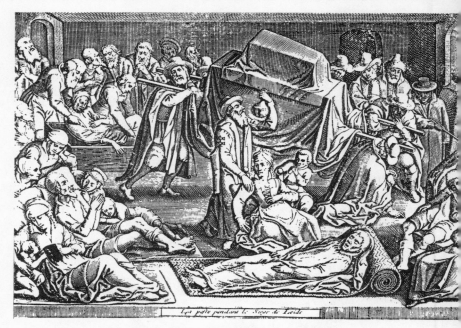

The plague in Leyden during the Spanish siege of 1574.

carriers and hosts. One has to contend not only with ordinary rats but also with at least forty other rodents who carry different species of fleas. Other mammals too are hosts of the plague bacillus— cattle, sheep, camels, dogs, cats and bats.

Here we enter the interesting and as yet obscure border country between genuine plague, so-called Manchurian plague, the plague of the Russian steppes and tularaemia which is dealt with below. In 1825 Chernobayev observed a small plague-like epidemic in Russia which was probably no more than tularaemia, and Zeiss maintains that a mild plague-like epidemic, a '*pestis minor*', in Astrakhan and its surroundings was tularaemia. During the First World War plague appeared in Paris and this too was probably a '*pestis minor*'.

Pseudotuberculosis

An anthropozoonic caused by *Pasteurella pseudotuberculosis (rodentium)*, a microbe related to the plague bacillus. It is really a hare disease and is briefly mentioned here as it occasionally strikes man in whom it can cause attacks of what appears to be appendicitis with swelling of the mesenteric lymph nodes. Only since 1950 has any substantial interest been taken in it (by Malassez and Vignal; Henschen; Strömbeck; Borg and Thal).

84

Tularaemia, hare plague

The microbe, *Bacterium tularense*, is transmitted by mosquitoes and ticks, and the host animals are principally rodents such as rats, squirrels, hares, rabbits, opossums, and possibly some other animals. Often it is associated with infected sores.

This very widespread infectious disease has existed for a long time, but was first described by McCoy in 1911, in a rodent of Tulare County, California. The first case in humans was also described in the USA (1914) and a considerable number of cases were soon registered in different states. In Japan, where the disease has long been known, it is called Ohara's disease. It is found in Russia and in northern parts of Norway and Sweden. Recent investigations by Jusatz and others show that it has an enormous distribution among European rodents, and that its transmission to humans is very similar to that of the plague. Jusatz considers that during the last thirty to forty years tularaemia has spread from western Siberia to European Russia, Central Europe and Turkey. The disease is to a certain extent an occupational disease, in that people who handle host animals—i.e. small furred animals and hares—like hunters, trappers, traders in pelts and edible rodents, game merchants and cooks, can be infected through small skin sores. Cases have also occurred among laboratory staffs.

Pertussis, whooping cough

The bacteria, *Haemophilus pertussis*, was described in 1906 by Bordet and Gengou.

The history of this disease can be traced only back to the sixteenth century, but everything goes to indicate that it is a very old disease. The earliest information is of an epidemic in Paris, described by Baillou in 1578, but this mentions that the disease is not new. We have German, English and Swedish (Rosén von Rosenstein) works on the disease from the seventeenth and eighteenth centuries. The disease seems to have become increasingly widespread. In the years 1749–64 in Sweden no fewer than 43,000 children are said to have died of whooping cough, although the possibility cannot be excluded that in many cases it was lung tuberculosis, as I found in certain countries on my visit to South America in 1948, where the latter disease occasionally figured in the official statistics as whooping cough. Whooping cough reached the Faroe Islands for the first time in 1778, Iceland in 1826 and Greenland in 1838, always brought from the mainland. In the previous century the disease had spread widely in Central Europe and in the British Isles mortality was high; in the Mediterranean it has always been rarer and milder.

The latest information on whooping cough still shows wide distribution in all countries of the world, but mortality is decreasing: in 1950 26,325 deaths in twenty-eight countries, in 1955, 10,376.

Brucellosis, Bang's disease, Malta fever, Mediterranean fever, undulant fever, in cattle, sheep, pigs and humans

These diseases are caused by three closely related bacteria, *Brucella melitensis*, principally in goats and discovered by Bruce in 1887, *Brucella abortus* (Bang, 1897) in cattle, and *Brucella suis* (Traum, 1914) in pigs. All are also pathogenic to humans.

Brucellosis seems to have been known in ancient times and is mentioned in the *Hippocratic Collection*. It is considered to have already appeared then on the island of Thasos and it was known in Asia Minor, India and China as a disease in goats and humans.

Gradually it became clear that the disease was very widespread in both domestic animals and humans. In many regions 20–30 per cent of the cows were infected. In the 1920s it seemed a dangerous threat, and at the time Nicolle looked upon brucellosis as an increasing disease which would perhaps replace tuberculosis. Rational measures however have averted the danger and at present both the cowsheds and the people of Denmark and Sweden are free of brucellosis. In countries where unboiled milk is drunk and hygiene offers no protection, it is quite widespread. In New Zealand in 1938 30 per cent of the cows were infected.

Haemophilus influenzae, influenza bacillus

This bacteria was cultivated by Pfeiffer in 1892–93 and was considered at the time to be the infecting agent of influenza. During the great pandemic in 1918 of 'Spanish 'flu', it was not usually possible to demonstrate it; in other epidemics it was found in the nose and throat. Its significance as a cause of disease is still being discussed.

Ulcus molle, soft chancroid

The microbe was demonstrated by Ducrey and bears his name. This disease was earlier often confused with other sores on the genital organs and glandular swellings in the groin. It was common all over the world, especially in harbour towns, but has as good as disappeared in countries with strict controls.

Malleus, glanders

The bacteria, *Pfeifferia mallei*, was cultivated in 1882–86 by Löffler and Schütz, from horses.

Glanders is really a horse disease which also attacks donkeys and mules. It appears in different forms, often with ulcers in different organs, and is considered to have been known since antiquity. The Latin name *malleus* is said to stem from the Greek *melis*, severe illness or epidemic, and to derive from Aristotle. The disease once had a wide distribution in cavalry horses and many men were also infected and died, partly through hand sores, partly through the consumption of the flesh of infected horses. The disease declined, but during the First World War it again spread in Russia and Germany and people were infected. In France in 1935–45 more than 5 per cent of the army's horses had to be slaughtered because of glanders. In Sweden, as in the rest of Scandinavia, glanders has long since been eradicated.

Gonorrhoea, ophthalmia neonatorum and other gonococcus diseases

The microbe, *Neisseria gonorrhoeae*, was first isolated by Neisser in 1879.

Few diseases can be traced so far back as this. In contrast to a number of other infectious diseases, it does not seem to have changed its character over the centuries, which is no doubt connected with the fact that there is no innate or acquired immunity to it. It is mentioned in the Ebers papyrus whose origins are supposed to go back several thousand years B.C. The Jews of the Old Testament knew that a pus-like discharge in the urethra occurs after intercourse with an infected woman. The disease is mentioned in the *Hippocratic Collection* and Aretaeus. In Pompeii instruments were found for the treatment of stricture of the urethra, presumably of a gonorrhoeal nature, and the method of infection was well known. Avicenna too knew the disease. A certain confusion in the teaching on gonorrhoea ensued at the beginning of the sixteenth century when it was classed with the new disease of syphilis, and it was a very long time before these two venereal diseases could be distinguished. During the Middle Ages all venereal diseases were in any case considered 'unclean', and doctors did not willingly concern themselves with them, leaving their treatment to barbers, bath attendants and army surgeons.

The white man took the disease to America and it is now widespread throughout the world. Reliable information on its frequency is on the whole lacking. In Israel it is supposed to have increased during the mass immigrations; an increase is also shown in countries where there has been no great movement of people. In certain African countries gonorrhoeal eye-diseases are common.

Epidemic cerebro-spinal meningitis (inflammation of the soft membranes of the brain and spinal cord)

The bacteria, *Neisseria meningitidis*, was isolated by Weichselbaum in Vienna in 1887.

This disease cannot be traced back further than 1805 when Vieusseux described an epidemic in Geneva. In the following year epidemics were observed in the Prussian army, in New England and a number of other countries, mostly where there were troops. In the 1840s epidemics appeared in Denmark but Sweden was spared until 1854. In many countries the disease has now almost completely disappeared, but it occurs endemically or epidemically in many non-European countries, where mortality is often very high. In 1935–40 China and Mongolia had numerous large epidemics, occasionally with a mortality of 20–45 per cent. It has particularly affected the Maoris in New Zealand. During recent decades there have been epidemics in many African countries, with up to 75 per cent and even 100 per cent mortality.

Pneumonia

The most important microbes causing these bacteriologically diverse diseases are the pneumobacillus, *Klebsiella pneumoniae* (Friedländer, 1883) and the pneumococcus, *Diplococcus pneumoniae* (Fraenkel, 1886). Pneumonias with a high mortality are often of a virus nature, such as the ornithosis virus, on which antibiotics have no marked effect.

With penumonias it is seldom possible to differentiate between different aetiological forms without bacteriological and other laboratory investigations. Primary and secondary, sporadic and collective cases have probably at all times been one of the most important immediate causes of death in all countries. Hirsch's classic work shows this, as does the modern *Global Epidemiology*. That pneumonia occurred in ancient Egypt has been confirmed by anatomical and bacteriological examination of a mummy in which diplococci could be shown. The doctors of Greece and Rome knew the disease.

With modern therapy, mortality in the bacterial pneumonias has declined rapidly where such treatment is used, but in large parts of Asia and Africa mortality was very high only a short while ago. In South-East Asia, in the Philippines, in 1937–38 71,000 fell ill with pneumonia and of these 64,000 died, i.e. about 90 per cent. Pneumonias in Africa show almost as high mortality rates, and in Egypt in 1933–35 about 70 per cent of those ill died, in former French West Africa 70–80 per cent. Modern chemotherapy and antibiotics have greatly reduced mortality, but in 1938 it was calculated that still about 260,000 people died in India of different forms of pneumonia.

Here in Sweden the previously common fibrinous pneumonias caused by pneumococci have practically disappeared from the autopsy tables.

Febris puerperalis, puerperal fever

By far the most important microbe here is the haemolytic *Streptococcus pyogenes*. The history of puerperal fever is lost in antiquity. The disease was known in ancient Greece, as were epidemics. Avicenna too described it. However, it was not until the fifteenth and sixteenth centuries that definite advances could be discerned. The name puerperal comes from Willis (1682). Terrible epidemics in recent centuries play a very great part in the history of puerperal fever. There are accounts extant from a great number of European cities, since the large Paris epidemic of 1664. Copenhagen had its first known epidemic in 1672, but there is no information from Stockholm before 1777, which does not mean to say that the disease was unknown earlier.

Very early on it was discovered that puerperal fever was primarily associated with places of confinement and it was soon evident that it was an infectious disease, a *'febris putrida'*, caused by a miasma or contagium. 'Nosocomial atmosphere', the lack of ventilation, was supposed to have played a decisive part. In Vienna, mortality rose from 1823 on and soon reached enormous heights. The moment for an awakening interest in pathological anatomy had arrived. 'In the course of anatomy,' wrote Semmelweiss, 'professors, assistants and students often have the opportunity to come into contact with corpses', and from these examinations they went straight to the maternity wards where women in labour were examined. It is to Semmelweiss's eternal credit (1847) that he showed the cause of this murderous disease and that he indicated the way to overcome it.

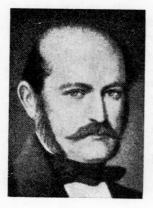

Ignaz Philipp Semmelweiss, the conqueror of puerperal fever, b. in Budapest 1818, d 1865. In pre-bacteriological times, he made fundamental investigations into the causes of puerperal fever and showed its infectious nature. The importance of his discovery was not appreciated until much later, after his tragic death.

Erysipelas

The cause of this disease is *Streptococcus erysipelatis*. The word erysipelas appears in the *Hippocratic Collection* as a name for different purulent and inflamed skin affections. The distinction between an 'idiopathic' and a 'traumatic' form was made early on. Earlier the disease occurred sporadically or epidemically, the latter mostly in hospitals, mental hospitals and children's homes, in which hygienic standards left much to be desired.

Scarlatina, scarlet fever

The microbe is *Streptococcus haemolyticus*.

Rhazes, Avicenna and other Arab doctors differentiate between smallpox and another acute-exanthematic disease which they call '*hasbah*', which could correspond to the rash diseases of scarlet fever, measles and German measles. Differential diagnosis slowly progressed thanks to the contributions of German and English doctors, especially Sydenham. The name scarlatina originally came from Italy. The origin of the disease and how it was, and is, distributed in different countries is not of any great interest; it seems as if

Emil von Behring (1854–1917), the discoverer of anti-diphtheria serum, was first an army doctor, then worked with Koch, and finally became professor in Marburg where the Behring-Werke, a factory for the manufacture of serum, bears his name. His discovery of the serum treatment for passive immunisation against diptheria and tetanus is his most famous achievement. Behring was awarded the first Nobel Prize for medicine in 1901.

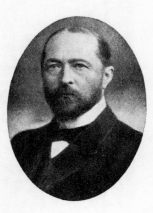

it was unknown in certain countries, such as Japan, for a long time. In North America the first epidemic was observed in 1735, in South America not until a hundred years later and in Australia first in the middle of the last century. This information should, however, be treated with caution.

Diphtheria

The microbe, *Corynebacterium diphtheriae*, was discovered by Löffler in 1884.

A disease, which may well have been diphtheria, is mentioned in the Ebers papyrus and the Egyptian word can be translated as '*cynanche*', inflammation of the throat. The *Hippocratic Collection* mentions different forms of throat inflammation accompanied by difficulty in breathing and swallowing, under the name of '*kunanche*'. The first clear description of 'croup' is found in Baillou (1576), and he also mentions fibrous membranes in the mucous membranes of the throat. The name croup was used before Löffler's discovery of the bacterium for different conditions of spasm in the bronchial tubes and breathing difficulties. It was founded on clinical symptoms and is now hardly ever used.

Before the introduction of the serum treatment discovered by Behring and of modern prophylactics, the disease had a vast distribution, especially in cold and temperate countries, but it is not unknown in warmer zones. Mortality was mostly high but varied

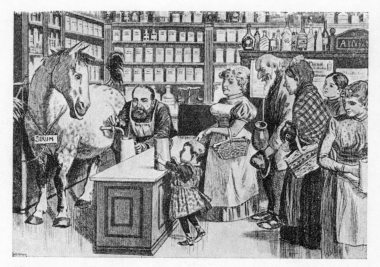

'Serum—straight from the horse' (*cartoon in* Lustige Blätter, *1894*). *The discoverer of anti-diphtheria serum, Professor von Behring, in an apron, is serving the serum* 'frisch vom Fass' *to the small-town public.*

considerably from country to country and epidemic to epidemic. In Egypt about thirty years ago, mortality was as high as 32–48 per cent. In Europe in 1948 119,000 cases were registered, ten years later the number had diminished to less than half and at the same time mortality decreased considerably.

Erysipeloid, in pigs and humans

The bacteria, *Erysipelothrix rhusiopathiae*, is transmitted from pigs and various wild animals, fish and shell-fish, via skin sores to those who come in contact with sick animals. No special geography is shown.

Anthrax, pustula maligna

The pathogenic significance of the anthrax bacillus was shown by Koch in 1877.

The early history of anthrax is obscure, but it is probable, according to Klemm and Klemm, that it was known in ancient Egypt and Mesopotamia 6,000–7,000 years ago. Moses warned Pharaoh about a severe disease in domestic animals, which could have been anthrax, and acute outbreaks still occur in Egypt today. In India the disease seems to have been known in 500 B.C. and in ancient Greece anthrax occurred in animals and in humans who used the flesh, skins and wool of infected animals. When the Huns advanced westwards, anthrax is said to have broken out among their horses and beasts and men too were infected; this epidemic is considered by some authors to have saved Europe. A severe epidemic in San Domingo in 1770 is very well known; there black and white colonists, during a period of famine, ate salted and smoked meat from anthrax-infected animals. No fewer than 15,000 died. In 1867–70 Russia suffered a severe outbreak of animal and human anthrax. Outside Europe there are huge areas where anthrax can be said to be endemic. During the First World War, in both America and Europe, people were infected by insufficiently sterilised shaving brushes made of Chinese horse-hair. In certain countries anthrax has the character of an occupational disease in workers who deal with raw hides, and in rag-pickers. It now seems to be on the decline all over the world.

Gas gangrene

There is a group of gas-forming anaerobic microbes, of which *Clostridium welchii, Cl. oedematiens* and *Cl. septicum* are the most important.

The sore-healers of ancient times almost certainly knew of the feared complications which these microbes cause. Ambroise Paré's descriptions of the wounded in the Siege of Rouen (1562) include cases which can be interpreted as gangrene. It was not until the middle of the last century that the concept of oedema and gangrene became clear.

Among related diseases in animals should perhaps here be mentioned a septicaemia with gas-formation in whales, which has been used since the Middle Ages to kill whales in a fjord on the coast of Norway. The fjord has a shallow opening. The whales, which come in at high tide, cannot swim out and when their backs rise above the surface of the water, they are shot with 'death-arrows', i.e. arrows whose points have been dipped in blood from whales which had died of septicaemia, rich in spores and preserved from year to year. When the arrow penetrates the skin, septicaemia and gas-formation develop and the animal dies; von Klinckowström has called this the oldest cultivation of bacteria in the world.

Botulismus, food poisoning

Van Ermengem discovered the microbe, *Clostridium botulinum*, in 1896 in a piece of salted ham, the consumption of which had caused three deaths and several cases of illness. In North America, especially in the winter, where preserves are extensively used and sterilisation was formerly imperfect, in the years 1899–1925 there were no fewer than 146 outbreaks of botulism with 504 cases and 337 deaths; the figures are, however, almost certainly too low. The disease has greatly receded now both in America and Europe. In Sweden also a few cases have been observed. The microbe is a saprophyte on dead tissue in which it develops extremely poisonous toxins.

Tetanus, lockjaw

The microbe, *Clostridium tetani*, was described in 1884 by the German Nicolaier, and was cultivated by Kitasato five years later.

There are accounts of this disease in the *Hippocratic Collection*, Galen, Aretaeus and Avicenna. It was also known to learned men of the Middle Ages. Reliable information on the spread and frequency of the disease in antiquity does not exist, but it was probably more common in hot countries than colder ones. Even in the 1880s Hirsch considered that changes in the weather formed the most important cause of tetanus, and he says: 'the assumption that the condition of the ground in itself exercises any influence on the occurrence of tetanus, is quite without foundation'. But experiences from the First World War tell another story about which one cannot be mistaken. In the forests and swamps of Russia tetanus was a rarity, but on the western front, where the fighting was in a terrain of highly cultivated, chalky, well-manured field and garden soil, cases were numerous. Horses droppings are rich in spores.

It has long been known that there are zones in which tetanus cases occur frequently. Chavannez mentions a number of such zones in France. Möse however, found no definite association with the number of horses or with the geology of the soil. On the other hand he thinks that areas with poor rainfall are richer in tetanus spores, for then the spores are not washed away or sucked up by the soil, but are left on the surface for longer periods.

Besides the form of tetanus which is complicated by dirt in sores, one should briefly mention the forms which occur in women in confinement or in new-born infants before the umbilical cord heals.

In countries with good hygiene such cases are nowadays rare, but they are still common in more primitive countries, as once in Denmark, Iceland and Sweden.

Since the Second World War tetanus has been rare in England, Scandinavia and, to a certain extent, Germany, with an incidence of

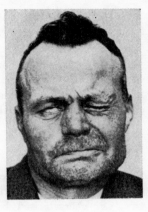

Tetanus in the head with cramp on the left side.

between 1·7 and 9·2 per million, but common in Austria, France, Spain, Jugoslavia (20–22 per million) and especially Hungary (50 per million). Much higher figures are found in many other countries, for instance, in Brazil (178 per million), San Domingo (475), former French Africa (650), Japan (1,161) and Mexico (no fewer than 1,934 per million).

Listeriosis

This anthropozoonic, still insufficiently understood, which was described in the 1930s in rodents and then in the 1950s in humans in several European countries, amongst others Sweden (P. Bergman *et al.*), is of no particular geographical interest, as far as is known. The pathogenic microbe, *Listeria monocytogenes*, is a gram-positive aerobic rod.

4 Tuberculosis, Leprosy and Fungus Diseases

For the sake of lucidity, certain microbes have been grouped here, which do not really belong to the genuine bacterias, but border on fungi—namely the tubercle bacilli, the leprosy bacilli and a number of pathogenic fungi. The so-called sarcoidoses, whose position is not at all clear, are dealt with in an appendix.

Tuberculosis

'Tuberculosis' nowadays embraces all tissue disturbances which are caused by the tubercle bacillus, whether they are chronic and productive, i.e. characterised by tissue-formation, or more acute and exudative, i.e. associated with a typical inflammation. The microbe, *Mycobacterium tuberculosis*, which was discovered by Koch in 1882 is, as the term goes, 'acid-fast' and occurs in different 'types', among which *Typus humanus*, *Typus bovinus* and *Typus avium* are of interest here.

Tuberculosis is in all probability older than the human race. The occurrence of tuberculosis in mammals, of tuberculoid changes with acid-fast bacilli in cold-blooded animals and of saprophytes (which live on dead organisms), similar to the tubercle bacilli and capable of producing tuberculoid changes in experimental animals, all point to tuberculosis in mammals and humans arising through the gradual adaptation of the saprophytic microbes to living tissue, to higher animals and to humans.

The earliest history of human tuberculosis is lacking in data and is principally based on a limited number of cases of bone tuberculosis. In certain respects, parts of the skeleton of a young man who died about 5,000 years B.C. near Heidelberg is regarded by some as a very early record. His cervical vertebral column shows disturbances which are considered by some to be healed tuberculosis, by others to be a healed fracture of the cervical vertebrae and by yet others to be a deformity. I personally am very sceptical about the diagnosis of

96

tuberculosis, but whether it is really a case of tuberculosis or an old fracture, this case shows at least that even at that time in ancient Germany a man with a severely injured cervical vertebral column was cared for over a period of many months.

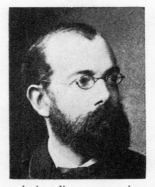

Robert Koch, discoverer of the tubercle bacillus, b. in Oberharz 1843, d. 1910. The photograph dates from before his discovery, which was made public in the spring of 1882, and aroused both great hopes and fierce opposition. He first carried out his famous investigations alongside his daily work as a country doctor. After 1880 he was active as a bacteriologist exploring distant countries. Many of his pupils bear world-famous names. He was Nobel Prize winner in medicine in 1905. He lies in a mausoleum in the Institut für Infektionskrankheiten in Berlin.

As far as the incidence of tuberculosis is concerned, we have no firm evidence before the time of the Egyptian Pharaohs. Eleventh and Twelfth Dynasty statuettes portraying typical hunchbacks and the mummy of a young Twenty-first Dynasty Ammonite priest showing damage to the twelfth thoracic and first lumbar vertebrae, as well as a large pus-formation or so-called abscess-cavity on the right side, which at embalming was filled with another substance, are evidence that the disease then already existed. At present it appears that only ten to fifteen cases of spinal and hip tuberculosis from ancient Egypt are known and one cannot really draw any definite conclusions from these few cases about the distribution and frequency of tuberculosis in the inhabitants; the lack of cases of tuberculosis of the soft tissues, especially tuberculosis of the lung, is to be especially regretted. The internal organs were nearly always carefully removed before embalming and the men who did this were only artisans who had no interest in the morbid changes they had daily opportunities to observe. Doctors scorned having dealings with the dead. In India lung tuberculosis is thought to have been known about 1,000 years B.C. and is described there as a wasting away. In

97

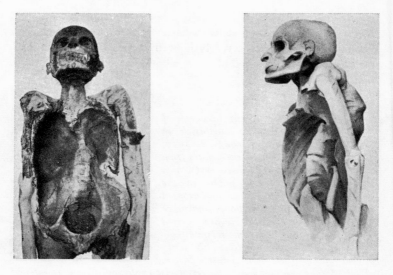

The mummy of a young Ammonite priest from the 21st Dynasty (c. 1000 B.C.) with spinal tuberculosis, damaged twelfth cervical and first lumbar vertebrae and a large so-called abscess-cavity with pus-formation, which in embalming was filled with another substance (after Elliot Smith and M. A. Ruffer, 1910.)

the statute book of Manu of 600 B.C., noble Indians of the three highest castes were forbidden to marry into families with consumption. Neander calls this the world's first legislation for race purity.

Greek and Roman doctors knew of lung tuberculosis, which they considered hereditary (*habitus phthsisicus*, see p. 11), as did innumerable later generations of doctors. If they ever had any conception of the appearance of disturbances in the lungs, they might, as has been pointed out, have acquired them from seeing lung tuberculosis in cattle. Arab doctors also knew of tuberculosis of the lungs.

Tuberculosis already existed in the New World before Europeans arrived. Means has found two cases of bone tuberculosis among 500 skeletons of Indians in Ohio, and recently Roney has reported a case of vertebral tuberculosis from California. Garcia Frias has shown in Peruvian Indian mummies both bone tuberculosis and a case of calcified tuberculosis of the right lung and corresponding lymph nodes. Peruvian pottery and Mexican art show the presence of tuberculous hunchback from pre-Columbian days. With the arrival of Europeans, the spread of tuberculosis among the native peoples of America rapidly increased.

In the Mediterranean countries, tuberculosis is said to have been widespread very early. In many places it was considered highly infectious, and the sick were isolated, but the teaching on tuberculosis as an infectious disease did not come until much later.

In Central Europe also tuberculosis was evident early on, though not among the overcrowded poor, but in the highest classes of society. A doctor in 1648 mentions that three young Brandenburg princes were infected by their tutor. In Sweden Linnaeus gave warning of the danger of having old women who coughed as

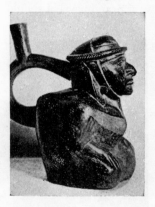

Peruvian ceramic from the pre-Columbian period (Mochica civilisation), showing a tuberculous gibbus or hump in the upper part of the thoracic vertebral column.

children's nurses: '*Vetulae laborant saepe phthisi.*' Another two cases of probable early tuberculosis infection can be mentioned. The Duke of Reichstadt, Napoleon's son, might have received tuberculosis from his father, who after autopsy was shown to have a tuberculosis cavity in his left lung. Oscar I of Sweden appointed as tutor to his sons, a Norwegian, Aubert, who died of tuberculosis. It does not seem unlikely that the tuberculosis from which his sons Carl and Gustaf died, and the mild chronic lung tuberculosis from which Oscar II suffered, stemmed from this tutor.

Tuberculosis probably came to Scandinavia quite late, when communications both in peace and war became more lively and foreigners arrived there. It does not seem improbable that the disease was at first characteristically one of the upper classes. The first mention in Nordic literature of what can be interpreted as tuberculosis is in Saxo who tells of a man of the priesthood in the reign of Canute the Great (d. 1086) who 'died consumed by lengthy prostration through a damaged lung'. Norway's early history includes a king, Inge Crookback (d. 1161), who possibly suffered from spinal tuberculosis. Even if both these cases are open to other interpretations, there is a skeleton of an eight-year-old Swedish boy from the twelfth century, which was found in one of the royal graves in Vreta Cloister, an unequivocal case of severe chronic tuberculosis of the spine. The child belonged to the Steinkel family and was perhaps the last male member of the oldest Swedish royal line (Fürst).

Before we leave the scanty information on tuberculosis in mediaeval Scandinavia, I should like to give prominence to the hypothesis

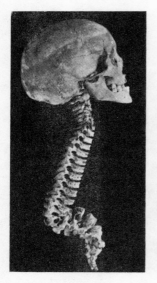

Skull and spine of an eight-year-old Swedish child from the twelfth century with tuberculous fusion of lower thoracic vertebrae, from Ragnvald Knaphövde's chapel in Vreta Cloister church, examined in 1919. C. M. Furst considers that the skeleton is probably of a child of King Inge the Younger and his Queen, Ulfhild, and that the child was perhaps the last male member of the Steinkel royal line.

that one of Sweden's loveliest folk-songs, 'The song of the dove on the lily-branch' (in which a noble maiden's illness and death is described in the style of the time), in fact refers to a case of pleural sac tuberculosis or some other form of pleurisy (inflammation of the pleural sac).

In Sweden the disease seems to a certain extent to have spread from the south northwards, although larger towns like Stockholm and Visby had probably already been relatively severely infected.

Tuberculosis in Swedish cattle, 1937–52. Thick line: infectious tuberculosis (clinically and bacteriologically established)— absolute figures (on right). Thin line: tuberculosis in slaughtered cattle as a percentage (on left.)

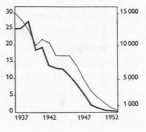

There was probably by then a considerable difference between country and town; thirty years ago, when tuberculosis was enormously widespread in Sweden, there were still distant corners of the countryside in which tuberculosis was as good as unknown.

Very little is known about the early history of bovine tuberculosis, which is of such importance to humans. In Scandinavia, as in many other countries, the primitive indigenous breeds of cattle were probably free of tuberculosis, but when pedigree animals were imported from stock centres in England and elsewhere, native breeds were soon infected and only the mountain breeds escaped. Nowadays, thanks to energetic measures, bovine tuberculosis has been eradicated from Scandinavia.

The history of tuberculosis during the last two or three hundred years is a very long and interesting chapter which nevertheless must be here dealt with very briefly. In many countries tuberculosis has for centuries been characteristically endemic, and only now has it been pushed back or virtually eradicated. In some countries it still retains its firm hold and in others it continues to advance. In this a number of internal and external factors combine, amongst which economic and social conditions and especially nutritional deficiency seem to play a decisive part. Isolation measures and natural, perhaps inborn, or artificially acquired immunity have also been of great significance. A very important factor has been the campaign against bovine tuberculosis and the control of meat and milk, even if this form of tuberculosis has been a very much smaller source of infection than human tuberculosis. The distribution and frequency of tuberculosis has therefore been subject to great historical changes. And even in countries with very little tuberculosis one cannot contemplate eradication as long as the country's borders stand open and people with infectious tuberculosis occasionally enter the country.

Today tuberculosis has an immense distribution. In many instances the disease has come to a country so recently that it is to a certain degree possible to study the time and the process of its occurrence. As far as one can see, tuberculosis seems to have afflicted the white races in particular, and it is still more widespread among them, while its frequency varies greatly within different parts of the areas of the world inhabited by whites. In large parts of Europe almost every individual who reaches maturity has been infected with tuberculosis, and this can be shown in several different ways, but there are also regions where tuberculosis is rare. Now it is advancing considerably in many primitive countries.

One should not think that the spread and character of tuberculosis in a certain population is constant over longer periods. Investigations in different quarters which have been carried out year after year, or at longer, say ten-year intervals, show that the frequency and general character of the disease can fluctuate appreciably. The reasons for these variations are many and cannot be completely gone into. An increase in tuberculosis in its more severe forms and particularly in children can be caused by a lowering of the general standard of living, especially a decrease in the supplies of high-value foodstuffs. Such a situation arose in Central Europe at the end of and after both world wars. A decline in the disease with a decrease in the number of early infections and better facilities for early cure partly depends on biological factors. A lengthy but not too severe infection in a community seems to be able to bring with it an increased resistance. To the biological factors can be added the resistance produced artificially by vaccination of one sort or another. But undoubtedly more important are factors such as improved public hygiene, increased understanding of the sources and infection routes of tuberculosis and most of all a raising of social and economic standards. In Norway, Scheel has shown that the decline of tuberculosis has run parallel with the rise of prosperity which he sees in increase in body-height, in consumption of certain luxury foodstuffs such as coffee, and in savings deposits, etc.

As it is impossible in this space to deal with the history and geography of each individual country, a few illuminating examples from Scandinavia are given here. As has already been said, tuberculosis presumably came to Sweden through travellers, either Swedes who visited the great cities abroad or merchants who came into the country. Foreign women and slaves, perhaps the spoils of war, were also possible carriers of the disease. At first cases were few and distribution probably limited, and one can presume that it was first found in the larger towns, Stockholm and Visby, which were seats of infection. In Visby and on Gotland tuberculosis was already quite widespread in the fourteenth century, which is shown in skeletons from the graves outside the ring wall round Visby which contain the remains of those who fell in the Danish attack in 1361, principally Gotland peasants. Later, tuberculosis seems to have been concentrated in Central Sweden, especially Stockholm. The disease spread, the number of cases increased and a new seat of infection appeared after the construction of a naval base at Karlskrona. The whole of poverty-stricken Blekinge was infected with tuberculosis, probably through the naval personnel who lived on the smallholdings. 1749 is an important year in the history of tuberculosis in Sweden, for it was then that the Swedish bio-statistics began and after that date one can be relatively sure of the spread and frequency of the disease.

The history of tuberculosis in Sweden during the last two hundred years is of great biological and epidemiological interest. Its development is considered to have gone as follows: from old centres like Stockholm, Karlskrona and Göteborg, the disease spread with growing violence over an increasingly wide area and seems to have reached its maximum c. 1820–40. It is calculated that at this time mortality in tuberculosis over the whole country rose to about 2·6 per cent, a very high figure. Many Swedes with famous names succumbed. At the end of the eighteenth century mortality in lung tuberculosis in Stockholm rose to about 7 per cent and in the second decade of the nineteenth century to no less than 9·3 per cent, a terrible figure. Similar figures could be produced for smaller towns in Central Sweden, such as Uppsala. How great the annual mortality from tuberculosis was at this time can no longer be established, but in all probability it involved very large numbers. After 1840 tuberculosis gradually began to decline but in the 1860s mortality still stood at about 4·3 per cent. Stockholm and large parts of Central Sweden had endured a lengthy and severe epidemic of tuberculosis. Poor economic and social conditions and widespread alcoholism had certainly contributed to a great extent to the high morbidity and mortality. One forgets only too easily in the welfare state of today that Sweden at the end of the nineteenth century was a poor and backward country.

At the turn of the century tuberculosis flared up again but this time in a completely different part of the country, in upper Norrland which had hitherto been largely spared, principally because of its geographical isolation. Here tuberculosis reached a new maximum in about 1915. Since then the disease has been on the decline all over the country and optimists have occasionally calculated that it will be possible to eradicate tuberculosis in Sweden—optimism which is almost certainly undue.

The four maps showing tuberculosis mortality in Sweden during the last 150 years (pp. 105–6) give a good idea of the interesting changes. Social and economic factors have principally been decisive here. The hundred years which separate the first two maps represent a period of successful development and economic renaissance. The great undeveloped 'colony' of Norrland was opened up, people came in from the south, the huge forests and rich mines began to be worked, and mining towns and industrial communities grew. But the immigrants were followed by tuberculosis. The previous inhabitants, who before had scarcely been infected, lacked resistance and sickened extensively, and hygiene unfortunately remained at a low level for a long time. During the last thirty years, however, conditions have been improved very satisfactorily and the economic circumstances of manual workers and the middle classes in particular have undergone immense changes, which have been a powerful additional cause of the swift decline of tuberculosis all over the country. The other two maps speak for themselves.

It is of interest that tuberculosis has declined at different rates in rural areas and in towns. Earlier the country had less tuberculosis than towns but in about 1932 the graph curve for rural areas crossed the urban curve and nowadays the urban position is slightly more favourable than that of the country.

In some counties such as Gotland and Blekinge tuberculosis declined more slowly than in others, e.g. Södermanland, Västmanland and Malmöhus, and also Stockholm city.

Largely similar conditions are to be found in Norway, while Denmark has gone one step further. During the years 1921–30, 84 people out of 100,000 died of tuberculosis. Now the figure has sunk to 5·1 in 100,000, an enormous decrease, and Denmark holds her own among the countries of Europe which have made the furthest advance. Sweden's figure is 9·5, Norway's 10·1, while Holland has managed to come down to 4·5. Finland, which fifty to sixty years ago had about double Sweden's mortality, after the war of liberation succeeded in taking a large stride towards sanitation. After the

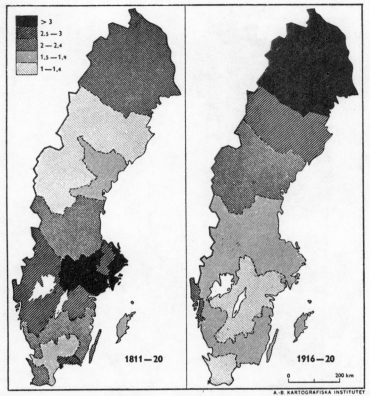

Mortality from tuberculosis per thousand in the counties of Sweden in
1811–20 and, 100 years later, in 1916–20 (after G. Neander). The
map on the left shows a maximum in Central Sweden, that on the
right in Norrbotten county.

Second World War the figure rose again and is now once more decreasing towards 35 per 100,000. Many European countries still show high mortality: Ireland 25·1, France and Austria just over 27, West Berlin 31·7. Worst among the countries which submit information to WHO is Portugal, where mortality in 1956 was 54·2 per 100,000.

Among non-European countries Canada has the remarkably low figure of 6·7 for 1956. In the United States the whites showed 7·1 in 1955 but the coloureds 8·6. Other parts of America had considerably higher figures. Among the few Asian countries that submitted information, Japan had a mortality of no less than 121·8 in 1950, a

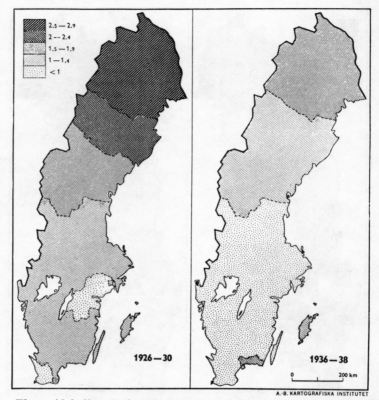

The rapid decline of tuberculosis over a period of about ten years. Since then the disease has become increasingly rare, but to think in terms of total eradication is almost certainly too optimistic.

figure which already after only six years is said to have come down to 42·4. In China tuberculosis seems to be increasing, at least that was the case fifteen years ago when at clinical examinations 35,000,000 had demonstrable tuberculosis and 92 per cent of all twenty-year-olds were tuberculin-positive, i.e. had been infected at some time. In Africa tuberculosis is still an immense problem, spreading from the coast to more or less untouched tribes in the interior. In Morocco mortality among Europeans was 59, among Jews 130 and among Muslims 222 per 100,000. Similar conditions existed a short while ago in the Union of South Africa, where whites showed 7·2, Asiatics 21·8 and negroes no fewer than 324·3 in 1950 and 176·1 in 1955.

It is unnecessary to emphasise that a low frequency of tuberculosis is in itself a highly advantageous and desirable state of affairs, but one must not ignore the fact that it also means a high degree of susceptibility. This was established earlier in Sweden, when young people from regions virtually free from tuberculosis came to Stockholm and were infected; the tuberculosis they contracted was often of an acutely progressive character.

Similar conditions are known from many other countries once free from tuberculosis, to which the disease came as a doubtful blessing. A similar mass infection of young people from previously free regions was observed for the first time when recruits from former Bosnia and Herzegovina were hauled into Austrian barracks. Similar unfortunate circumstances are known from all over the world. Kalmuck children who left the steppes to go to school in Astrakhan generally did not manage to finish their schooling but fell ill at 15–16. Many of them died of tuberculosis. Eventually these children of the steppes were forbidden to go to Russian schools. A number of years ago 2,000 natives from some tuberculosis-free Pacific islands were imported for certain work in Peru. After several months, no fewer than 1,500 were dead or dying of the disease. Nubians and negroes who have come to Europe for employment, or as soldiers in the French Army, have succumbed heavily to acute tuberculosis. Similar acute tuberculosis raged among the negro troops which France sent, mostly as occupation forces, to Germany after the First World War. Change of climate, unfamiliar food, barrack and trench life all prepared the way for what the tubercle bacillus completed, and three to four months after the appearance of the first signs of the disease, a large number of these coloured people who had been brought over 'to defend civilisation' had died of acute tuberculosis. These are only a few examples of what lack of resistance can mean if individuals without tuberculosis come into a densely infected environment.

Leprosy

The microbe, *Mycobacterium leprae*, was discovered very early, in 1873, by the Norwegian leprosy specialist Armauer Hansen. The microbe is present in immense numbers in the leprous scabs, a fact which naturally facilitated the discovery.

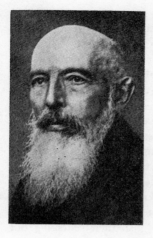

Armauer Hansen (1841–1912), the discoverer of the leprosy bacillus. The microbe had already been shown by him in 1873, i.e. long before the true bacteriological era.

Formerly leprosy was a collective name, much like the name plague, and embraced the most heterogeneous chronic skin diseases: apart from genuine leprosy, it included venereal and tuberculous diseases (scrofula and lupus), yaws, scabies, psoriasis, eczema and skin cancer. According to Kraus, leprosy originally meant a scaly crustean disease, as for instance psoriasis. The Hebrew word for leprosy, *saraat*, really means rash. Other names with a somewhat blurred demarcation are *elephantiasis graecorum* and *lepra arabum*. The Scandinavian name *spetälska* and *spedalskhed* are derived from the word for asylum.

Leprosy is one of the most interesting diseases from a historical,

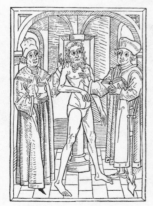

Two doctors examine a leper. Woodcut from Regimen sanitatis, *printed by Conrad Dinckmut at Ulm in 1482.*

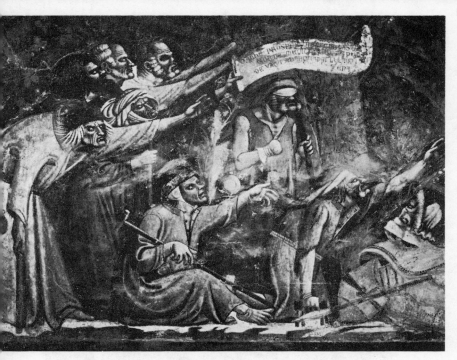

Group of lepers. Detail from the famous monumental painting The Triumph of Death *in the Campo Santo in Pisa, attributed to Andrea di Cione, called Orcagna (died c. 1370).*

cultural and geographical point of view. It has played a very great part in men's lives, perhaps even more in their art and imagination, and the word leper still has a malignant ring to the ears of many people today. The disease was endemic in Egypt many thousands of years B.C. It is mentioned in the Exodus of the Israelites from Egypt, and Moses, who no doubt had come to know the disease in Egypt, issued edicts against it. A victim was declared unclean and was to be hunted out of the camp with torn and dirty clothes, his head bare and a veil over his mouth, to remain an outcast until another examination should proclaim him safe. If he were declared healed, sacrifices of atonement were made; otherwise he would be rejected for ever and his clothes and chattels thoroughly cleansed and burnt.

Leprosy is said to be of equal antiquity in India, where its name was *kustha*, and in China. In Persia it is thought to have been known five or six hundred years B.C. Leprosy came from the Orient to Greece and in the *Hippocratic Collection* it is called *leuké*, but whether this was real leprosy is very uncertain. Secluded holy places were instituted in Greece for lepers—types of leper colony or leprosarium under the direction of a priest. Leprosy was brought to Rome by, amongst others, soldiers returning from the Orient. From Rome it soon advanced into the rest of Europe. In the first century A.D. the Gauls are thought to have set up special sanctuaries for lepers, which are now said to have been discovered. In the eighth to tenth centuries leprosy was already widespread in many southern European countries and special ordinances against it were in existence.

In the north the disease spread rapidly in the eleventh and twelfth centuries—according to many, coming via the Crusades, brought either by those returning from the Holy Land or by generally livelier communications. During the middle and later mediaeval period leprosy ravaged practically all the countries of Europe. One gets some idea of its extent from the fact that in 1200 there were 2,000 leprosaria in France alone, and about 19,000 institutions in the whole of Christendom. These usually lay outside town boun-

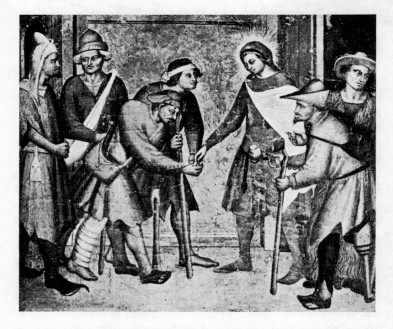

A saint distributing alms to lepers, from a painting in the Uffizi, Florence, by an unknown master of the Tuscan School, late fourteenth century. It shows many realistically portrayed pathological features.

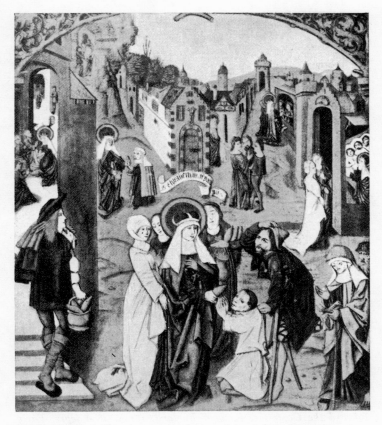

St Elisabeth of Hungary curing lepers, from a late fifteenth-century painting in Cologne Museum.

daries. Lepers were rigorously isolated and separated from the community by religious ceremonies, which virtually meant a death sentence—proclaiming them dead as citizens, forbidding them marriage and ordering them to wear special clothing. In many places they had to warn others of their approach with a special 'Lazarus rattle'. In 1313 Philip the Fair wanted quite simply to burn all lepers, but fortunately this effective if somewhat radical measure was forbidden by the Church. Lazarus, who lay at the rich man's door covered with sores that the dogs licked, soon became the patron saint of lepers.

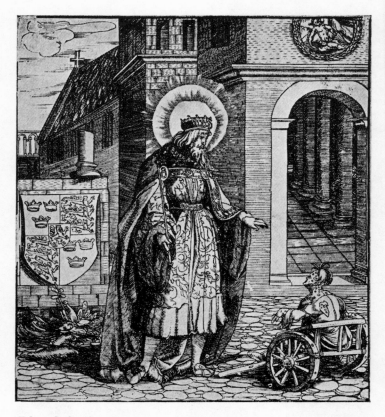

*Edward the Confessor, King of England, speaks to a leper. Early
sixteenth-century woodcut by Hans Burgkmaier. The royal coat of
arms with three crowns and leopards can be seen on the wall behind
the king.*

The first leprosarium is supposed to have been constructed
at Châlons in 580; in 1067 there was one in Spain; in Venice one
was founded on the island of San Lazzaro, and in Paris the twelfth-
century St Lazare hospital was for lepers. In Great Britain, northern
Germany and Scandinavia leper hospitals were dedicated to St
George or St Göran, like the one in Lund of 1248. Many extant
hospitals can probably be traced back to old leprosaria. Outside
Stockholm there was a leper hospital, St Göran's—on Norrmalm,
according to Klockhoff, perhaps where the present Drottninghus

stands. At the end of the Middle Ages there was an asylum on Gråmunkeholm, now Riddarholm, but it is not known whether it was ever used for lepers. King Gustavus Vasa had the Gråmunkeholm patients moved to Danviken together with the lepers from St Göran's. He complained that 'a powerfully evil stench lay over Gråmunckeholm and the water which runs thereabout, in which the sick wash themselves and their foul clothing, is drawn by the current round the castle and the city; therefore I wish these same lepers to be taken to Danviken with all speed' (Martin Olsson, *The Church on Riddarholm*). The hygiene of Stockholm's waters was obviously of topical interest even four hundred years ago.

In the latter half of the Middles Ages Sweden had twenty leper hospitals, but the number of patients is not known. Some idea of how the lepers lived, and especially of their food and drink, can be found in a mediaeval Latin statute for the leper hospital in Enköping, issued by Archbishop Birger of Uppsala at the end of the fourteenth century. First, all persons of both sexes suffering from the disease were to be diligently sought out in 'the whole diocese of Uppsala' and if they were poor they were to be received into the asylum gratis. The goods and chattels of the wealthy were to go to the sick or to charitable institutions. The poor were to have daily two corn loaves and well-cleaned milk, and on the eight enumerated saint's days a 'pure wheat loaf'. They also had plentiful 'good ale', a group of ten, for example, would have half a bowl of ale, and a group of twenty a whole one. During fasts the diet was somewhat changed and each then received two herrings. On the eleventh day of the fast they were given plenty of dried cod and pike, one cup of peas and two salmon. If a person's weakness demanded it, it was incumbent on the warden to increase his portion. Every seventh day, apart from fast days, each received half a pound of butter and half a pound of pork or smoked ox meat. In the summer, every fourth day, they were given a pail of sour milk or if the number of sick were greater, seven-day-old ale. In addition the statute mentions lentils, at Michaelmas three pounds of salt for every eight sick and on St Martin's feast, eight yards of homespun cloth for each patient. If there was no fish for fast days, egg custard was served every other day. Detailed regulations about the household utensils of the poor, especially those for food, were also given. No one, however powerful, would dare, once he had dedicated himself to God and the asylum, to leave its enclosure and go to church, on a visit or to accept any

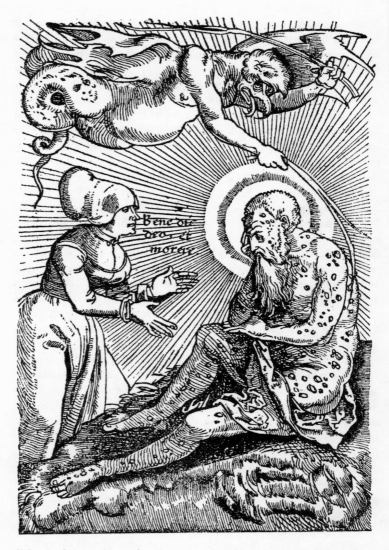

Job as a leper—sixteenth-century woodcut from Gersdolf's Feldtbuch der Wundarzney. *Job has been left to the mercy of Satan and is now afflicted with sores 'from the soles of his feet to his forehead'. His wife is standing in front of him, deriding her sick husband and saying 'Praise God and die.'*

other invitation, unless he wished to expose himself to severe punishment because of the danger of infection. One must admit that this programme, if it really could have been carried out, appears, for the conditions of those days, to be a very good one.

Very little is known with certainty of the number of lepers in Sweden during the Middle Ages and the next two hundred years, nor of the location of the largest seats of infection. It is likely that the numbers of sick very soon decreased, but cases were probably spread all over the country. Huss says that at the end of the eighteenth century there were many to be found in the county of Bohus and also that 'round the banks of the river Dal, especially by and above the outlet, leprosy has been endemic since times of old'. It was especially common at the river mouth, hence the name 'Elfkarleby-disease'. It has, however, gradually declined. Because of the fear of infection, Älvkarleby parish in 1755 requested the Lieutenant of the county to forbid lepers to take Holy Communion together with the healthy, and to assign them a special place in the church so that they did not disturb those sitting near with the stench they spread round them. In Hälsingland leprosy was called 'lump-sickness' and it was especially common near the rivers Ljusna and Ljunga, but it declined. According to Huss the records of leprosy in Hälsingland go no further back than the beginning of the eighteenth century, but before that many people had died of 'malignant scabies' which was probably leprosy. In Hälsingland the disease was not considered infectious, but hereditary, particularly through the father, and it spared neither rich nor poor—'the richest farmer in the whole district is a leper'.

Leprosy continued to recede and in 1873 only 173 cases were registered, although the number of cases, if the mildest are also included, was probably much greater. Of these 173 cases, 103 were in Hälsingland, where our last leprosarium stood in Järvsö. I performed an autopsy there on a victim who had died in 1907. In 1923 only eleven patients were to be found in the whole country, and now there are probably only two or three left.

During the Second World War a couple of cases came from the Baltic, among them the former senior naval medical officer of Estonia, who had considerable facial changes and was very hoarse.

In Denmark during the Middle Ages there were at least thirty-five leprosaria; one of the churchyards which preserves their bones (Naestved) has been the subject of a very detailed, interesting and

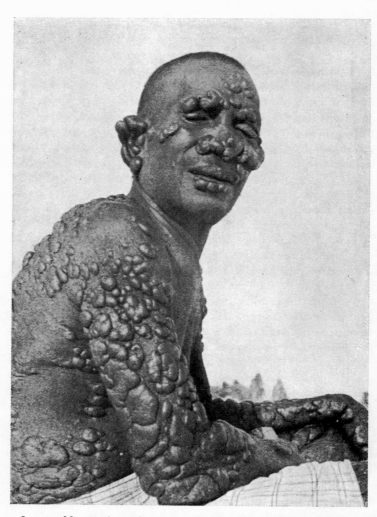

38-year-old man from the Loyalty Islands with tuberous leprosy of about ten years' duration.

productive investigation by Møller-Christensen. The country has now been free of the disease for a long time. A hundred years ago, Norway had 2,858 lepers, i.e. 1·9 per 1,000 of the whole population; now only seven are left. The main seat of infection lay round Bergen. In Iceland leprosy once was very widespread and in 1768 it was calculated that there were 280 victims, i.e. 7·4 per thousand of the population. Now there are only a couple of cases.

Leprosy has declined all over Europe. In France there was a considerable distribution at the end of the eighteenth century and even today leprosy is not a great rarity there. Spain a few decades ago had about 10,000 lepers and Portugal no fewer than 13,000–14,000. In the Balkans and Russia leprosy is not uncommon, and the number of lepers in the whole of Europe is now calculated to be about 20,000. In Asia leprosy is still a very great problem in many countries. The number of lepers in India is calculated to be over a million. China a short while ago held a quarter of the total number of the world's lepers, and the disease is common in Korea, Japan, Burma and the East Indies. In Africa the number of lepers is calculated at 1·6–1·7 million, of whom 400,000 live in Nigeria and at least 200,000 in Ethiopia. In West Africa there is the highest frequency in the whole world, but on the other hand relatively little tuberculosis, and there is some talk of a kind of antagonism between the two diseases, in which tuberculosis is said to give a certain immunity to leprosy. In North America there was formerly no leprosy, but now there are scattered cases totalling about 1,500–2,000. One suspects that immigrants from Norway and Iceland brought it with them, but the importation of negro slaves was probably more significant. The disease has a large distribution in South America, especially along the coasts. There too negro slaves are supposed to have brought leprosy with them from severely infected Africa. Australia, which was once free, was infected through imported Chinese coolies during the exploitation of the gold-fields, and islands in the Pacific have been infected by cheap labour from Asia. The total number of leprosy cases was previously reckoned to be 5–10 million and many now favour the still higher one of 12–15 million, a figure which includes quite mild cases.

Leprosy is not limited by geographical and climatic conditions but it appears to be more common in warm damp climates and less so in dry, steppe and desert regions. It seems that skin affections increase its frequency, and dirty dwellings, poor hygiene, social distress and over-population play a very great part.

There was once a great deal of confusion about the transmission of the disease from individual to individual. When it was found that the mucus in the nose of victims contained large quantities of leprosy bacilli, it was thought that the respiratory passages were the place of entry. Nowadays opinion has to a large extent gone over to the theory that vermin, especially fleas and lice, are the most important transmitters of the infection. In this context perhaps a remark by a Batak warrior in the Dutch East Indies might be repeated, from Thierfelder, as it seems to show that the idea of the significance of vermin in the transmission of leprosy is an old one: 'In earlier wars we let lice bite lepers and then spread them in the enemy's camp. Many were infected with leprosy in this way. But since the wars have ceased, leprosy has declined and for us natives life has now lost all its excitement.'

There has also been talk of unsuitable foodstuffs, which contain large quantities of saponins, being of some significance. In Scandinavia *Agrostemma githago* and in the tropics *Colocasia antiquorum* are said to be of importance; it is not, however, possible to go into this matter here.

Mycoses, fungus diseases

The great wealth of different forms and the often very inadequate botanical diagnosis make a scientific exposition and classification of the very common and significant fungus diseases, especially of the tropics, somewhat hazardous. A good description of the pathogenic fungi is given in the handbook by Conant, Smith, Baker, Callaway and Martin (1954).

Actinomycosis, ray-fungus disease

Actinomycosis in humans, caused by an anaerobic fungus, *Actinomyces hominis*, which is probably identical to the common *A. bovis* in cattle, is of little significance in Sweden. In cattle, on the other hand, it is quite common in the tongue and the sinuses. The fungus lives like an ordinary saprophyte in the human mouth and can in rare cases penetrate through abrasions and cause severe disturbances in neighbouring soft parts and also deeper in the body. In certain regions as many as 10–20 per cent of the cattle can be infected.

Madura foot

This disease is caused, according to Castellani, by a number of related species of fungi, among which *Streptothrix madurae* is probably the most important. Madura foot is mentioned in the most ancient medical writings, and according to some, it has perhaps only one rival in antiquity, namely *Dracunculus medinensis*, the long guinea worm, which will be dealt with later. (In cuneiform medical texts Madura foot probably corresponds to 'Kabrtu disease' and dracunculosis to 'Sangalla disease', which really means 'long sinew' and would correspond to the worm.) The fungi of Madura foot produce a shapeless swelling of the foot with formation of abscesses and fistulae. The disease is named after the town of Madura in south India. It is found in large parts of India, in Africa and also in North and South America, but rather rarely.

Histoplasmosis

The fungus, *Histoplasma capsulatum*, causes fever, enlargement of the liver and spleen, and anaemia. The disease centres on the Mississippi basin and in Ohio where no fewer than 80 per cent of the inhabitants show a characteristic skin reaction for this fungus, when tested with histoplasmin produced from an extract of the fungus.

Other mycoses

In tropical and sub-tropical countries with hot damp climates, fungus diseases, especially of the skin, play a role which in northern countries one can hardly begin to imagine. At least twenty different forms are known, but most can probably be ignored. One of the most important is so-called paracoccidioidomycosis, which occurs in south-west USA, Mexico and large parts of South America. It is caused by *Blastomyces brasiliensis* and is focused in the central and southern parts of Brazil. A North American skin blastomycosis, which is distinct from the latter and causes disturbances in the skin and many internal organs, is also well known.

Sarcoidosis

One other disease will be dealt with in this chapter, one which has been associated, and still is by some researchers, with tuberculosis, but whose aetiology and systematic position is still as yet extremely obscure.

The disease, which is also known as Besnier's, Boeck's or Schaumann's disease, after a Frenchman, a Norwegian and a Swede who have given great service to research into it, is nowadays usually called sarcoidosis. It is a systemic disease which can be found in all organs. Previously considered to be a rare disease with bad prospects for health, it has now, since its acute stages have become known, shown itself to be quite common and relatively benign. It seems to occur all over the world, but present information seems to point to its being more common in Sweden than in any other country, a fact which could perhaps be explained by the widespread and thorough mass chest-radiography surveys which have been made. Its frequency in the whole of Sweden is calculated at 40 cases per 100,000 inhabitants, with a maximum in Jämtland of no fewer than 140 per 100,000. In Sweden it is more common in women than men. The fact that tuberculosis has declined so rapidly has in this context also roused some notice and has been interpreted in different ways.

In the USA the average frequency is lower than in Sweden, but the south Atlantic states and those round the Mexican Gulf form an exception. Strangely enough negroes show a considerably higher frequency than whites and in them it is found 7–20 times as often. Among soldiers of the Second World War sarcoidosis was found in 40 negroes per 100,000 but in 3·3 whites per 100,000. In Switzerland a number of cases can be found in the markedly dry areas. There those who work with wood and paper show the highest frequency. It has been asserted that there is a connection with pine-tree regions, but this has not been confirmed, and the real nature of the disease is still the subject of a great deal of research.

5　Spirochaetal Diseases

Spirochaetes, literally spiral threads, are thin spiral flexible microbes without cilia. Some of them are harmless saprophytes.

Febris recurrens, relapsing fever

Microbe: *Borrelia recurrentis* (*Spirochaete obermeieri*) and other related forms.

Carriers: in the epidemic European form, lice, *Pediculus corporis* and *Phthirus inguinalis*; in the Asiatic, African and American forms, mostly ticks.

This disease, which is characterised by periodically recurring attacks of fever, can, according to Hirsch, be traced back no further than the beginning of the eighteenth century, but it is probably a very ancient disease. The first definite epidemic was observed in Dublin in 1739–41. Later larger epidemics occurred in Ireland, Scotland and England as well as many other countries. A Swedish North Sea naval squadron was infected in 1769 and brought the infection back to Göteborg. A new epidemic flared up in 1788 when the crew of a Russian ship, captured at Hogland, came into contact with Swedish sailors. Relapsing fever came to Denmark at the same time as to Göteborg, in 1769 (Hult). Ireland had its last big epidemic in 1868–71. With improved hygiene and the eradication of lice, it has declined over nearly the whole of Europe, but it kept a hold on Ireland and Russia for a long time. When the Russian Red Army defeated the counter-revolutionary White generals, they had nearly 100,000 cases of relapsing fever to contend with. The disease was also common in Russia during the Second World War (Schlossman).

Relapsing fever is endemic in many non-European countries and is very widely distributed. Egypt in 1946 is said to have had over 100,000 cases and there the infection is said to be transferred by lice. In Algeria in 1947–48 no fewer than 400,000 cases are said to have been registered.

Stomatitis gangrenosa, noma, angina vincenti

In the presence of poor mouth hygiene, a harmless saprophyte, *Spirochaeta denticola*, lives in the mouth. Pathogenic spirochaetes are to be found in large numbers in all kinds of gangrenosae in association with necrotic ulcerous sores in the mouth, gums, tonsils and cheeks; these disturbances were formerly very common in hospitals and elsewhere with the poor hygiene and unbalanced diet of the time. Diseases of this kind have been known since Graeco-Roman doctors and Avicenna. Mediaeval doctors such as Paracelsus also described the disease which corresponds to gangrenous stomatitis. In Sweden it is nowadays seldom seen, although a number of mild cases did occur twenty-five years ago among the inhabitants of the outer archipelago of Stockholm, after bad winters and unbalanced diet. In tropical regions, like Madagascar, gangrenous processes in the mouth occur among children, with very high mortality.

The following three forms of spirochaetes are grouped under the name treponematosis: framboesia (yaws), syphilis and Mal del Pinto. Common to these three diseases is the fact that the microbes do not require carriers, which has almost certainly facilitated their spread.

Framboesia (framboise = raspberry), yaws

The microbe, *Treponema pertenue*, is transmitted by direct contact and dirty clothes and probably also by flies. It is very widespread in all tropical countries and seems to occur only among coloured people. The infection usually occurs in childhood, which not infrequently creates immunity against syphilis. The disease is a very ancient one; Stewart and Spoehr have found the remains of human skeletons on Tinian, one of the Mariana islands in the west Pacific, the age of which by the C^{14} method was decided as 854 ± 145 by our calculation of time. The cranium showed a periostitis with corrosion of the skull-cap bone reminiscent of the skull changes caused by syphilis. A skull with a similar lesion has been found in Iraq, probably dating from the first 500 years A.D. Arabian doctors seem to have been familiar with yaws. No syphilitic changes of an even remotely comparable age are known, but yaws and syphilis are closely related and both give a positive Wassermann reaction. It is a case of two diseases which were perhaps originally identical and caused by the same microbe.

It is possible that a disease described by Avicenna and Ali Abbas was yaws. It existed in Central and South America before the arrival of Columbus in the West Indies. Oviedo came to know it in Hispaniola, now San Domingo.

The disease occurs in southern China and is more common in Cambodia and Malaya. In tropical Africa it was once very common but seems to have become rarer. In 1934–43 Uganda had an annual average of 47,741 cases, in 1947 only 37,803. Previously in Tanganyika 90 per cent of the natives were infected, in 1938 there were 132,469 cases, ten years later only 51,259. In Madagascar the disease is endemic, and yaws are also often seen in tropical South America, the West Indies and the Pacific islands.

Syphilis

The microbe, *Treponema pallidum* (earlier *Spirochaeta pallida*), was discovered in 1905 by the Germans Schaudinn and Hoffmann. Two years earlier Metschinoff and Roux had succeeded in transferring the disease to apes.

History. From a historical point of view, syphilis is among the most interesting diseases, not only because of the lengthy arguments about its origin, but also because of the considerable influence it has had on the general view of morality and on hygiene.

For centuries researchers have been divided into two camps, Europeanists and Americanists. According to the former view the disease has existed in the Old World since time immemorial. The evidence lies solely in written records. In the brothel regulations of Queen Joanna I of Naples there is a clause which could be put forward as evidence to support the incidence of the disease before 1492. Similarly Peter Martyr's letters, the court protocol of Dijon, and the text of an edict in the health regulations in Worms are said to show that syphilis was already known in the Middle Ages. A pair of apparently valuable documents originate from Denmark, one an Italian manuscript with prescriptions against 'mal franzoso', the other a remark in Roskilde's *Aarbog* (Year Book) that 'in 1483 came the severe French sickness and fever called *poch* [syphilis] among Christian folk'. None of these documents is considered to have any decisive value by the Europeanists' opponents.

The skeletal changes produced as evidence in support of the incidence of the disease in Europe before Columbus have been completely uncharacteristic. About thirty years ago came the sensational news that syphilis had been shown in a Stone Age skeleton in France. However, it soon turned out that this Frenchman had had some bone disease other than syphilis, and anyhow it was not a case of skull changes which are specifically syphilitic but of morbid changes in the long bones with periostitis (inflammation of the bone membrane) which is very similar to syphilis. The well-known English anthropologist Elliot Smith, who examined about 25,000 Egyptian crania, found not a single case of characteristic syphilitic periostitis; a suspected case was shown to be insect or worm damage which had occurred after death. Nor have X-ray examinations of Egyptian mummies shown any definite syphilis, though certainly other skeletal diseases which we still come across today.

What then is the position as regards pre-Columbian syphilis in America? Thirty or so years ago the Americanists could not produce any decisive evidence showing syphilitic changes. Peruvian mummies which were examined certainly showed some skeletal changes, but no definite syphilitic periostitis, and there were no skeletons of value from the West Indies, which can probably be explained by the fact that the hot damp climate there is extremely unsuitable for the preservation of superficially buried bodies. It was not long, however, before critical examination of bone remains, especially skulls, showed that syphilis had had a considerable distribution in North, Central and South America before the arrival of Europeans. It is changes in the bones of the forehead which are especially typical, and an American researcher, Williams, has said that they are just as definite as a Wassermann reaction ($+ + + +$). (One normally uses only three pluses.) I have myself had the opportunity of examining crania from Peru and the latest finds from Mexico, which, in my opinion, definitely indicate severe tertiary syphilis.

Nevertheless, the problem of the true origin of syphilis is not finally solved. Is it a disease originating in America, or was it, as Russian researchers assert, imported from the extreme north-east of Siberia, where there are said to be tribes who in fact should be described as ancient Americans as they are quite distinct from other Asian peoples (Boas)? These pre-Mongoloid (Horkheimer) or Americanised tribes migrated, it is thought, probably in different

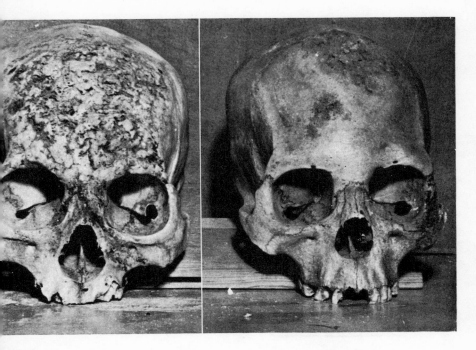

Two crania of pre-Columbian Indians buried in the Calendaria cave in northern Mexico. The examination was carried out by A. Romano, who in his publication of his finds in 1953 comments, with caution, on 'remarkable affections which seem to be bone changes caused by syphilis'. (When I examined the crania in 1954, I came to the same conclusion.)

waves, over the dried-up or very narrow Bering Straits. If syphilis is a primary autochthonic American disease, then its age goes back some tens of thousands of years, inasmuch as America is thought to have been colonised possibly as late as 15,000 years ago. If it was imported, then its origin vanishes into a much more distant Asiatic remoteness. One need hardly concern oneself with the theory, current among lay South Americans, that the Indians acquired the disease from the lamas which are their food, clothes and women.

Whatever the sources and origins of syphilis, the written records and skeletal changes from the last years of the fifteenth century clearly cannot be misinterpreted. Syphilitic bone lesions earlier than 1493 have never been demonstrated in Europe, but numerous typical syphilitic skulls and long bones of after that date have been unearthed in the churchyards of nearly all European countries. The disease spread widely and extremely swiftly after Columbus's return from his first voyage in March 1493, and the doctors were helpless in the face of this new disease which corresponded neither to any mentioned by Galen and Avicenna nor to any they themselves had seen.

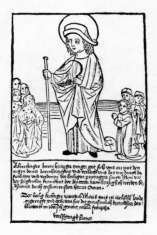

St Minus, patron saint of syphilitics, from a late fifteenth-century German woodcut. Those who had contracted the disease turned in their need to this saint or to St Denis, who after his execution walked with his head in his hand. St Minus is also portrayed in late mediaeval wood-engravings with a text below including a prayer for protection against syphilis.

There is a great deal of contemporary literature referring to the early spread of syphilis in Europe and other parts of the Old World. Its advance through our part of the world, which had not previously been infected, can be followed step by step from the first seats of infection in Spain shortly after Columbus's landing in Palos, his stay in Seville and his visit to the court in Barcelona. Good descriptions are to be found of the first Spanish period of the disease. The small sores of primary infection and the skin rash of the secondary stage were not considered of any importance.

The campaign which the young French king, Charles VIII, led against Naples in 1494–95 was of devastating significance to the rapid spread of the disease. His army of 30,000 men was composed of French, German, Swiss, English, Hungarian, Polish, Italian and Spanish troops, and there were Spanish troops among the defenders of Naples. Knowing the life in army camps of that time, where excesses '*in Baccho et Venere*' made a welcome change from more martial exercises, and loose women went from one side to the other, it is easy to imagine how the new disease rapidly spread from already infected soldiers to the rest of the armies. The celebrated anatomist Fallopius (1523–62), whose father was in the citadel of Naples during the siege, tells how the defenders 'finally with violence drove their harlots and women out of the citadel, and especially the most beautiful ones, whom they knew to be suffering from the infectious disease, on the pretext that the food had come to an end. And the French, gripped by compassion and bewitched by their beauty, took them in . . . .' *'Die Freude an den schönen Dirnen war gross, sie waren für die Soldaten eine willkommene Beute.'* The historical fact is that during this campaign the French were surprised by a new and terrible disease which broke out in their camps during the winter and spring of 1495. Charles had to abandon the siege and retreat through Italy under great difficulties, his army disintegrating into lawless bands which scattered into France, Switzerland, Germany, the Netherlands and Poland, taking the new disease, the Neapolitan disease, later called the French disease, all over Europe. Charles VIII himself died of it in 1498 at the age of twenty-eight.

Many contemporary records speak of the explosive spread of the disease. Severe skin cases were first sent to leprosaria, but the lepers refused to mix with them, and in some places special establishments were built for them, *Blatternhäuser* or pox houses. In Paris about one-third of the inhabitants are said to have been infected. Francis I of France, who on the strength of what he considered to be his rights had taken *'La Belle Ferronière'* (widely known through Leonardi da Vinci's portrait, which in fact is of an Italian lady), was infected by her. Her husband, enraged by the king's action, had infected both himself and his wife. A number of famous historical personalities contracted the disease. Much points to Francis I's contemporary in England, Henry VIII, having syphilis: his queen's many miscarriages and stillborn children, his own chronic leg sores and a suspected nerve syphilis towards the end of his life are all thus best explained.

During the first great syphilis epidemic in 1493 and for the next few decades, the connection with sexual intercourse was not understood, nor was it realised that the severe disturbances in the internal organs of the so-called tertiary stage of syphilis belonged to the same disease as the apparently harmless rash. Moral judgements on those infected showed the same tendency; syphilis was a punishment sent by God, and theologians proved that the general godlessness was the cause of the scourge which had struck Christendom. Syphilitics had their own patron saints, St Dionysius and St Minus, to whose graves pilgrimages were made. Long descriptions of the new disease appeared and the poets sang of it. One 'Ballade sur la grosse vérole', held to be in the handwriting of François Villon, describes the disease with astonishing accuracy and the author mentions that he was infected.

Academically trained doctors refused to have anything to do with the new disease and handed the sick over to barbers, bath attendants and charlatans, who successfully tried their old remedy against scabies, a grey ointment prepared from mercury. Ulrich van Hutten gives a terrible picture of the suffering he had to endure during his quicksilver cures. Many died of mercury poisoning, while others preferred to forgo treatment rather than be smeared to death. Another much sought but not very effective remedy was a concoction of guaiac wood, the 'holy Indian wood', which was imported in great quantities from western India. The importers made large sums of money in the transaction and it can be especially noted that the fortunes of the Augsburg banking house of Fugger were partly founded in this way.

One of the earliest and best descriptions of the new disease is given by Jean de Béthencourt. He called it *morbus venereus* or *lues venera*, which shows that, in contrast to many of his contemporaries, he saw that the infection was transmitted through sexual intercourse. The name syphilis, by which the disease was later known, was first suggested in 1530 by Girolamo Fracastoro, famous as doctor, astronomer and poet, in honour of a herdsman in a poem by the name of Syfilus. As soon as it became clear how the disease was generally transmitted, moral judgements on it became inextricably tangled with preaching on sexual and marital morality. The name *mal vénérien*, sexual disease, became common and sufferers were by many considered sinners and criminals, who must be both treated and punished. Fasts, purgings and penances supported the treatment, which the terrible sweat-forcing quicksilver in fact made a suitable punishment. But condemnation of the victims was generally restricted to 'the people'. Among the aristocracy, the upper priesthood and in the French, English and Spanish courts, where syphilis soon became extraordinarily widespread, sufferers were not so severely judged, and it was even considered a sign of poor upbringing not to have contracted the new 'gallant' disease. Erasmus mentions that a nobleman who had not yet had the disease was looked upon as '*ignobilis et rusticanus*'. Syphilis became the best possible

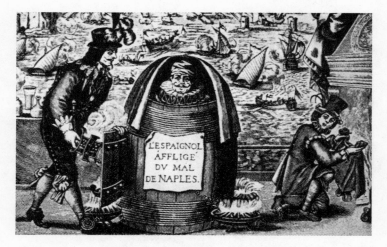

Treatment of syphilis at the beginning of the sixteenth century. The patient is sitting in a barrel which contains cinnabar (mercuric sulphide) which was then heated. On the barrel is written: 'The Spaniard afflicted with the Neapolitan disease.' (Seventeenth-century engraving.)

evidence of chivalrous behaviour in this era of amorous adventures.

The disease reached Scandinavia quite quickly, as is witnessed by, amongst other things, typical severe skull changes which have been found in Danish graveyards of the last years of the fifteenth century and also in the old churchyard in Lund. These finds admirably supplement medical and historical accounts of the time. As in large parts of Europe the new infectious disease, which here was at first called pox, meant a revolution in many living conditions. Troels-Lund has pointed out that when the disease acquired an increasing hold and showed itself to be so infectious, this led to the closing down of the public bath-houses which in the Middle Ages had played such a great social and hygienic role. Many of them were never reopened and individual cleanliness thus considerably deteriorated. In the case of Sweden the disease was thought to have primarily been brought in by the Danish armies, which during the last stages of the Union several times advanced towards Stockholm. Christian II's army was especially notorious.

In 1499 syphilis spread via Poland into Russia where the disease is supposed to have appeared first in Smolensk in a particularly severe form.

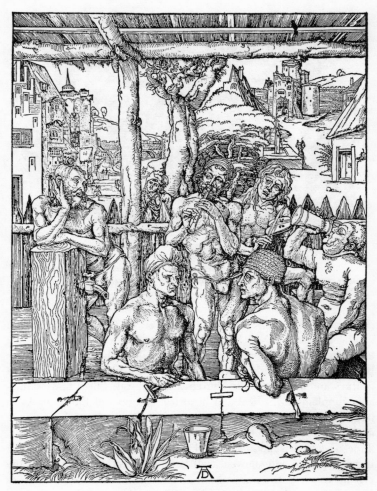

Social life in the bath-house. Wood-cut by Albrecht Dürer.

The first eastward spread of the disease is not known in detail, but much points to Vasco da Gama's men taking it to Calcutta in India, from where it spread to the Malay peninsula, then, as now, an important trading centre, and at the beginning of the sixteenth century to Canton. In China it was called Canton disease, and when it reached Kyoto in Japan it received the name *karakasä*, Chinese pleasure disease.

The Conquistadors carried syphilis to those parts of America which were probably not infected before. Castillo, one of the followers of Cortez, noted in his diary the advances of the disease among the soldiers who captured Mexico.

The Rococo period made no secret of the disease. 'Cupid's arrows' were poisoned. Voltaire wrote a poem on Francis I's syphilis, mentioning his *'corona Veneris'*, the syphilitic rash on the forehead, and he dedicated the following lines to a beautiful actress who had the disease:

> Belle Duclos,
> vous charmez toute la nature!
> Belle Duclos,
> vous avez les dieux pour rivaux
> et Mars tenterait l'aventure,
> s'il ne crainiait le dieu Mercure,[1]
> Belle Duclos.

But with the French Revolution a new era began, the age of the bourgeoisie, and there followed a reversal of opinion. Syphilis became a shameful disease which one avoided mentioning. Finally, in our time, the disease is no longer just a private affair, but can be a social menace, and the state grudges no expense in fighting it. Legislation, prophylactics and therapy have tackled the problem extremely successfully.

Geography. The distribution of syphilis today cannot be dealt with in a few lines. It is practically global with only a few islands free of it. Nevertheless, wherever legislation and medical measures have gone hand in hand, it is on the decline and in many European countries, like Sweden, new cases of syphilis are rare. However, a few Swedes returned from the Spanish Civil War with the infection. In many ports in the Mediterranean and the tropics, it is still very common, in contrast with favourable developments elsewhere. Syphilis still has a very wide distribution outside Europe. It is difficult to judge the frequency in figures, partly because differential diagnosis between syphilis and yaws is so difficult.

There are especial difficulties with the singular endemic 'non-venereal' form of treponematosis which some authorities regard as syphilis, others as yaws, and others as a third form or middle form.

[1] Alluding to the painful mercury cure.

Many cases of syphilis in Jugoslavia, Bulgaria, South Russia, Arabia, Iraq, Persia and India, are said to be of an extra-genital nature. According to Hudson (1937) this form, occasionally called *bejel*, is a special form of treponematosis. It is said to begin in childhood among North African Bedouins, among whom, on the other hand, genital syphilis is said to be almost non-existent.

Information on the frequency of syphilis in Africa shows huge numbers of infected people treated annually. In Algeria in 1847 40,000 cases were treated, in Egypt in 1942, 30,000. In the Sudan at that time certain tribes were infected up to 40 per cent. In Ethiopia syphilis is a huge problem, 30–50 per cent of the population being considered infected. A Swedish surgeon, Hanner, who prac- tised there thirty-five years ago, gave everyone who was to be operated prophylactic anti-luetic treatment. In Madagascar in the 1940s about 160,000 cases were registered annually; in the ports of Africa and Asia syphilis is enormously widespread; but in many places it is impossible to find exact figures as all the venereal diseases, syphilis, soft chancroid, climatic buboes, lymphogranuloma inguinale and gonorrhoea, are put together.

In recent generations the disease has to a certain extent changed character, at least in many places in Europe and North America. Severe cases of skin and bone syphilis, of syphilitic gummata in the muscles, liver, testicles and brain, which only fifty years ago in Sweden were not all that infrequently seen, have become rarities. On the other hand there are relatively more cases of syphilitic damage to the central nervous system in the form of meningitis, tabes dorsalis and G.P.I. (general paralysis of the insane), and it is said that the spirochaete seems to have become more inclined to attack the nervous system. Why this is so, is not easy to explain, as there are so many factors involved—improved methods of treatment which nowadays give freedom from recidivism, changed virulence and altered conditions of environment. The severe forms of syphilis which one once came to know in Europe and North America are nowadays only found in remote countries where the disease is still widespread and treatment is ineffective or non-existent.

Pinta, Mal del Pinto, carate, spotted disease

Microbe: *Treponema carateum.*

The name 'Pinta' or 'Mal del Pinto' is used in the tropics for several skin diseases with spot formation, but should be reserved for the infectious disease caused by *T. carateum*, which like yaws and syphilis gives a positive Wassermann reaction. It has been indigenous to Mexico and parts of South America since ancient times. More than 600,000 cases are known.

Another spirochaetosis is dealt with below, which, however, belongs to a different group of microbes from the previous ones. It bears the name leptospirosis.

Leptospirosis ictero-haemorrhagica, Weil's disease

The microbe is represented by three main forms: *L. ictero-haemorrhagica*, *L. canicola* and *L. pomona*. The host animals are rats and dogs.

During the American Civil War of 1861–65 more than 70,000 sickened of fever and jaundice. Whether these were in fact Weil's disease or perhaps more likely virus hepatitis (see p. 237) is uncertain. In any case Uhlenhut and Fromme consider it was a case of leptospirosis, as do Topley and Wilson. According to these authorities the disease occurred during the First World War on both sides of the western front. Epidemics have also been described in the 1920s and 1930s in different parts of the world.

In the 1930s France, Holland and Great Britain were especially affected. The disease was endemic among sewer workers and fish handlers in England. This leptospirosis has been especially common in Japan, Korea and China. The form caused by *L. canicola* is common in Indonesia and Sumatra. Weil's disease is also common in India with its vast numbers of rats. Infection is by dirty water; in an epidemic in Lisbon with 130 victims and about 25 per cent mortality, the source of infection was the waste water from a rat-infested sewer.

6 Protozoal Diseases

Protozoa, unicellular animal organisms, are here divided into four groups, which will be called in the following accounts Rhizopoda (Sarcodina), Flagellata (Mastigophora), Sporozoa and Ciliophora (Infusoria).

Rhizopoda

This group is represented by the amoebae, among which one, *Amoeba histolytica*, is a very important pathogenic microbe, especially in tropical and sub-tropical countries.

Amoebiasis, amoebic dysentery

This parasite, which in warmer climates is extremely important, causes a special form of dysentery. In Scandinavia it is only an occasional visitor, brought into the country via seamen or other travellers. In Germany, amoebic dysentery was not uncommon after the First World War, especially in Hamburg, and there were also quite a few cases among the British and American forces of occupation. In Tiflis, pus-formation in the liver was once common in amoebic dysentery. In Central and South America, about half the cases of dysentery are the result of amoebic infection, and the same applies to amoebic infection in tropical Asia and Africa. In 1938 in India 1,500,000 cases of dysentery were treated, of which about two-thirds were amoebic dysentery. Of those treated, about 300,000 died and about 11,000 had liver abscesses. Among the Asiatic countries, Japan is an exception. There the bacillary form of dysentery predominates (see p. 75).

134

Flagellata

To this group belong four families of pathogens, among which Trypanosoma are incomparably the most important. The others are Leishmania, Lamblia and Trichomonas.

Trypanosomiasis

There are three species which are pathogenic to humans, of which two are African, *Trypanosoma gambiense* and *T. rhodesiense*, and one South American, *T. cruzi*. There are also numerous species pathogenic to animals, the best known of which is that which causes so-called stallion disease in horses. Another species was extremely common, at least thirty years ago, among the rats of Stockholm.

Trypanosomiasis africana, African sleeping sickness, is a terrible chronic fever which leads to death after increasing wasting and somnolence interrupted by outbreaks of rage. The discoverer of the disease was the English colonial doctor Winterbottom, who in 1803 described it in negro slaves imported into Cuba. The two species of Trypanosoma which cause the disease are transmitted by different species of the tsetse fly, Glossina, of which some so need shade and humidity that they only thrive in hot humid river valleys with shady trees and bush vegetation. If the river banks are stripped bare the fly disappears. Other species of Glossina are less particular and even appear as high as 1,000–1,500 metres above sea level.

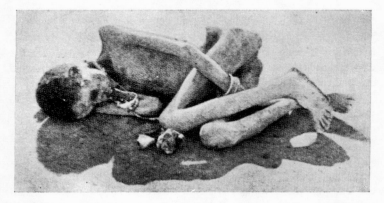

Final stage of African sleeping sickness (after M. Mayer, Exotische Krankheiten, 1924).

So there too humans are menaced with trypanosoma infections. It is principally people who move along rivers and go from caravans to fetch water and so on, who are attacked by the fly. Coloureds are more susceptible than whites. The fly can transmit the parasite direct from person to person, but usually the parasite stays in the body of the fly where it reproduces itself. It can also adapt itself to domestic animals, such as ruminants and pigs.

In many African countries, African sleeping sickness has declined, thanks to the campaign against the Glossina, but in others one still has to contend with an increase in the number of cases, as in Kenya, Tanzania and Mozambique. Considerable advances have been made in Uganda where at the beginning of the century about 200,000 cases were treated annually, in 1940 only 425, and in 1947 only 100. In the Congo great advances have also been made: in 1928 among two million natives, up to 30 per cent were infected, in 1948 only 0·77 per cent.

South American trypanosomiasis, which has the name of Chagas disease after its discoverer, is caused by *T. cruzi* and has an extremely peculiar course. The parasite is transmitted, usually at night, by lice of the Panstrongylus species and other small lice. The disease has an acute form in children and is chronic in adults, causes enlargement of the thyroid gland and leads to death. Strangely enough, the parasite is found in lice which live outside the regions in which the disease occurs. Apart from humans, certain mammals, rodents and armadillos are carriers of the parasite.

Leishmaniasis

Among the Leishmania species which are pathogenic to humans, two deserve special mention here, *L. donovani* which causes the tropical disease kala-azar, and *L. tropica* which causes the so-called oriental sore.

Kala-azar is a particularly malignant fever which is similar to tropical malaria and causes anaemia, enlargement of the spleen and wasting. The parasite is transmitted by different species of the sand-fly, Phlebotomus. The disease occurs in the Mediterranean and southern Russia, in the valley of the Ganges where it was first described in 1869, in many other places in India and in the valleys of the Yangtze and Hwang Ho rivers where in 1949 there were calculated to be 500,000 cases. Peking, once considered the most highly infected city, is now said to be free of kala-azar. In Mesopotamia,

Arabia, Iraq, North Africa, Kenya, Madagascar and Brazil cases are not infrequently seen.

Oriental sore, which also takes the name of certain cities and is then known as Aleppo sore, Delhi boil, Biskra button, Baghdad boil or Lahore sore, is an endemic disease in the Orient, but has spread to the Mediterranean countries and many South American states. In Aleppo 70 per cent of the population was previously infected. The parasite, which is transmitted by a sand-fly, Phlebotomus, causes boils and sores on the skin, face, arms and legs. This leishmaniasis has a relatively mild course, and one can be vaccinated against it.

L. braziliensis, which occurs in Central and South America and is also transmitted by a Phlebotomus, causes large sores in the nose and mouth.

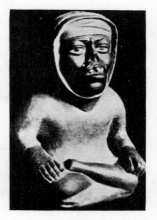

Peruvian terracotta figure (Mochica civilisation) with facial disfiguration caused by scar-atrophy of the nose and mouth, probably due to South American leishmaniasis of the skin and mucous membrane, possibly a tertian form of framboesia. Left leg amputated at birth(?).

Lambliasis

Lamblia intestinalis is an intestinal parasite which was discovered by Leeuwenhoek in 1681; in many cases the infection runs its course without any symptoms and it is therefore difficult to define its distribution. In Bonn it was found, in an investigation some ten years ago, that 23 per cent of all those examined had the parasite, in England it was almost 40 per cent, mostly children, and in USA 48 per cent among children. In Egypt it seems to be less common, an investigation showing 4–16 per cent. In Sweden the parasite is seen now and again but is not thought to be of much significance as a cause of disease.

Trichomoniasis

Symptoms do not necessarily appear, either, with infection by the intestinal and vaginal parasite *Trichomonas intestinalis* and *vaginalis*. In the USA it was found in 30 per cent of those examined and during a dysentery epidemic, in the Andaman islands it was found in 80 per cent of the evacuations examined.

Sporozoa (previously haemosporida)

The most important representatives of this group are the malarial plasmodia, of which four species are pathogenic to humans, namely *Plasmodium vivax*, which causes third-day fever, tertiana, *P. malariae* which causes fourth-day fever, quartana, *P. falciparum* which causes summer-autumn ague and *P. ovale* which like *P. vivax* causes tertiana. Apart from these four, there are a number of species of plasmodia which are pathogenic to different animals, such as apes, rodents and birds, but not to humans. The four species of plasmodia which can live in humans are transmitted to the blood by species of the mosquito family Anopheles, of which about seventy different species are involved as carriers.

Malaria

History. Malaria has been one of man's worst enemies since the beginning of human life and its influence on historical and cultural development cannot be exaggerated. Its earliest history is hidden in obscurity but it has certainly existed in the warmer parts of Africa and Asia since time immemorial. Some consider that the great migrations were partly due to the need to find new lands so that the people should not succumb to this invisible enemy. It seems that the disease was not known in ancient Egypt before Hellenistic times or in pre-historic Greece, or anyhow that it was of no great importance there. Possibly the disease that, according to the Iliad, afflicted the Greeks at the siege of Troy was malaria. Certainly malaria occurred in Asia Minor at a very early date, and the *Hippocratic Collection* contains observations on attacks of fever and their connection with the seasons. It is also thought that the campaigns of Alexander the Great, like so many other wars, contributed to the spread of malaria, and, according to Sorre, Alexander himself fell victim to the disease —a statement which is doubted by others.

Active communication with the Orient meant that Greece became increasingly infected. The disease became endemic and chronic cases appeared together with malaria cachexia, severe attacks of inertia, wasting, etc. The disease soon spread to Magna Graecia, the flourishing Greek colonies in southern Italy. According to Jones (1907) it is not unlikely that malaria brought with it a general deterioration of physical and intellectual strength, a more pessimistic view of life and a resignation very alien to earlier generations of Greeks, which finally led to political decadence and general economic and cultural decline in the prosperous cities of the mother country as well as in the colonies. The epidemic spread northwards into Italy where the Etruscans' high standard of agriculture had previously prevented it from gaining a foothold. When the drainage systems used during the later Roman Imperial period fell into disuse and the fields were transformed into swamps, and when the Goths invaded, malaria increased rapidly. Powerful popes could counteract the epidemic up to a point, but for many centuries, well into the nineteenth century, malaria was a feared enemy along the coasts of Italy. To travel in Italy entailed risks, as is shown by the malaria to which Albrecht Dürer succumbed.

Malaria was disseminated throughout Europe by the returning Crusaders, but in more peaceful conditions it declined and in many countries disappeared altogether. At the outbreak of the First World War, Great Britain, which had earlier been free of it, was once again infected. During the Second World War even Finnish troops fighting on the Karelian isthmus became infected.

With the introduction of insecticides began a new era in the history of malaria.

Aetiology. Ancient Roman writers such as Varro and Columella thought that malaria was caused by small living creatures. In his *De re rustica*, the former speaks of 'the marshes, where there live little animals which cannot be seen by the human eye, but which penetrate via the air into our bodies and cause severe sicknesses.' The statements of Lancisi, doctor to popes and kings (1717), are most remarkable: mosquitoes spread malaria 'not only by stinging and biting but principally by injecting their own malignant juices into our blood.' But Lancisi goes even further, and here his words have a ring of inspiration: 'I should be a poet, a prophet, if, with no experimental basis, I should presume that certain living creatures penetrate into the blood of malaria victims and there circulate.' To

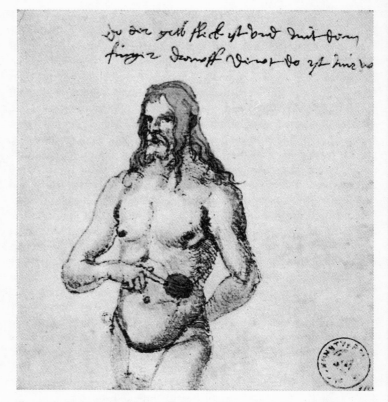

Part of a letter from Albrecht Dürer to his teacher. Above the drawing one can read, not without some difficulty, 'Do der gelb Fleck ist und mit dem Finger drauf deut, do ist mir weh' (where the yellow spot is and where my finger points to, there it hurts). The spot is yellow in the original and corresponds to the spleen.

solve the problem he suggests that one should examine the blood of patients time and time again (!) under the microscope, but this, however, was not allowed. But Lancisi's clear view of the method of infection was forgotten and even at the beginning of the 1880s his theory of infection was still considered unlikely. It is possible that the Africans of Tanganyika instinctively believed in a connection between malaria and mosquitoes, which is indicated in a note of Robert Koch, who says they used the same name, *mbu*, for the disease and the mosquito. The discovery of the plasmodium was made on

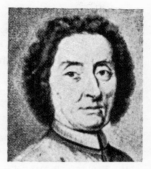

Giovanni-Maria Lancisi (1654–1720), whose remarkable comments on the cause of malaria are mentioned in the text.

6 November 1880 by the French army doctor Laveran, for which he was awarded one of the first Nobel Prizes for medicine in 1907.

It was soon possible to show that the different clinical forms of malaria corresponded to different species of the plasmodium: third-day fever, tertiana, to *P. vivax,* fourth-day fever, quartana, to *P. malariae,* and the malignant tropical fever to *P. falciparum* (*praecox*); and in addition there were the mixed forms. The fourth species of plasmodium, *P. ovale,* which occurs in the Congo and South America, gives the same symptoms as *P. vivax.*

Geography. Warmth and access to water are the necessary conditions for the malarial mosquito's survival and the plasmodium's ability to live in the body of the mosquito. Therefore the mosquitoes prefer low-lying regions near rivers and freshwater lakes, but minimal accumulations of water are also sufficient for the development of the larvae. Many species of Anopheles can live quite high up in the mountains, in the French Alps up to 1,650 metres, in

Charles-Louis Laveran (1845–1922), an army doctor in Constantine, Algeria, the discoverer of the malaria plasmodium; awarded the Nobel Prize in 1907.

141

the mountains of Morocco up to 2,000 metres and in Guatemala even up to 3,500 metres. The coldest parts of the world do not suit the mosquitoes and even if they can survive there, the plasmodium must have a summer temperature of at least 15–16° C. to develop. It has been observed that in parts of the world where the summer temperature is usually too low for the plasmodium, a hot summer can bring occasional outbreaks of infection. Sometimes it happens that malarial seats of infection appear in regions which have long been spared, and this is sometimes difficult to understand. It happened, for instance, in France, when long free areas were again affected in 1914 and 1918; possibly soldiers on leave brought the plasmodium with them.

Once, before its eradication was seriously undertaken, malaria had an enormous distribution. About three-quarters of the inhabitants of the world live in regions which can be infected. It is calculated that until about 1948 a round figure of about 300 million sickened annually of malaria and 3 million died. Countries, which are now free, a few generations ago had malaria annually, often with clear maxima and minima. The whole of southern Asia, from Asia Minor to Japan, had malaria. Malaria was India's main disease and at the end of the 1930s the number of sick was estimated at 13 million, with up to 4 million deaths per year. In Ceylon in 1942 there were nearly 3 million cases of malaria, in China in 1949 those infected with malaria were calculated to number 30 million, in Indo-China one-fifth of the population always had malaria and it was calculated that every native at the age of 25 had had malaria once or several times. It is obvious that the vitality and capacity of a whole population must be lowered by such conditions. Similar infection of the native population was prevalent in Africa.

The age of malaria as a disease in America has not yet been decided, but after the arrival of Europeans and the importation of slaves from Africa it spread swiftly to all regions where the humidity and temperature allowed the mosquito and plasmodium to survive. The tropical parts of the continent suffered in particular.

It is not possible to go into the geographical distribution of all the different species of plasmodia. Temperate zones almost always have cases of tertiana and quartana. In the tropics, especially in Central Africa, southern Asia and the East Indies, the malignant form was once very common, occasionally with severe kidney damage and blood in the urine, so-called Blackwater fever, almost exclusively connected with falciparum malaria. (An interesting detail which has been recently discovered is that negroes who have the curved form of red-blood corpuscles known as sickle cells, drepanocytes (see p. 207), showed increased resistance to malaria.)

In the spring of 1955 WHO began a systematic campaign to eradicate malaria. The results were everywhere encouraging and are a challenge to renewed efforts so that what has been accomplished is not wasted. Of the 2,768 million people in the world, about 1,071 million live in regions where malaria has never been endemic or where it has disappeared without specific measures being taken. In that year about 1,052 million people lived in malarial regions and about 645 million in countries from which there is no reliable information (China, North Korea, North Vietnam). Certain parts of the world, with about 300 million inhabitants, which earlier were severely infected, are now free of malaria and it is planned at present to eradicate malaria in countries inhabited by 700–800 million people. Despite this there are still population groups totalling about 150 million in regions which suffer from the disease. According to Schöne (1960), five species of Anopheles act as transmitters of malaria in China. In October 1959 there were still in the southern and central parts of the country large endemic malarial seats of infection and Canton, Kwantung and the island of Hainan were especially affected. The feared tropical form was to be found in southern China, as well as tertiana. The problems in the eradication campaign are of many kinds. It is not only the indifference and resistance of the inhabitants that are obstacles, but just as much the resistance of the mosquito to insecticides, which have therefore to be occasionally varied.

In Sweden malaria was once endemic in many places, and many older people to whom I spoke told me of their attacks of ague, especially in the spring. According to G. Berman, who has studied the history of ague in Sweden, the disease is recorded in the thirteenth century, but it probably existed much earlier. Deaths after lengthy attacks of ague are recorded in the monastery journals. Bishop Israel Erlandsson, when he went to school in Linköping in the 1200s, 'there contracted the severe sickness which is called quartana for three and a half years.' In the fifteenth-century statutes of King Magnus Eriksson and in a manuscript of the same period, there is mention of a remedy for 'cold-sickness', which is malaria. Peter Månsson's medical work and the Benedictus Olai 'book of healing', both of the sixteenth century, comment on malaria under the name of 'shivering sickness'. The ague formed an important part of Swedish folk-diseases and was known by a number of provincial names among the people. A number of academic disputations and other works on malaria have appeared during past centuries in Sweden.

According to Huss, the northern-most point for ague in Sweden, was the mouth of the river Ångerman where the Lo sawmill and Nylands loading-wharf, which lay opposite one another, were attacked by 'alternate-day ague, seldom by every-day ague, and never by third-day ague.' The disease was to be found in the Hudiksvall region and in Gästrikland, especially at the mouth of the river Gävle and fifteen to twenty miles inland. Especially notorious were the Mälar islands (Svartsjöland ague) and Drottningholm, where the pools made excellent breeding-grounds for the mosquito larvae, but in the eighteenth century health improved there as it did round the great Lakes Hjälmare and Väner (Lake Vätter's shores were practically free of malaria). Many river mouths, like those of the Em, the Helga and the Göta, were notorious. From these almost permanently infected regions, the ague spread in the form of epidemics with varying distribution and mortality. In general one finds a distinct parallel between the great epidemics of Europe and those of Sweden. Those who were infected were mostly outdoor workers or countrymen. During the extensive construction of the railways in the 1850s and 1860s, malaria raged among the navvies. The following table shows how the average mortality from malaria in Sweden has decreased.

1861–70	119	1911–20	3·5
1871–80	34	1921–30	2·5
1881–90	10	1931–40	—
1891–1900	9	1941–50	—
1901–10	6	1951–60	—

It is not surprising that malaria has occurred significantly in Finland with all its water-courses and lakes. According to R. Sievers, the disease, which had been known there for centuries, occurred in severe epidemics in 1846–48 and 1853–62, the worst years being 1860–62.

Finally, it is perhaps worth mentioning that the disappearance of malaria from northern regions such as Sweden is not due to any change in climate, as one sometimes hears, but to other, not wholly explained circumstances. Anopheles, the mosquito which transmits the plasmodium, is just as common as before and found as far north as 80° N, but the infection has disappeared.

Toxoplasmosis

This sporozoa can be only briefly mentioned here as its geography is still insufficiently known. It seems to be more common in hot humid climates and its distribution in Europe and North America is being investigated with a serum test. It is estimated that there are many different forms in humans, among others a form which is inborn and localised in the central nervous system. Dogs and cats are considered to be the host animals.

Coccidiosis

The coccidia, long known in animals, in recent years have also been shown in humans. An Isospora species has been described in the Netherlands and South America.

Piroplasmosis

The Babesia family also belongs to the sporozoa, and in Sweden is represented principally by *B. bovis* which causes piroplasmosis in cattle, a disease, very important from an economic point of view, and associated with fever, destruction of the red blood corpuscles and anaemia. It is principally found in south-east Sweden and is transmitted by the tick *Ixodes ricinus*. At mass immunisations against piroplasmosis, it is considered that there is a risk of the leucosis virus (see p. 63) being transmitted to the cattle.

Ciliophora

The most important representative of this group is *Balantidium coli*, discovered by the Swede P. H. Malmsten in 1857, a relatively large protozoon which lives in the large intestine of pigs, apes and humans. The disease, which is characterised by severe diarrhoea, was once very widespread in Europe, and in Sweden also cases were observed by many doctors, but now it has become rare in all countries with better hygiene, and in northern Europe it has as good as disappeared. It is not so common in Italy, more so in the Balkans. It is widespread over southern Asia, and especially common in a number of Pacific islands.

7   Worm (helminth) Diseases

As this chapter concerns diseases caused by worms, it is better to use the term infestation rather than infection.

That worms cause diseases is almost certainly one of man's earliest medical observations, and according to some medical historians it is no coincidence that the staff with a snake coiled round it has been for centuries the symbol of the art of healing. The snake is said to be none other than a Medina worm rolled round a short stick; *Dracunculus medinensis* already in prehistoric times was a parasite of humans in large parts of the Orient, from where such a

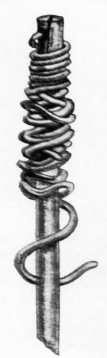

large proportion of our medical knowledge and ideas originates, via Egypt and Greece. But even if a great deal points to the snake being a symbol of healing, there is by no means a lack of other explanations. The snake has always played a prominent part in ancient myths and religions. It is of course impossible here to go into the literature which deals with the snake symbol, and it can only be pointed out that the snake of healing in both Egypt and Greece occasionally appears without being coiled round a staff. Zeus Meilichios appears in the form of a snake and the snake cannot be regarded generally as a symbol for the art of healing.

Worm diseases occur in the ancient Egyptian myths of the gods. The sun god Ra fell ill when a worm infested (by penetrating?)

The Medina worm, Dracunculus medinensis, rolled on to a short stick. Could this be the origin of the Aesculapian staff with a snake coiled round it, the ancient emblem of the art of healing?

146

his ankle. Bilharzia eggs have been found in mummies from different dynasties, but it is doubtful that the Egyptians knew of such intestinal parasites as the schistosome (cause of bilharzia) and hookworm, or that they realised their importance. Nevertheless, the females are 18–22 mm long and the males 10–12 mm, and are not difficult to see. In Mesopotamia also worms were known as causes of disease and the ancient Indians are said to have known twenty such diseases. At all events, knowledge of the biology of worms, and especially their microscopic forms, metamorphosis, intermediate hosts and pathogenic significance, belongs to the last 100–150 years.

From a global viewpoint, the importance of worms as causes of disease is much greater than one might think in temperate and cold climates and in good hygienic conditions. In these conditions, from a pathogenic point of view, worms come a long way after viruses and bacteria. But in the tropics the order is reversed and there worm diseases have a tremendous distribution. In many tropical countries 50–100 per cent of the inhabitants are affected by one or often more worm diseases. In the tropics the worm or its larvae generally penetrate through the skin, while in temperate regions the mouth is the most important place of entry.

A closer zoological classification, which in any case varies from author to author, will not be made here. Worms will be divided into three main groups: nematoda (round and thread worms), trematoda (flat or sucker worms) and cestoda (tapeworms).

Nematode diseases

Filarial diseases

Wuchereria (*Filaria*) *bancrofti* and *malayi* as adults live in humans in the lymph vessels and lymph nodes of the lower half of the body and gradually cause the well known and often enormous swelling of the legs, scrotum and labia which goes under the name of elephantiasis. The microscopic form of the larva lives in the blood and is taken up by the mosquito Mansonia, which transmits the larvae to others. In China larvae are also transmitted by *Anopheles sinensis*, a malarial mosquito. Formerly in Egypt up to 25 per cent of the inhabitants of certain districts were affected. A short time ago in the Sudan 2,500–3,000 cases were treated annually and in Tanganyika about a third of the native inhabitants have worms. Similar conditions prevail in other places in Africa. This filarial disease is also common in the whole of southern Asia as far north as Korea; it is also found in the Pacific islands and sometimes in South America.

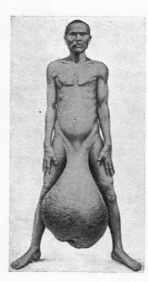

Man from the Samoa islands with enormous swelling of the scrotum, the result of lymph blockage caused by the small round worm Wuchereria (Filaria) bancrofti, *which lives in the lymph cells.*

Loa loa is another form of filaria from which inhabitants of the humid forest regions of Equatorial Africa often suffer. It causes limited swellings in the subcutaneous tissues and can also take root in the conjunctiva of the eye. In this case also a small mosquito transmits the microscopic larvae from person to person. Another small worm, *Onchocerca volvulus*, which is transmitted by a small fly, Simulium, penetrates into the front part of the eye. It is estimated that in Ghana and Nigeria about 30,000 people are blind because of it.

Dracunculus medinensis, the Medina or Guinea worm, is the largest of all the filaria. The female can be over one metre long, a single person can have four to five worms, and a number of domestic animals are also worm carriers. *Dracunculus* was once very common in certain parts of Africa, and not so long ago in the Sudan about 2,500 cases were treated annually. Cases also occur in Arabia, Persia, east of the Caspian Sea and in India, and this giant filaria has been seen even in South America. The worm lives below the skin and in the muscles, and when it bores its way to the surface, it gives off its microscopic larvae, which in fresh water are absorbed by a small shell-fish. If this water is drunk, there is a risk that the larvae are also consumed. When the worm shows itself in a little sore to lay its larvae, the carrier has the opportunity of getting hold of the end of it with a cloven stick and he can then, by daily winding up the worm once or twice, gradually pull it out, which takes about a month. If the worm is broken off, an unpleasant inflammation sets in.

Learned men of antiquity discussed whether a worm or a nerve was involved.

Trichocephaliasis, whipworm infestation

This small worm lives in the large intestine and is often quite harmless, but can cause diarrhoea. After the First World War it was very common in Central Europe—in Germany 2–40 per cent, in Paris 30–40 per cent, among Russian prisoners-of-war 43–65 per cent, in Rumania 72 per cent and in Baku 95 per cent. It is also quite common in America and an investigation in the USA showed that 11 per cent of children were infested.

Trichinosis (preferably trichinellosis)

Trichinella spiralis was once a very common parasite in most countries but is now more or less eradicated in countries that have compulsory control of pork. An oversight can result in minor epidemics, as happened recently in Blekinge in Sweden. Apart from pigs, other animals play a lesser part. In Sweden bear-meat has caused minor epidemics, which have even had fatal results. Foxes from fur-farms have also, during recent times of crisis, been the source of small epidemics. In Stuttgart a few decades ago, a slaughtered bear caused a severe epidemic with many deaths. Besides pigs, dogs can be worm hosts in places where dog-meat is consumed, and even rats are considered to be carriers. In Stockholm, however, I could not find a single case among one hundred wild rats examined. *Trichinella* seems finally to have been eradicated. In Greenland six epidemics have been known since 1947, and in the first, which involved 300 Eskimos, thirty-three died. There polar bears, walruses and seals are the sources of infection—dogs are not eaten. In the USA, where pork is not always controlled, infestation of humans is not all that rare. In 1894 no fewer than 14 per cent were found to be infested at autopsies, and in 1901 still 5·3 per cent.

Very little is known about the distribution of trichinosis in remote countries where pork is eaten, but presumably it is very common.

Ancylostomiasis, hookworm disease

Both the main representatives of the hookworm, *Ancylostomum duodenale* and *Necator americanus*, are among the most common and most important of all parasitical worms. It is estimated in round figures that 500 million people are carriers of either one or the other, often in large numbers, but infestation does not in itself mean that the carrier is very ill. Both worms look alike and it is thought that *Necator americanus* was originally an African parasite which negro slaves took to America. The distribution of the two worms varies, in some places only one is found, in others both at once. The larvae live in damp earth and in dirty food or water and are either directly absorbed with the food and water or perforate the skin of people who walk with bare feet and legs in mud and water containing the larvae.

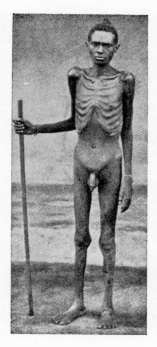

East African Negro with high degree of emaciation from hookworm disease, ancylostomiasis (after M. Mayer, Exotische Krankheiten, 1924).

As the larvae need a certain temperature, they can only develop in humid warmth, mainly in the tropics, but otherwise only in warm tunnels and mines. In 1880 a terrible epidemic (*malattia dei minatori*) broke out among the men working on the St Gotthard tunnel, so that work on the last stages of construction had to be postponed. Similar outbreaks took place in the mining districts of the Ruhr where in 1903 23,000 workers or 13 per cent of the employees fell ill. The mines were sanitated, with good results, and in 1914 only 0·14 per cent of the miners were infested. Similar conditions existed in the mining areas of Liége where formerly 25–50 per cent of the miners were infested, but in 1923 only 0·3 per cent.

Each worm's relative share in infestation varies, as I have said. In Madras, *Necator* constitutes over 90 per cent of cases, in China *Ancylostomum* is 80 per cent, in some parts of Africa *Necator* is found in nearly every case and in others in barely half. The frequency of the disease is often extremely high. In Helouan, near Cairo, worms were found in 90 per cent of those examined, in other parts of Egypt only in 50 per cent. In parts of Africa practically the whole of the population is infested. In some places energetic efforts have been made to eradicate the worm, for instance in the South African gold mines, where in 1925–36 the miners were still widely infested, and where now the parasite has almost completely disappeared.

Ascariasis, roundworm infestation

Until a few decades ago the relatively harmless worm *Ascaris lumbricoides* had a universal distribution and in 1947 it was estimated that about one-third of mankind was infested. In countries with relatively good hygiene, like Sweden, the worm is now seldom found, but earlier it is said to have been common in children, especially in Småland (it seems to be most common now in upper Norrland). During and after the First World War the worm was found in 12–63 per cent of combatants, in Vienna at that time 35–40 per cent of those examined were affected by *Ascaris*, in Bonn 40 per cent, and in 1929 in Zurich 48 per cent. In large parts of Africa, Asia, the Pacific and America, the worm is found in 40–100 per cent of those examined. In rare cases one can find dog-, cat- and pig-ascaris in humans but only in the form of larvae which cannot develop into adult worms.

Oxyuriasis, pinworm (Oxyuris vermicularis and other small intestinal worms)

This quite harmless worm is a parasite in the large intestine and is also not infrequently seen in the *processus vermiformis* (worm-like appendage) or appendix, where according to some authors, no doubt inaccurately, it causes appendicitis. It has a universal distribution.

Trematode diseases

Fasciola hepatica, a very common liver parasite in cattle, found in parts of Sweden too, is very seldom seen in humans. I myself have seen only one case, an Estonian who had come to Sweden. In the veterinary world it is known as liverfluke.

Two distantly related flukes, Paragonium and Metagonimus, play an important part in the Far East as there they are very common. Another trematode, *Opistorchis felineus*, is, as its name implies, predominantly a parasite in cats, but occasionally infests humans. In Tomsk it was found in 6 per cent of those examined. Before the two world wars its western limit lay in the region of Königsberg, where about forty cases were observed in humans.

Clonorchis sinensis is particularly common in China, where wretched hygienic conditions favour its reception in humans. In Kwantung from 25 to almost 100 per cent of those examined are infested, in Tonkin 50 per cent. Also in Japan, Formosa and Korea nearly three-quarters of the population may be infested.

Schistosomiasis or *bilharziasis* are names for diseases caused by the two very similar suckerworms, *Schistosomum haematobium* and *Sch. mansoni*. The disease was common in ancient Egypt and eggs have been found in mummies, even in those of Pharaohs. Even today bilharziasis is economically one of the most important diseases in Egypt. Year after year workers in the flooded fields of the Nile delta are infected and cases of severe disturbances in organs are regularly returned among autopsy results.

The parasite was first discovered in 1852 by the German doctor Bilharz who was then working in Cairo. Later, in 1907, it was shown that in fact two closely related species of worm were involved. As with ancylostomiasis, there are some tropical and sub-tropical areas where only one occurs, and others where both are found. *Sch. haematobium* is largely confined to the Old World, principally Africa, whereas *Sch. mansoni* is found not only there but also in Central and South America, for instance in Venezuela.

In Egypt, where *Sch. haematobium* predominates, it was estimated in 1949 that 14 million or two-thirds of the population were infested and that 5–10 per cent of all deaths were due to this worm disease. Since then, however, an improvement has been made, but it is still estimated that about 12 million are infested. The annual financial loss through loss of manpower is estimated at no less than

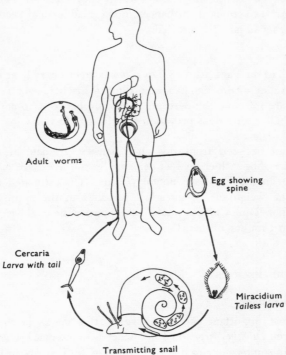

Adult worms

Egg showing spine

Cercaria
Larva with tail

Miracidium
Tailess larva

Transmitting snail

The life-cycle of the Bilharzia parasite. The egg leaves the rectum and bladder and develops into larvae when it reaches fresh water. These larvae, miracidia, after further development in a small snail which lives in the vegetation of the flooded fields, grow into small, torpedo-like, highly mobile larvae, cercariae; these bore through the human skin and circulate in the blood. The adult worm lives principally in different veins where the long thin female lies inside the sword-shaped male (Tropical Products Institute).

153

80,000,000 Egyptian pounds. In Tunis worm eggs were found in the urine of 20–86 per cent of the men but only 0–72 per cent of women and children. In Algeria 43 per cent of the men had worm eggs in their urine. The disease is more or less common over the whole of Central and South Africa and the number of those infested not infrequently rises to as much as 60 per cent.

The eggs in urine and stools enter fresh water and are absorbed by a small snail in which they develop into small torpedo-like larvae, which easily bore through the human skin to the surface capillaries and then go to the lungs from which they circulate. The adult worm causes serious disturbances in the bladder and rectum, but many other organs are affected.

Schistomiasis japonica

In much of the Far East, *Sch. japonicum* is an ordinary liver parasite. In the valley of the Yangtze, according to Fischer, over 11 million people are infested, the percentage varying between 10 and 70 per cent. Similar conditions prevail in the Hwang Ho valley.

As can be seen from this short survey, trematodae, and in particular those which live as parasites in the liver, are extremely common in the Far East, notably China. It is estimated that the sum total weight of all intestinal parasites in the approximately 700 million living Chinese would correspond to the total weight of no less than 2 million of them!

Cestode diseases

Bothryocephalosis

The most important representative of this genus is the broad tapeworm, *Dibothryocephalus latus*, which is found nearly all over the world. In some countries it is very common, for instance in Finland, where it is estimated that up to one-fifth of the inhabitants have this internal parasite. In some cases it produces a disease-picture very reminiscent of pernicious anaemia, which vanishes when the worm is expelled. According to W. Nyberg and others, the anaemia is due to a lack of vitamin B_{12}, caused by the worm. The broad tapeworm was very common in northern Sweden, especially a hundred years ago. On the coast of Norrbotten it has been known from time immemorial, according to Huss, and is considered to 'run in the family'. The cause of its appearance is not known, he goes on to say, but 'the old teaching about self-generation (*generatio aequivoca*) has been completely reversed, since we know its development from the egg outside the animal organism, as well as some of the different changes of form it undergoes before it appears as a fully developed tapeworm'. In old St Petersburg 8 per cent of the people were infested, in Dorpat 10 per cent, in Archangel 40 per cent. In western Switzerland the worm was very common once but is now quite rare. In the USA it is especially found round the Great Lakes and it is presumed that it was brought in by Finnish and Swedish immigrants.

The small intestinal parasite, Hymenolepis, is related and is the only cestode which prefers tropical and sub-tropical zones. It occurs with varying frequency in the Mediterranean; in Algiers in 20 per cent of those examined. In Florida it has been found that up to 39 per cent are infested.

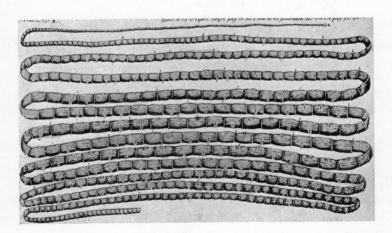

Louis XIV, a heavy eater, complained of almost permanent indisposition which to a large extent tallied with his diet and way of life. His doctor purged him and bled him, and one could say he became a victim of the medical practices of his day. After a strong laxative, a long tapeworm appeared, a Taenia. The one portrayed here is from a somewhat later date.

155

Taeniasis

The two main representatives of the Taenia, *T. solium* and *T. saginata*, occur all over the world, but in countries with good hygiene both forms have rapidly declined and *T. solium* has almost completely disappeared. In China tapeworms of different kinds are still very common and it is estimated in round figures that 90 million Chinese have one or more.

Echinococcosis (hydatid disease)

Two forms are differentiated: *Echinococcus granulosus* and *E. multilocularis* (*alveolaris*). The former occurs all over the world where large herbivores and large carnivores live together. The latter become infested by eating infested meat. The adult worm is only a few millimetres long, and lives mainly in the duodenum of carnivores. *E. multilocularis* has a more limited distribution and occurs principally in the mountainous countries of Europe, in Russia, north-east Asia and Alaska. The proportional occurrence of both forms cannot be given exactly. In all countries which have efficient meat controls the disease has declined rapidly, in Iceland for instance, where it was once widespread. In Lapland, where only a few years ago reindeer were badly infested, occasional cases were seen in humans who had been infested through intimate contact with infested dogs which had been present at the slaughter of reindeer. During the years 1920–46 I personally saw only two or three cases in about 15,000 autopsies on humans in Central Sweden. In Transcaucasia and also particularly in those parts of South America and Australia where sheep breeding goes on, echinococcus is quite common even in humans. In Uruguay, with its 2 million inhabitants and 8 million cattle, 25 million sheep and 500,000 horses and donkeys, this disease is of the greatest importance in pathology and the country has the greatest occurrence in the world of this parasite. The known frequency is rising, partly, presumably, because of better diagnosis and partly in actual fact, because of the sharp increase in number of domestic animals. It is said that 'hydatidosis follows cattle like a shadow following the body'. In more primitive countries such as northern China and certain parts of Africa, hydatidosis or bladder-worm disease is common, especially in nomadic tribes.

8 *Arthropod Diseases*

Arthropods, invertebrate animals, can themselves cause diseases, but their chief significance lies in that to a great extent they act as transmitters or vectors of many pathogenic forms of virus, rickettsia, bacteria, fungus and protozoa. As such, they have, as Bates points out—however strange it may sound—largely influenced the destiny and development of mankind. As in the case of worm diseases, this is not the place for a systematic classification.

The poisonous spiders which are common in hot countries, among others the Black Widow spider of the USA, tarantulas and scorpions, can here only be mentioned in passing.

Ixodes, ticks, play little part as direct causes of disease but they are, as will appear in the following, very important as vectors.

Trombidiosis which is caused by trombiculae, autumn mites, plays a not unimportant role as the cause of skin affections in bathers. These mites occur as far north as Denmark where between 8,000 and 10,000 people are annually affected. Their significance as transmitters of scrub typhus has been mentioned on p. 67.

Scabies

The scabies parasite, *Sarcoptes scabei*, is found all over the world and especially in places where hygiene is very poor, in large armies, in refugee camps and where people of diverse origins are crowded together in confined living spaces. Sexual intercourse strongly favours the transmission of the parasite. Scabies, which in English generally goes by the name of Norwegian scabies, was formerly very widespread in Sweden. Probably the *'radesyge'* so often mentioned by writers in the past, which was found principally along the coast, for instance in the county of Bohus, was mostly scabies. In the middle of the last century Huss graphically described conditions in Västergötland: on the plain, especially in the Fal district, scabies in association with eczema was seen in every third or fourth person;

157

all ages and both sexes were affected, 'and most of the young men in the militia from the plain district have scabies'. Dr König says that:

> the peasant most probably considers it as a condition of good living. It has been known in these regions since time immemorial and will probably remain there, at least until the inhabitants learn to realise that domestic contentment is possible without scabies. The people's reluctance to relinquish this disease is probably due to a traditional belief that scabies wards off other diseases and that if it is got rid of, others more dangerous will follow, or, as they say, the scabies will strike. The inhabitants in these regions where scabies reigns supreme live and are content to live, with few exceptions, in a high degree of squalor.

In some of the counties of Norrland, scabies is still not unknown as a skin disease.

The following figures from Stockholm, otherwise relatively scabies-free, which Hellerström has put at my disposal, are illuminating in that they show how external circumstances, such as war with its flocks of refugees, affect the frequency of scabies. The number of cases increased from 1935 when the refugees began to arrive, a maximum was reached in the years 1941–46, and then the number of cases again decreased. The following figures came from a Stockholm hospital:

Year	Men	Women	Total
1935	448	390	838
1937	555	489	1,044
1939	693	960	1,653
1941	1,486	2,296	3,782
1943	3,981	3,683	7,664
1945	1,484	2,079	3,463
1947	754	973	1,727
1949	480	471	951
1951	237	197	434
1953	265	302	567

During the middle and late 1950s cases of scabies decreased rapidly and nowadays it is a relatively rare skin disease in Stockholm.

Scabies is extremely common in all Asian and African countries as well as in South America, and in many places it is the most important skin disease.

Dipterous arthropods, flies and mosquitoes are important causes of disease in tropical and sub-tropical countries, quite apart from their significance as vectors, carriers and transmitters of different pathogenic microscopic organisms. They occur in the skin and subcutis as well as the intestines and nose, and even the large body openings can become the sites for their larvae. Even in Sweden cases of fly larvae in the intestine have been described.

Siphonaptera, fleas

1. The sand-flea, *Pulex* or *Tunga penetrans*. The sand-flea has been known for more than a hundred years as an unpleasant parasite in South America and western India. It was brought with sand ballast to the west coast of Africa in about 1850 and gradually spread across Africa, till in the 1890s it was found on the east coast and in Madagascar. From there it was not far to India. The sand-flea, which likes warm, sandy soil, is found between 30° N and 30° S of the equator.

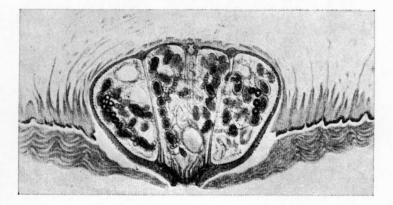

Section of the skin of the sole of the foot including section of a sand-flea which had penetrated the epidermis; it is filled with eggs which pass out through a small opening (after M. Mayer, Exotische Krankheiten, 1924.)

It penetrates the feet, especially under the toe-nails, of those who walk bare-foot and causes inflammation which leads to sores—so-called chigo sores—and even to the loss of toes. In some parts of Africa its ravages are so extensive as to be a national scourge. In Uganda more than half the inhabitants of some villages are incapacitated and in some places there is not a single man, woman or child free of chigo sores.

2. The common flea, *Pulex irritans*, has in itself little pathogenic significance, but it can serve as a transmitter of microbes, among which the plague bacillus and probably also the leprosy bacillus should be especially mentioned

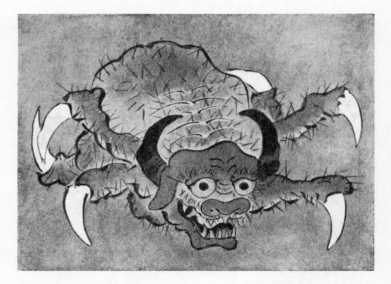

Old Japanese coloured woodcut representing Phthirus pubis, *one of the human body lice.*

A table grouping the most important infectious diseases transmitted by arthropods and showing the geography of the vectors follows on the opposite page.

The Role of Arthropods as Transmitters of Diseases

Vectors	Geography of vectors	Viruses	Rickettsia	Bacteria Spirochaetes	Protozoa Helminths
Mites					
Allodermanyssus	New York		Rickettsial pox		
Ticks					
Ixodes species	eastern USA	equine encephalitis			
	Asia, Europe	meningoen- cephalitis			
	Australia		Australian rickettsiosis		
	universal			tularaemia, relapsing fever	
	universal				piroplas- mosis in cattle
Dermacentor	USA	Colorado tick fever			
Dermato- centroxenus	N., Central and S. America		Rocky Mountain spotted fever		
	v. widespread USA		Q-fever	tularaemia	
Haemophysalis	v. widespread		Q-fever		
Ornithodorus	Africa			relapsing fever	
Autumn mites					
Trombicula	eastern Asia		Japanese river fever, scrub typhus		
Lice					
Pediculus corporis hominis	universal		epidemic typhus	relapsing fever	
	Balkans, etc.		trench fever		
Phthirus pubis	Balkans, etc.		trench fever		
	universal			relapsing fever	
Panstrongylus	S. America				S. American trypano- somiasis
Rhodnius	S. America				,, ,,

Vectors	Geography of vectors	Viruses	Rickettsia	Bacteria Spirochaetes	Protozoa Helminths
Mosquitoes *Phlebotomus* species	Europe, Africa, Asia, S. America	Papataci fever			
	Mediter- ranean, S.W. Asia, S. America				verruga peruviana? oriental sores cutaneous leishman- iasis
	Mediter- ranean, Africa, Asia, Central and S. America				kala azar visceral leishman- iasis American visceral leishman- iasis
Culicine mosquito	various places Africa, S. America	encephalitis			acantho- cheilonema
Anopheles species	USA	St Louis encephalitis			
	universal Africa, Asia, Pacific				malaria *Wuchereria bancrofti*
Aedes aegypti	eastern USA, Venezuela	equine encephalo- myelitis			
	Africa, America	yellow fever			
	Mediter- ranean, Asia, USA	dengue			
Culex species	western USA	equine encephalo- myelitis			
	USA, Japan, Australia	meningo- encephalitis			
	Scandinavia and elsewhere			tularaemia	
Mansonia	Africa, Asia, Pacific				*Wuchereria bancrofti*
Haemagogus	tropical S. America	jungle yellow fever			

Vectors	Geography of vectors	Viruses	Rickettsia	Bacteria Spirochaetes	Protozoa Helminths
Simulium species	tropical Africa and America				*Onchocerca volvulus*
	USA			tularaemia	
mosquito?	Central Africa	malignant lymphoma in children			
Flies					
Tabanus	humid tropics			plague, anthrax	
Chrysops	W. Africa, Congo				Loa loa worm
Musca domestica	universal	trachoma		plague, tuberculosis, yaws	
Glossina species	tropical Africa				sleeping sickness
Fleas					
Pulex irritans human fleas)	universal			plague, leprosy	
Xenopsylla (rat fleas)	Africa, Asia, America		murine typhus		
	various places			plague	

Non-Infectious Diseases.
Diseases of Organs

1   Quantitative and Qualitative Nutritional Disturbances

Hunger, usually with vitamin deficiency

In the past, protracted periods of hunger and years of famine were very common in nearly all countries. The reasons varied: crop failures, devastating wars and all-embracing epidemics with such high mortality that the fields could not be worked, nor could stock be cared for but had to be slaughtered. Only a few generations ago, shorter periods of starvation were not uncommon in western Europe, even in countries which are now regarded as highly developed. Even then crop failures were largely responsible, but additional causes were poorly organised distribution and inadequate supplies from more favoured countries. Among European countries which have suffered severely from food-shortages, one should especially mention Ireland, where famine came repeatedly between 1800 and 1826 and especially in 1845–46, when hundreds and thousands of Irish died of starvation after the failure of the potato crop. But as late as 1894–97, the shortage of foodstuffs was still appalling. Germany, Belgium, Bohemia and Russia suffered severely from famine in 1846–47; in some parts of Russia there was still famine at the end of the century. Hunger oedema was already known at that time, but the first modern experience of oedema in association with severe shortage of food comes from the internment camps which the English set up in the Boer War.

During and after both world wars, Germany and other Central European countries suffered from severely disrupted food supplies. The terrible malnutrition in Germany after the First World War was also witnessed by neutral doctors. The Swedish physiologist J. E. Johansson spoke of 'the slow but sure effect of the shortage of foodstuffs', and he continued: 'Those who saw how every year the shortage took its victims from lower and lower among the younger age-groups, naturally could not help seeing in the continuation of the blockade a measure aimed directly at the country's continued existence.' At the end of the Second World War, chronic malnutrition had caused 'an advanced physical deterioration of the people'.

The majority of the population 'lived on rations which contained only one-third of the internationally agreed minimum', which substantially reduced their spiritual and physical productivity. Large parts of Russia suffered similar extremely severe conditions of famine at the end of the First World War and after the revolution in 1921–22, when the worst consequences of famine—serious crime, murder and cannibalism—occurred (Rosenstein). The psychology and psychopathology of extreme hunger has been described by, among others, Dante, Byron and Hamsun.

A great deal could be said about lengthy periods of severe hunger in parts of Africa and Asia in ancient and more recent times; for instance how Negro tribes try to deaden the pangs of hunger by eating grass, mud and the like. In such conditions it is not uncommon for dysentery, typhus, malaria, etc., to appear. Among the few systematic investigations which hitherto have been made, that of Darby in Ethiopia should be mentioned. Supplies of food were generally below subsistence level, the inhabitants were very thin and body-weight was 80–70 per cent of the 'normal'. Hunger oedema and anaemia were found, especially in the malarial regions.

Apart from these severe states of hunger and their serious consequences, one should also mention here the common but much lesser nutritional disturbances which have occurred and which still do occur even in relatively highly organised countries, especially in isolated areas where there are transport difficulties and severe climatic conditions. North Sweden is an example, where even during the 1920s and 1930s, minor disturbances, with vitamin deficiencies, abnormal thinness, anaemia and achylia (lack of gastric juices) were observed (Odin; Westin; and others). Gerbasi in 1956 gave an account of deficiency diseases in Sicilian children.

One not infrequently gets horrific accounts of present-day conditions in the great overpopulated countries of southern Asia, describing the undernourishment and pronounced famine which all form part of the pattern of constantly recurring misery. This applies especially to India and China, but to other countries too, like Formosa, and, a quite recent example, Indonesia. Large parts of Africa also still suffer from shortages of the most essential foods and the population is to a great extent undernourished, in particular during lengthy spells of drought which in many places is an annually recurring evil. In Somaliland, Kenya, former French West Africa, parts of the Congo and Mozambique, hunger oedema is not at all a rarity. Da Costa has described the consequences of deficient diet among Negro workers. Higginson and others have told of heart affections among South Africa's urbanised Bantus as a result of chronic undernourishment. A peculiar disturbance, which is associated with undernourishment and faulty diet, is siderosis— severe deposits of iron—which has been observed among the Bantus in South Africa and is associated with a sclerosis in certain organs (Higginson; Brugel; Bothwell; and others). As it is also occasionally seen in well-nourished Negroes, an abnormally rich iron-content in the food is said to be an important factor. Periods of famine among the Indians in parts of South America are not rare either (de Castro), and in Brazil this is one of the most important socio-medical problems. In Mexico conditions are 'broadly speaking fairly satisfactory' (Dávalos Hurtado), but in 1955 Henriques Inclán and others reported numerous cases of different vitamin deficiencies.

Avitaminosis

A short survey of the forms of vitamin deficiency which occur in different countries and of the diseases which result from them should here be sufficient.

Avitaminosis A

Fincke in the late eighteenth century told of night-blindness in China. Night-blindness—xerophthalmia (withering and glazing of the conjunctiva of the eye) and keratomalacia (ulceration of the cornea)—is still mentioned in India. This avitaminosis A is said to have been described in ancient Egyptian papyri and has also been known for a very long time in India, China and Japan. The *Hippocratic Collection* also mentions this eye disturbance.

Huss wrote in 1852 that the complaint was found in the 1830s in troops manning the fortress of Karlsten in Marstrand, Sweden, but that by the middle of the last century it had almost disappeared. According to Dr Marin, medical officer to the pioneer corps, 'A considerable number of the men belonging to the corps more or less completely lost their ability to see when dusk began to fall.' This state is called night-blindness or dusk-blindness (hemerolopia). The strength of the corps was three hundred men and of these as many as sixty suffered daily from this disease—only those who were completely night-blind were included. As soon as dusk fell, they became more or less blind and the blindness continued during the night and disappeared after the day had fully dawned the next morning. 'It is not rare to see these sick men on summer evenings being led home or with difficulty fumbling to find their living quarters.' They walked like blind men. 'They fall and stumble over the slightest obstacles in their way and bump into walls.' And so on. 'Their eyes are glazed, dull and immobile, with the eyelids wide open.' At first the men were believed to be malingering. The disease was found only in the pioneer corps, not in the troops manning the fortress, and it gradually disappeared, with only two cases left in 1850. A similar disease occurred in July and August in the German fortress of Ehrenbreitstein, where no fewer than 138 soldiers were affected.

In Africa, night-blindness is said to be particularly common in the Congo, but also occurs in Tanganyika (now part of Tanzania), Malawi (Nyasaland) and Kenya. The formation of sores on the cornea can lead to blindness, and in Madras and Calcutta more than 8 per cent of the cases of blindness are said to be traceable to damage to the cornea. Block and Widmark demonstrated in 1919 that skimmed milk alone could lead to a withering of the cornea and that non-separated milk gave protection.

Avitaminosis B

Beriberi is one of the avitaminoses of which our knowledge goes a long way back. Hirsch, who naturally did not know its cause-complex, devotes no less than twenty-five pages to it. Its symptomatology varies and disturbances in the nervous system are especially prominent. The disease can probably be traced back to about 200 B.C. in China, where it is mentioned under the name of *Kak-ke*, and to the ninth century in Japan, where a dry form with paralysis was distinguished from a wet form with oedema. Pontius, who in the seventeenth century saw the disease in the East Indies, called it beriberi and Tulp, another Dutch doctor, observed it at about the same time on the east coast of India. In the western hemisphere it was observed considerably later. It was not uncommon on long sea voyages, in prisons and internment quarters, barracks, mining colonies, plantations and among railroad workers with an inferior and unbalanced diet. Beriberi has also sometimes been seen in French and German mental hospitals. There were numerous cases

of beriberi in Ireland during the famine years 1894–97. The disease
is now on the decline, since its causes have been learnt, especially
the danger of an unbalanced diet of polished rice, but in the 1940s
it was still very common in South East Asia. In 1939 in Burma
4,000 were hospital cases, of whom 250 died. At about the same time
there were 6,500 hospital cases in French Indo-China and 50,000
in India. Beriberi was then very common in southern China in the
towns, but less so in rural areas with a bigger variety of foodstuffs.
The inhabitants of the Philippines and other islands were also
severely affected.

The disease which is nowadays called pellagra was probably first
observed in 1735, by Casal in the Asturias in northern Spain. Somewhat later it was described in Lombardy, from where the name
pellagra (*pelle agra*, sour, coarse skin) comes. There followed a
swift succession of reports from other parts of northern Italy,
Portugal, Dalmatia, France, the Tyrol, the Balkans, Poland and
Bessarabia. In Russia pellagra appeared after the First World War;
Hamperl mentions an epidemic in Georgia in 1930 in which 30,000
fell ill and in one village 7·4 per cent of the inhabitants were affected.
It has been very common in Egypt and also in Central and South
Africa, in certain Negro tribes. In the Far East it is common in India
and China but not so in other parts. Cases are also known from
Central and South America. Remarkably enough, it was very widespread in the USA in the years 1905–20. During that time it was
estimated that there were 500,000 cases, mainly of a mild nature
but with numerous deaths, mostly in men. Pellagra was formerly
said to be due to an unbalanced diet of damaged maize, but the real
reason was a lack of nicotinic acid, one of the substances belonging
to the vitamin B complex. The symptoms are various; skin and
intestinal disturbances, loss of strength, nervous symptoms and
even psychoses. Nicotinic acid usually produces rapid improvement.

Avitaminosis C

Scurvy is a very ancient disease. According to Swanson, it existed
among the ancient Hebrews, but all the old accounts, even those of
Hippocrates, Celsus and Avicenna, are much too vague for certain
identification of genuine scurvy. The disease has always found
victims on board ship during lengthy sea-voyages and in war when
it was considered inevitable that diet should consist mainly of salted

meat with no, or very few, vegetables. It is thought that the Nordic peoples, especially the Vikings, knew how to prevent scurvy by eating cloudberries and the scurvy herbs, *Cochlearia officinalis*, a method which later fell into disuse. Presumably the disease raged among the Crusaders. In the ranks of Vasco da Gama's and other expeditions of exploration, there was usually a terrible number of deaths, and it is hard to imagine today the price paid by warships and merchant ships in the past, in the form of disease and death. The log-books of Drake, Hawkins and other sea heroes give some idea of the ravages of the disease. It was not unusual for half, even four-fifths of the crew to die during a single long voyage. Captain Cook, during his voyage round the world, was one of the first to equip his ship with the necessary materials to combat scurvy. The British naval surgeon James Lind had published in 1753 *A treatise on the scurvy*, in which he demonstrated experimentally that scurvy could be prevented and cured by the administration of fresh oranges, lemons and green vegetables. But as recently as the 1870s and 1880s it was one of the worst enemies, especially to Arctic expeditions. By contrast, Nansen's great expedition in the *Fram* should be mentioned, in which not a single case occurred.

On land too, the disease made terrible ravages in besieged fortresses and in prisons. In the *Chronicle of Erik*, there is an account of a disease which in 1299 or 1300 raged in the fortress of Landskrona, built by the Swedes at the mouth of the Neva. The walls of the castle were new and damp, the food rotted, flour heated and was spoilt, and the malt lay too tightly packed and burned. All this brought ruin to many; they sickened with severe scurvy (and probably other deficiency and toxic diseases). They sat at table, seemed quite healthy, ate and drank, and then their teeth fell out on to the table. Who could withstand this? So many died that the castle was virtually doomed. (From C. Cederschiöld, *On the 'Chronicle of Erik'*.)

In Russia scurvy broke out especially severely in Troitskaya Lavra, the famous fortified monastery in the vicinity of Moscow, which endured a long siege by Polish forces and rebellious Russians in 1608.

Scurvy took many victims in Ireland during the famine years of 1846–47, and several decades later it appeared periodically in Russia, Rumania and northern North America, as well as in some parts of Africa, Asia, especially India and northern China, and New Guinea, These were mainly the most severe forms of scurvy. If one takes into consideration the milder forms, perhaps ones which the victim himself does not notice, then the disease, even in countries with high social and economic standards like Sweden, was by no means as rare a few decades ago as many may imagine. The form of scurvy characteristic to children, called Møller-Barlow's disease, was also not infrequently seen fifty to sixty years ago, when the milk in children's hospitals was boiled for a long time for fear of tuberculosis and consequently the vitamin C content was destroyed.

The symptoms are, as the name implies, mainly bleeding and inflammation of the gums and loss of teeth, but further bleeding, oedema and damage to the teeth and bones were also symptoms in adults. Although it was known for centuries that inadequate supplies of fresh food from the plant and animal world were the main reasons for the disease, it was research into vitamins that first made it clear it was essentially due to a lack of vitamin C. The green vegetables which in Sweden are considered especially valuable include parsley; in the form of parsley-butter it was included in the daily issue of food ordered by Dr Sjöborg at Ronneby Well in about 1800.

Avitaminosis D

Rachitis (rickets), literally 'back disease' and in Swedish usually called 'English disease', is a children's disease, probably of very great age, at least in those parts of the world with little sunlight. By contrast, it seems to have been unusual in such countries as ancient Egypt and pre-Columbian Peru, as far as can be judged from the very few finds of child skeletons with rickets. The first certain written account of rickets dates from the middle of the eighteenth century when Whistler, and, a little later, Glisson recognised the characteristic skeletal changes in English children. The disease was very common in northern and central Europe, and in Stockholm typical skeletal and tooth disturbances were often seen, but our knowledge of cod-liver oil and other preparations and foods rich in vitamin D and the addition of vitamin D to vitamin-deficient foodstuffs have almost completely eradicated this avitaminosis. However Rominger and Roemer mention rickets in 1953 and 1954 in Kiel, and it appears sporadically in most northern countries.

Reports of the earliest incidence of the disease in southern countries are scanty and often contradictory. That sunlight plays a very important role is evident from the fact that rickets was formerly much more common in Egypt among children of the wealthier classes, who were protected from the sun, than in poor children, who were constantly out in the open. Over large areas of the tropics the disease simply does not exist. A study of over 5,000 children in Borneo made by Dutch doctors gave negative results. That the disease occasionally does occur in tropical countries is mentioned in a publication by Stransky and Dizon in 1956. It also occurs in Japan, according to Sano (1956). Broadly speaking, however, it is rare in Central Africa, Australia, Central and South America, but occasionally seen in North America.

Other nutritional disturbances

Kwashiorkor

During the past thirty years a great deal has been written about a chronic nutritional disturbance, mainly in fast-growing children, which bears the Ghanaian name kwashiorkor. The disease, which is considered to appear as a sequel to deficiency in several essential foodstuffs, especially proteins and which is associated with a number of clinical disturbances, has been mainly observed in tropical and sub-tropical countries of Africa and Asia. It has also been observed in Central and South America where it is called '*sindrome pluri-carencial infantil*' (multiple-deficiency syndrome in children). It has some bearing on the condition described as '*Mehlnährschaden*' in Central Europe after the First World War, which however, disappeared after 1925. It is considered to be due to extensive deficiency of first-class proteins, and the name kwashiorkor is gradually being supplanted by the term protein malnutrition.

It is, however, evident that the disease also occurs in southern Europe, in Greece, Sicily, Spain and southern France. On the other hand, there have hitherto been no known cases from the northern countries, Great Britain and Central Europe or from Canada, Australia and New Zealand. In Central and South Africa the disease is associated with a very high mortality, in the Congo almost 100 per cent and in Johannesburg and Pretoria 30–40 per cent.

'Hunger osteopathy'

As the name implies, this disease is mainly a matter of disturbances in the skeleton, especially an increasing brittleness of the bones. It is best dealt with in connection with diseases of the skeleton.

174

The same applies to the singular disturbances in the vault of the skull and the eye sockets which for a long time have gone under the name of cribra cranii et orbitalia, i.e. a colander-like change with the appearance of minute holes in the compact bones.

Oedema

The first definite observation of this nutritional disturbance is said to have come from St Helena, where the British had interned Boer prisoners in 1902 during the Boer War. In the latter part of the First World War and during the period just after the Armistice, oedema was very common among the populations of the Central Powers as well as in other countries which suffered severely from under-nourishment, Finland, for instance, in 1918, and Russia. Even in Sweden scattered cases were observed. The disease appears particularly in association with an inadequate supply of calories, protein and fat, together with a plentiful supply of water and a salt-rich diet, for example an unbalanced diet of swedes, which leads to the disappearance of fat and lipoids, other fatty substances of varying composition, severe dispersion of the albumin in the body and discharges from the body openings and subcuticle. Oedema is also seen with other nutritional disturbances such as the wet form of beriberi, scurvy and severe anaemia.

2 Poisoning and Occupational Diseases

Air pollution

With the increase of urbanisation and industrialisation, air pollution has become a rapidly growing problem, although in many areas and in certain cities and factories it has in fact existed for a long time. Smoke from the giant chimneys of industry and the coal stoves of the home, exhaust fumes from the internal combustion engine in traffic and in industrial concerns, and the increase of smoking in poorly ventilated premises are the most significant sources of aerial pollution. If wind or ventilation do not carry away the harmful substances in the air, an accumulation of those substances can become so concentrated that human beings and animals sicken and die.

This is not the place for an account of the many different substances involved in air pollution, for they are very varied, both chemically and physically. Nor is it possible to do more than touch on the old questions of concentrations of bacteria in tunnels, places of assembly and aircraft cabins.

The first great disaster of this kind is probably the one which occurred in the Meuse valley, near Liège, in December 1930. The gases from the iron, zinc and glass works and other chemical industries accumulated into a five-day poisonous fog which caused hundreds of cases of severe illness and cost sixty-three people their lives. Many animals had to be slaughtered as well. Under similar circumstances, in Denora, an industrial town of 14,000 inhabitants near industrial Pittsburg in the USA, one-tenth of the population was taken ill in November 1948 and nineteen people died.

Even worse is the London fog, often called smog, which in four days in December 1952 caused thousands of cases of illness and cost no fewer than 4,000 their lives, mainly elderly people with heart and lung affections. Such large numbers of Londoners had not died over a period of a few days since the cholera epidemic of 1866 and the worst ravages of Spanish 'flu in November 1918. The London fog of 1956 was not quite so severe, but nevertheless 1,000 people

176

died in Greater London from air pollution. London had its first taste of smog in the 1880s.

Other cities and regions with similar accumulations of gases are, for example, Los Angeles—but only in certain special weather conditions—and Poz Rico in Mexico, where sulphur dioxide in the air can accumulate in poisonous quantities. In many European countries such as Germany, Holland, Switzerland, Sweden and Finland, the problem has arisen in similar but less acute forms, and one must consider whether the inhabitants of large cities do not in fact gradually become poisoned by all the exhaust fumes, mostly from motor engines of different kinds.

According to Hentschel, the danger of an accumulation of poisonous fumes is greater when the air pressure is high, for, he says, the mass of air lies horizontally in layers and the interchange between the layers becomes reduced; at low pressure the air moves constantly and is thus renewed.

One should distinguish between this mass pollution from accumulation of poisonous fumes and the minor pollution of air that occurs in many industries and certain mines. In tunnels too accidents can happen as, for example, when a coal-fired locomotive stops unexpectedly; in an Italian tunnel in 1944 521 people were suffocated by coal-smoke from the locomotive. Pollution of inhaled air by minute floating particles of dust, silicon, asbestos and glass can in susceptible individuals produce chronic lung damage, so-called pneumonconiosis or lung-dust disease—this will be dealt with below.

Other forms of poisoning

Metal and metalloid poisoning

Only a few examples can be given here.

Lead poisoning was formerly a common occupational disease among typographers and painters. The lead in exhaust fumes is also considered capable of causing poisoning.

Mercury poisoning (quicksilver poisoning) was once not uncommon when mercury was the sovereign remedy for the treatment of syphilis. As the ointment was smeared on, considerable amounts of the fugitive metal were breathed in. Also the absorption of mercury preparations and injections of equivalent substances sometimes led to mercury poisoning. In the middle of the last

177

century metallic quicksilver treatment was still used in the treatment of ileus, intestinal obstruction, as it was believed that the heavy liquid metal would force a passage through the intestine at the intestinal kink, volvulus. Professor G. Retzius informed me that his father, Professor A. Retzius, was said to have died of this treatment, prescribed by one of Stockholm's most dependable doctors. A. Retzius's porter, who drank spirits laced with mercuric chloride, at that time used for preserving anatomical specimens, apparently came to his professor and complained of severe inflammation of the mucous membrane in his mouth and a loosening and loss of teeth—this was a typical stomatitis from mercury poisoning.

Recently a singular nerve disease, Minamata disease, with disturbances of intellect and disposition, and organic brain damage, has been described in Japan. It is said to be due to poisoning by an organic mercury compound which was allowed to run out into the sea from several factories and was absorbed by fish and other edible sea creatures. Food cooked in such sea-water is also said to give rise to these symptoms.

The very high silicon content in drinking water in certain parts of Japan is estimated to be of great significance in the incidence of brain damage and disturbances of the circulatory system. According to Akiya, the high silicon content in the arteries is one of the factors causing arteriosclerosis.

Fluoride poisoning is known in Iceland and elsewhere after volcanic eruptions, when farm animals can be poisoned. Similar conditions are known in the USA in cattle which graze on land with a high selenium content, from which the plants absorb the selenium in toxic quantities. The discoverer of selenium, Berzelius, was himself poisoned by it in his laboratory.

The threatened increase of radioactive substances in human and animal bodies and crops cannot be discussed here.

Plant poisons

Among bacterial and fungus poisons, botulism has already been dealt with in an earlier section. The most important in this group of diseases is ergotism, rye-spore poisoning, which was in all probability known to Roman authors like Pliny and Galen. The disease is caused by *Claviceps purpurea*, a fungus on the rye. There are definite reports of ergotism from the early Middle Ages; it is mentioned in chronicles under the name of *ignis sacer* or *ignis Sancti*

Antonii ('holy' or 'St Anthony's fire'), a strange epidemic disease with spasms, violent pains, gangrenous sores and occasionally terrible mortality. According to Hirsch, ergotism was particularly common in France where it was mentioned as early as 591 and later in the

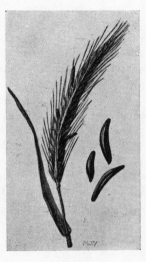

Ear of rye with several spore mycelia of Claviceps purpurea, *enlarged grains. To the right are three such grains, approximately life-size.*

tenth and eleventh centuries. It is estimated that during the seventeenth, eighteenth and nineteenth centuries France had about twenty severe epidemics. In Germany ergotism was known from the ninth century and occurred sporadically in the Middle Ages. During the last four centuries there have been an estimated sixty severe epidemics. There were also occasional epidemics in Holland, England and Italy. More recently similar outbreaks occurred in Russia, Switzerland, Sweden, Flanders and Spain, while Great Britain seems to have been relatively spared. It is not known how long the disease has been in Sweden but the first more detailed accounts date from the eighteenth century. Three famous doctors, Linnaeus and the brothers Rosenblad and Rosén von Rosenstein, took an interest in the disease, which in Sweden is known as 'spasm disease' on account of the characteristic spasms. It appears to have occurred particularly in the south, but Närke and Dalarna in the north were also affected. The last recorded epidemic took place in 1867–68 in Kronoborg county. In my own childhood in the 1880s

179

and 1890s one saw the spores in large quantities in every field of rye in Västmanland. In Finland in the 1840s and 1860s there were widespread epidemics and others took place in Norway. An epidemic occurred in Russia as late as 1926–27, with over 11,000 victims.

Among poisons from higher plants the only ones I will mention here are *Agrostemma githago*, which is remarkable for its high saponin content and causes gitagism, and *Colocasia antiquorum*, which grows in the tropics. Dried flowering heads of *Cannabis sativa*, hemp, contain a poison which can cause cannabism—generally known as hashish or marijuana. The leaves of the coca plant cause cocainism which mainly occurs in South America.

Poisoning by pricks, stings or bites, so common in tropical countries, can only be briefly mentioned here. Poisonous insects play an important part, likewise fish and especially snakes. The victims of poisonous snakes in the tropics are estimated at about 10,000 a year. Fonseca estimates the number of those bitten by snakes in Central and South America in 1949 at 35,000. An ancient Egyptian myth tells how Horus, son of Osiris and Isis, once fell ill

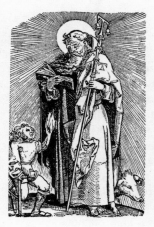

St Antony, patron saint of ergotism, which often occurred in the Middle Ages and was sometimes called 'St Antony's fire'. The victim, one of whose legs shows a contraction or spasm, is stretching out his burning hand towards the saint. The original is a woodcut in Gersdorf's Feldtbuch der Wundarzney *(1540).*

after being stung by a scorpion. The scorpion has, of course, given its name to one of the signs of the Zodiac.

Finally, there are artificially produced poisons, of which huge quantities are now produced. They have practically no historico-geographical significance in this context.

Occupational diseases

Diseases which are peculiar to certain occupations form a special group of their own. Among them is a disease among lacquerers in Japan, known since the seventh century; formerly at least, 'lacquerer disease' or *shisso* was a very common chronic skin inflammation. Other such skin affections are known in European industries —in the analine and raw paraffin industry, among cotton spinners, in London chimney sweeps from coal soot, and also caused by splashes of lubricating oil. Examples could be multiplied, but some of these skin affections will be dealt with later in connection with cancer and pre-cancerous diseases.

Pneumoconioses, lung-dust diseases, one of the most significant groups of occupational diseases, will be dealt with later under lung diseases. Sigerist maintains, probably rightly, that Egyptian stone-cutters, who were slaves, suffered from similar lung conditions. Occupational diseases were described in the Middle Ages, for instance by Ulrich Ellenbog, who in 1473 wrote of some, particularly in goldsmiths. Paracelsus and Agricola gave an account of miners' lung disease in *De re metallica*. Similar diseases were described in the seventeenth century by Martin Pansa and others.

Linnaeus in 1741 drew attention to so-called Orsa disease in his remarkable inaugural lecture at his installation as Professor of Medicine at Uppsala University, and put the question: 'Why do all men in Orsa die of phthisis before they are thirty?' (He was referring to pneumoconiosis and its association with lung tuberculosis.) A horrible account of this silicosis, characteristic of Orsa where it was called 'chest-sickness', 'grindstone disease' or 'Orsa disease', is given by Magnus Huss, based on accounts from a pastor, Sernander. With grim realism it presents a picture of health and social conditions in Orsa at the beginning of the nineteenth century. Boys quite often began to work in the grindstone mines as young as 12–15, though some began later. The former were affected much more quickly. By the time they were 18–25 they were so ill that they had to stop working and most died before they were 35. The latter might reach the age of 45–50, even 55. The work was as follows: from 1 October to the middle of November the workers stayed in the mines where they lived almost entirely on salted and dried food—fish and hard bread. They consumed 'corn-brandy with industry, many to excess', and as drinking water they had only what water was to be found in the mine, of which they drank a great deal, partly because they needed to cool themselves for they sweated a great deal in the course of the heavy work, and partly because the dry and salty food demanded it. The water tasted good but when it stood in a glass a deposit of salt would cover the glass. When work in the mine was completed and the blocks had been brought out, then the so-called 'chopping' began, at which they continued from the beginning of December to the end of March. This chopping took place in *small* (Huss's italics) 'chopping huts', especially built for the purpose, in which eight to ten men sat together. Because of the cold these huts were kept closed up and the air became very dusty. 'The fine dust hangs in these huts like smoke.' Later on dust was kept down by using water while work progressed. The most industrious workers began as early as three or four in the morning and worked until ten or eleven at night. When they rested during the day, they did so in the same dusty hut and usually lay down among the stone chippings on the floor. From April until the end of September the stone-cutters became farm workers like others who lived in Orsa.

Chest troubles began as early as one, two or three years later. Breathing became short and panting, the voice rough and hoarse, the appearance changed, the face became sallow and haggard as the man grew thinner. Breathing became more difficult and the victim could not lie in bed but had to sit up. Soon his feet and legs began to swell, then liquid accumulated in the lung sac and the lungs and he suffocated to death. Those who could no longer manage the work in the mine, continued to work as long as possible in the 'chopping huts'. Huss adds, quite rightly, that the disease was of such interest that it deserved investigation by a knowledgeable person. 'Even then an investigation would be required on the part of the State,' he adds. And one must agree with him on that!

Pneumoconiosis, especially silicosis, is now much rarer in Sweden than it was even thirty years ago. As medical officer in charge of autopsies at St Erik's hospital at that time, I saw—and it was even more frequent five years before that—many distressing cases among Stockholm's old makers of tiled stoves and Rörstrand's porcelain workers, usually combined with lung tuberculosis. But since tiled stoves have to a large extent been superseded and more effective protective measures introduced, these occupational diseases have practically disappeared.

Finally it is worth mentioning that the extremely fine dust in desert sandstorms can cause considerable pneumoconiosis in the nomads who live there permanently.

3   Endocrine and Metabolic Diseases

Diseases of the thyroid gland

Goitre and cretinism

By goitre is meant an enlargement of the thyroid gland. This can be of many different kinds: diffuse or nodular, hormonally active or inactive, malignant or non-malignant. Congenital and acquired lack of thyroid gland secretion give rise to cretinism and myxoedema respectively. Simple goitre will be discussed here first, together with its connection with the incidence of cretinism.

Simple goitre and cretinism

Enlargement of the thyroid gland and cretinism are diseases which aroused comment probably much earlier than most. Hettche traces the history of goitre back to the time when man went over from hunting to keeping stock. Dwarfs play a considerable part in the art and religion of ancient Egypt, and some of them would have been cretins. In India goitre is said to have been known for at least 4,000 years. Roman writers such as Pliny, Vitruvius, Juvenal and Ulpian mention its occurrence in the Alps where it has constantly been prevalent. Marco Polo saw people with goitres on the high plateaux of Asia. In the fifteenth century, French and Italian authors mention that the disease was to be found in the Foix area and in the province of Lucca. Paracelsus devoted much space to goitres and cretinism he saw in the region round Salzburg. Sixteenth- and seventeenth-century accounts of both conditions are found from the Alps, the Pyrenees, the Atlas Mountains of North Africa, the mountain regions of Peru and Guatemala, and Sumatra.

The history of research into goitre is full of hastily drawn conclusions and downright mistakes, but discriminating voices were heard early on. In a conversation in Göttingen between the famous Swedish traveller Biörnståhl and the celebrated Swiss physiologist A. von Haller (d. 1777), the latter admitted '*offenherzig, dass er nichts wisse, welches die wahre Ursache der Kröpfe und Cretinen sey*'

183

(frankly, that he did not know what was the true reason for goitres and cretins). Probably no cause of a disease has attracted so much discussion as that of endemic goitre (Galli-Valerio). The old water theory seems now to have the soundest basis but it is not altogether

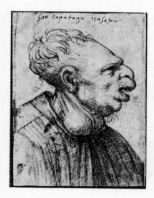

Goitre in a grotesque figure drawn by Leonardo da Vinci. The strange shape of the head is said to occur in goitrous cretins in the Alps.

satisfactory and there is no agreement on the nature of the harmful factor. The iodine theory has shown itself to be inadequate, and it is worth mentioning that the ancient Chinese doctors knew that sea creatures contained a substance which gave protection against goitre. According to Galli-Valerio and others, there is obviously a substance which causes goitre and is still not known, and another which counteracts goitre, namely iodine.

During the years of hunger in Germany after the Second World War one could see conditions caused by deficient functioning of the thyroid gland. The transient rise in the frequency of goitre which was observed there has been associated, by several German doctors, with the steep drop in supplies of vitamin A. This vitamin deficiency has also been given by Eggenberger as a factor in the incidence of goitre.

Goitre and cretinism are two diseases with a marked geographical distribution and it is therefore natural that one has great hopes of solving the problem of goitre through geo-pathological research. Today we are quite knowledgeable as regards the distribution of the disease, its geology and hydrology, its water and general hygiene, the conditions of nutrition, the division of goitre into age and sex, its incidence in animals, etc., but nevertheless many questions still remain to be answered.

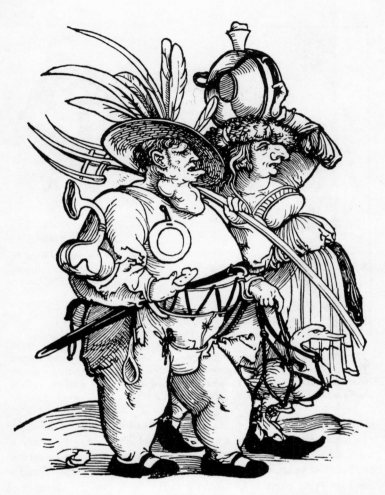

Grotesque caricature of a German married couple. Woodcut by Hans Weidlitz, about 1521. The man has a large nodular goitre.

The geography of goitre and cretinism in modern times. In the four Scandinavian countries, Finland's most eastern regions show a moderate incidence of goitre; the areas north of Ladoga (now lost to the USSR), with their poverty and low social standards, are particularly affected. In Norway the best-known goitre centre lies

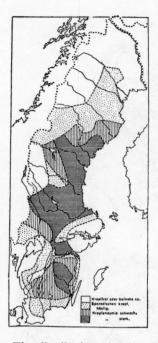

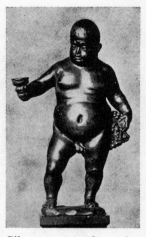

Silenus portrayed as a boy with myxoedema. Renaissance statuette, Louvre, Paris.

The distribution of goitre in Sweden at the end of the 1920s, after J. A. Höjer (1931). The white areas, free or almost free; dotted areas, sporadic goitres common; vertically hatched areas, mild endemic goitre; horizontally hatched areas, severe endemic goitre.

in the region of Drammen, south-west of Oslo. There the incidence of goitre, which is often seen in school-children, was formerly as high as 30–60 per cent, but, through prophylaxis with iodine carried out over five years, this has decreased to 3·5–13·3 per cent. In Sweden the high-lying parts of Götaland and Småland, and the counties of Kopparberg and Gävleborg are quite severely affected by goitre. In Dalarna goitre was called 'throat-tumour', 'throat-lump' or 'Falu-lump', as it was very common in the Falun district. Huss says that in Falun, Sundborn and Aspeboda one in thirty of young women has, or has had, goitre. According to Höjer's investigations at the end of the 1920s, which involved 11,800 people, goitre (including the very mildest grades) was to be found in up to 50 per cent of the age-group between ten and thirty. In the goitre area 5–10 per cent of the male and 20–30 per cent of the female population had severe goitres and the number of cretins was one per thousand. Denmark has very little goitre.

Great Britain has not much goitre, apart from a few groups of cases on the plains of the south-west and in the valleys of Derbyshire. Conditions in Holland are of particular interest as goitre there is said to be gradually becoming more common, on the basis of accounts from 1918–52. Recently, in the region of Utrecht and in Gelderland, 45–50 per cent of school-children had enlarged thyroid glands, despite improved supplies of water and foodstuffs and iodine prophylaxis. Hettche's investigations of 1952 have shown that one cannot consider the iodine content of drinking water to have any decisive importance, as many goitre-free areas had very little iodine, whereas many goitre areas had plentiful supplies. According to Hettche, goitre occurs only in areas of intensive stock-rearing—this should be a subject for further investigations. Goitre is not uncommon in the higher areas of Belgium.

In France the goitre areas are mainly located in the Massif Central, Savoie and the Vosges. In Robertsau, near Strasbourg, in 1927 22·2 per cent of the school-children had goitre. There on the Ill plain the subsoil water lies only 2·5 metres down, 66 per cent of the school-children drank well water and 90 per cent had intestinal worms, all of which points to poor hygiene. Goitre centres in Spain are mainly found in the Pyrenees and the Asturias, where many cretins are also seen. Galicia is less affected. Marañon gives an account of a remote goitre region, Las Jurdes, with 8,000 inhabitants, of whom 25 per cent were severely goitrous, dwarfs or idiots. In Italy certain parts of the Alps have been known since the time of Pliny as goitre regions; Piedmont, Aosta and Savoy have been known for centuries as goitre areas (Kreissler, 1780). There is also a great deal of goitre round Genoa and in Sicily.

In Switzerland goitre is very extensively found, despite prophylactic iodine treatment, especially in the northern and central regions, whereas it is quite rare in the north-west, in the Juras, where cretinism is unknown. In the canton of Berne (according to Walthard) the number of cases has decreased and congenital goitre in particular has become rarer. In Austria there are large areas severely affected by goitre, and the disease has the character of a folk-disease. Zondek says that in 1945 40–50 per cent of school-children in the Tyrol and southern Bavaria had goitre and that in certain parts of Steiermark he found a cretin to every hundred inhabitants!

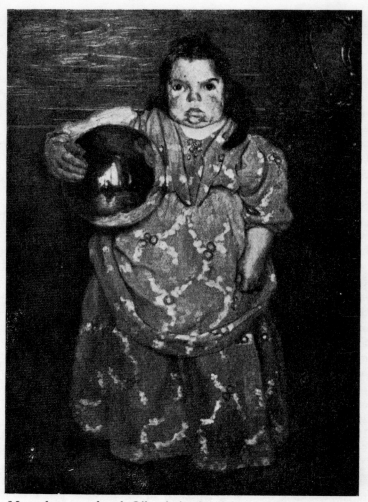

Myxoedematous dwarf. Oil painting by Zuloaga, Musée du Luxembourg, Paris.

In Germany, in 1927 extensive studies were made of the incidence of goitre. In the Memel area 5–10 per cent of school-children were goitrous, in the Danzig area 15–19 per cent, in the region round the Oder up to 25 per cent. In Berlin Goebe, among 27,000 hospital patients, found enlarged thyroid glands in 18·6 per cent, of whom

188

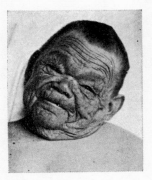

Typical cretin. 69-year-old man from Switzerland.

six-sevenths were women. In certain mountainous areas, such as the Sudeten, up to 25 per cent of the population had goitre, but in Alb, near Sigmaringen, only 6·6 per cent. In some parts of the Taunus area, Gersbach found enlarged thyroid glands in up to 90 per cent of school-children. Cretinism occurred almost exclusively in the areas most affected by goitre, regardless of whether they were in low-lying or mountainous parts of the country. It is perhaps worth mentioning that the great variation in figures to some extent may be due to the different techniques used and to a certain amount of subjectivity in the diagnosis of goitre. The Baltic states seem to be relatively free of goitre, and in Poland and Hungary conditions vary greatly. In northern Hungary there are areas with 60 per cent of the population goitrous. In Rumania there is said to be a great deal of goitre and cretinism in rural districts.

In Asia, goitre areas have been known for hundreds, even thousands of years in places such as Galilee, the Lebanon, Oman, the Caucasus and Altai, the region round Teheran in Persia. In the valley of Amur-Radja in north-east Afghanistan 50–60 per cent of the population are goitrous. In India, there are goitre areas both in mountain regions, such as Bengal, and in the flatter parts, as round Madras and Bombay. The Himalayas were known of old as a goitre district. Tibet and Siberia have a great deal of goitre and even low-lying northern Siberia is affected. In central Ceylon goitre is not uncommon and Burma also is quite severely affected. In China, goitre is often found in the Yunnan and Kveishov. North Borneo is one of the largest centres of goitre in the world. In Dutch New Guinea, cretins with congenital defects of the central nervous system have been described.

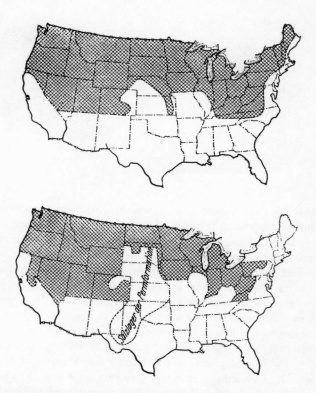

The distribution of goitre and the iodine content of water in the USA about 1920 (after McClendon and Hataway). The upper diagram shows goitre frequency, white 0–5 thousand, hatched 5–11·1 per thousand. The lower shows iodine content of drinking water, white 0·23–184·7 iodine, hatched only 0·01–0·2 iodine per litre of water.

Not much is known about conditions in Africa. In some Egyptian oases practically all the inhabitants are affected by goitre and 10 per cent are cretins. In Algeria and Morocco there are goitre centres in the mountain areas; also in Ethiopia, Liberia and Madagascar. In former Equatorial Africa a great deal of goitre is seen in many river valleys. In the Congo the region north of Stanleyville is goitrous. Many interesting details must be passed by here. In Zambia, along the border of Angola and the Congo a large proportion of the inhabitants are said to have goitre, and in the Union of South

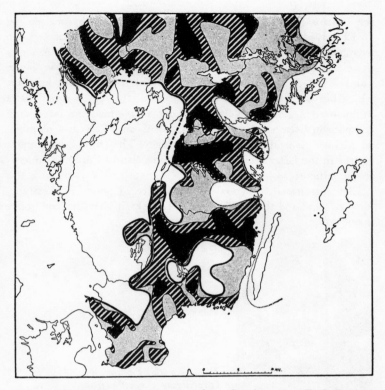

Distribution of thyrotoxicosis in southern Sweden, after T. Sällstrom (1935). The black areas show a frequency of more than 1·5 per thousand, the hatched areas a frequency of 1·5 per thousand, in the light grey areas only scattered cases. The black line marks the border of the true distribution of the disease.

Africa goitre epidemics appear to occur both in high- and low-lying regions.

In North America goitre occurs in the Hudson Bay area. Comprehensive investigations into conditions in the USA are available. Two maps (on p. 190), which were compiled by McClendon and Hataway and are often reproduced, show the distribution of goitre and iodine content of the water in about 1920. The evident similarity between the two maps cannot fail to emphasise the importance of the iodine content of drinking water. In Central America there are many goitre areas which have not been investigated, such as Guatemala where the Indians in the mountains often have enlarged thyroid glands. In El Salvador no fewer than 119,000 school-children of 673,000 examined—i.e. more than one-sixth—had goitre. In South America there are also many known areas with goitre which are as yet uninvestigated, for example one in southern Brazil and another, which has been described by Mazzocco, in the region round Salta in northern Argentina. Welsh and Correa have made an interesting comparison between New Orleans, USA, and Cali in Colombia, an area with considerable iodine deficiency. They found many more goitres in the latter area, where the goitre also had different microscopic structure.

Clements has investigated the incidence of goitre in Australia, New Zealand and the Pacific Islands (1954). In New Zealand goitre is not rare.

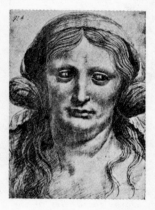

Woman with exophthalmos (protruding eyes) from thyrotoxicosis, mild goitre. Drawing by Leonardo da Vinci, Louvre, Paris.

Thyrotoxicosis is usually known as Basedow's disease in Sweden and Graves' disease in the English-speaking countries.

Its most conspicuous signs are protruding eyes (exophthalmos), but a number of other important symptoms in the nervous system and metabolism are of equal significance. It is said to have been first described by St Yves in 1772 in a work on eye diseases. Nine cases of thyrotoxicosis were described in 1796 in a posthumously published edition of the work of C. Parry, and Graves reported three cases in 1834–35. Basedow's work did not appear until 1840.

Unfortunately there have as yet been few investigations into the geography of thyrotoxicosis, its occurrence and frequency, and into the interesting question as to how far the distribution areas of

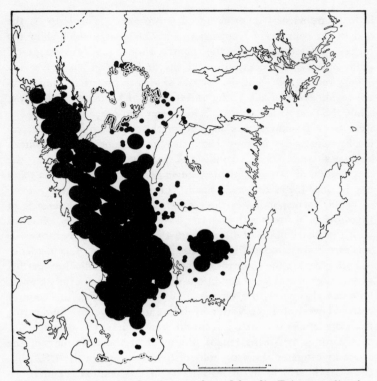

Distribution of bog heather (or crossleaved heath), Erica tetralix, *in south Sweden. This map is drawn on the basis of an extremely thorough inventory of the habitats of this plant in Sweden. A similar inventory has been made of* Ledum palustre *('Labrador tea'). Both plants only grow to a very limited extent in the same area. A comparison between this and the map on p. 191 shows a remarkable correspondence between the distribution of bog heather and those parts of the country which are free of thyrotoxicosis. The islands of bog heather in Småland should be particularly noted as they practically correspond to a limited area where thyrotoxicosis is virtually non-existent. (After T. Sällstrom, 1935.)*

thyrotoxicosis and goitre correspond. Holst found latent thyro-toxicosis in goitre-free areas on the Norwegian coast. The first person to study these questions in more detail was probably T. Sällström, who in 1935 investigated conditions in Sweden. He could show that areas with a high frequency of thyrotoxicosis often coincide with high goitre frequency, but that occasionally one finds relatively little thyrotoxicosis in pronounced goitre areas. The latter is the case in the counties of Kopparberg and Gävleborg, which show the highest goitre frequency in the country. From a purely geographical point of view, the distribution of thyrotoxicosis in south Sweden is very remarkable. The disease was shown to be strictly limited to the region east of Lake Vätter and to parts of Värmland and Skåne, while the land to the west of Lake Vätter and other parts of Skåne were free. To find an explanation for this interesting geographical localisation, Sällstrom investigated, in vain, a number of geographical, geological and climatic conditions. Finally he showed that the distribution of two wild plants, *Ledum palustre* ('Labrador tea') and bog heather (or cross-leaved heath), *Erica tetralix*, accurately, even in detail, corresponded to the respective incidence and absence of thyrotoxicosis. Areas with high frequency of thyrotoxicosis coincided with the distribution of *Ledum*, and the areas where thyrotoxicosis was rare corresponded with the distribution of *Erica*. The incidence of both plants in the countryside should in all probability be regarded as a pointer to ecological conditions which are as yet not fully known. One can also point to a further dissimilarity between the country east and west of Lake Vätter in different blood-groups, indicating two populations originating from different sources (Flodström).

According to Means (1948), Plummer at the beginning of the 1920s investigated the geography of thyrotoxicosis in the USA, but the work is said to be of no interest in this context. Pendergrast has recently investigated the relationship between thyrotoxicosis and goitre in the US.

Means associates the problem of the geography of thyrotoxicosis, probably rightly, with hereditary and psychological circumstances. The occupation of Denmark and Norway by German troops during the Second World War is said to have led to an increase in the number of cases of thyrotoxicosis. The significance of psychical trauma is suggested by both American and German authors. Gudent, in an investigation of 1950, has emphasised the high frequency of the disease in the Mark of Brandenburg in East Germany, where nearly every other girl and every tenth youth then had thyrotoxicosis. There were hardly any normal thyroid glands there at all (Hettche). Perhaps the difficulties of the postwar period are reflected here, not least from a psychological point of view. Decourt's investigation of the circumstances surrounding the incidence of this disease in France is also of great interest.

On the other hand, it must equally not be forgotten that during the hungry years in Germany during and after the Second World War, several metabolic diseases, among them thyrotoxicosis, declined. The incidence of thyrotoxicosis in distant countries is more or less unknown. Buer has described cases in Korea.

Diabetes mellitus, sugar diabetes

Diseases which have been interpreted by modern authors as diabetes mellitus have been known for a very long time. According to Barach, the history of the disease goes back to the Ebers papyrus, in which enormous quantities of urine are mentioned. In the *Hippocratic Collection* there is no account of any disease which could have been diabetes mellitus, but Celsus mentions cases of a very strong flow of urine. The term diabetes seems to originate from Aretaeus and really means abundant flow of urine, but indicates nothing whatsoever about sugar in the urine. Galen speaks of 'diabetes or violent thirst'. '. . . diabetes', he says, 'is a genuine kidney disease' with unquenchable thirst. In my opinion it is uncertain whether these authors really had diabetes mellitus in mind, mainly because although thirst is certainly an important symptom, it is not always so striking and in many cases is so little in evidence that it does not generally arouse special notice. Also none of these writers says a word about sugar in the urine and, in addition, Galen, although his books repeatedly mention 'diabetes' and violent thirst, in fact saw only two cases of the disease in the whole of his undoubtedly very large practice. The sweet taste in the urine, blood plasma and sweat, which is so characteristic of diabetes mellitus, seems to have been observed very much later in the West, probably first, as Hirsch maintains, by Willis in 1673. Barely a century later, in 1776, Dobson demonstrated that the patient's urine contained a sugar-like substance which he had determined by fermentation experiments.

On the other hand, Chinese, Japanese and Indian doctors knew that a diabetic's urine was sweet, before the first century A.D. Chang-Ke (A.D. 229) mentions that the urine was so sweet that dogs liked it. Furunculosis (boils), which occurs with diabetes, was also known at that time. Hindu medical works mention diabetes under the name *madhumea*, honey urine, with symptoms of thirst and a sweet taste in the urine like a sugar drink; diabetes is called a disease of the rich. The Indians are said to have found out about the disease when flies and ants made for the sweet urine.

From the above it seems correct to doubt that the 'diabetes' mentioned by Galen and other Western doctors was in fact diabetes mellitus and not, as in Galen's two cases, the rare diabetes insipidus, with the unquenchable thirst and abnormal flow of urine which are its two predominating symptoms.

In the more recent history of diabetes mellitus, one should mention here Claude Bernard's discovery of its connection with the gall bladder, Minkowsky's work, the discovery of insulin by Banting, Best and McCleod and finally the sulphonylureas which in many cases are active oral preparations.

Finally, it is of great historical interest and of considerable importance for the understanding of the disease that the number of cases decreased greatly in Germany and elsewhere during the last war and the years of crisis connected with it.

In the case of a disease like diabetes mellitus, where the number of patients in the whole of the world is estimated at 20 million and in the USA alone at 3 million, and in which heredity and way of life evidently play a large part, it is not easy to show any special geographical distribution. One should preferably talk of a *social* distribution which is characteristic of the disease. As far as the complicated and yet unexplained hereditary aspect is concerned, Lamy and others put forward interesting hypotheses in 1959. Other studies have been made by Steinberg, by Barta and by Johnson (1959–61), but the results appear uncertain and contradictory. Steinberg considers that predisposition to diabetes can probably be hereditary but of a recessive character. Barta finds no definite evidence of a hereditary course. An investigation made by Seftel and Schultz into urbanised Africans in Johannesburg shows that diabetes is more common in women than in men and that the disease often begins in obese individuals after the age of 40. What particularly favours the occurrence of the disease is an increase in the standard of living and urbanisation.

According to Danish research, the O-blood group is said to be greatly in evidence.

In the USA the frequency of the disease was formerly estimated at 0·5 per cent of the population, but this figure is considered by many to be much too low. A recent study of the incidence of diabetes among US employees (Pel and D'Alonso, 1960) shows 4·8 per

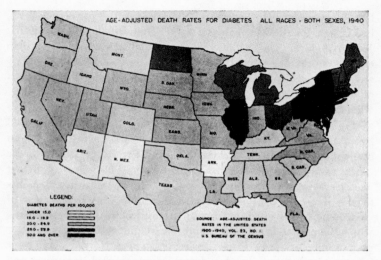

Diabetes mellitus deaths in the USA in 1940, of all ages and both sexes. The key gives the relative number of deaths per 100,000.

thousand in men and 2·7 per thousand in women. Lamy gives the frequency in France as 1 per cent, a figure, however, which the geneticist Hanhardt considers at least five times too high.

A study in 1958–60 at Blekinge, Sweden, of the incidence of diabetes mellitus in the population aged over 10 has attracted wide attention abroad. The frequency it gives for Blekinge is 1·5 per cent, which would mean that there should be about 100,000 diabetics for the whole of Sweden. At all events, the report is of great interest.

It is an old theory that certain races, or perhaps one should say certain specialised populations, have a higher incidence of diabetes than others, but one must not therefore exclude the possibility that it is not so much the population's hereditary tendencies but more their way of life and occupation which are the essential factor in the manifestation of the disease. For example, in the opinion of many, Jews have a special predisposition to diabetes. According to Strauss, in Frankfurt-am-Main before the last war the disease was six times more common among Jews than among non-Jews. In Budapest it was estimated that in the early 1930s, deaths from diabetes mellitus among Catholics were 5·9 per 100,000 but among Jews no less than 21·4 per 100,000. In New York diabetes is said to be three times as common in Jews as in non-Jews. According to some authors, hereditary tendency to diabetes is between 44 and 48 per cent in Jews, but in non-Jews between 10 and 25 per cent. Similarly it is said that Jewish children and adolescents have diabetes more often than others. On the other hand there are diabetes researchers who deny any special predisposition in Jews. Among the poor Jewish inhabitants of what was formerly Galilee, diabetes is said to have been rare, whereas rich Jewish merchants and stock-exchange speculators are said to have a great deal of diabetes. The disease is found in harassed business men and politicians who perhaps end their day with an opulent meal. 'When shares fall on Wall Street, the sugar in the blood rises,' Dr Emil Kleen says pointedly. The information that diabetes is apparently relatively frequent among train-drivers points to the importance of psychical momentum. The significance of environment and nutrition is also prominent in the investigations which Cohen published in 1960 into the frequency of diabetes among poor immigrant Jews from the Yemen and Kurdistan, and their fellows who had long lived in Israel. Newly arrived Yemenites and Kurds very rarely had diabetes, while as much as 2·8–2·9 per cent was found in those who had lived in Israel for a long time.

The frequency of diabetes in other countries has already been touched upon briefly. From the USA there is an investigation of 1940 in which it is shown that mortality in diabetes is especially high in many of the north-eastern states, but especially low in some states in the south and west. This points to the important role played by environment. In many countries the disease seems to be more common among townspeople than country people. In Germany before the war it was said that Württemberg and Thüringen had proportionately more diabetics than the rest of Germany, but experienced specialists doubt this. Investigations in Leipzig, published in 1960, show a frequency of 5·14 per thousand in men and 7·09 in women. In the British Isles the disease is evidently most common in England, less common in Scotland and rarer still in poorer Ireland. In France, especially in Paris, diabetes seems to be very common, as it is also in Italy and Istanbul. Interesting figures from the early 1930s come from Egypt where the disease is very common among the less numerous upper and middle classes, but rare among the poor and practically unknown among the Berbers who live a nomadic life and have little food. The frequency is said to be especially high, both in men and in women, in rich, well-known Coptic families with numerous intermarriages and a static way of life. Similar reports come from India where diabetes is said to be especially common in wealthy Hindu families, while Muslims seldom have the disease and the ancient Buddhist Jain sect, whose adherents live on milk, butter and vegetables, is said to be free.

The incidence of diabetes in certain tropical countries has aroused new interest in recent years. De Zoysa found in 1951 that diabetes was common in Ceylon but mostly in a mild form, rarely with coma. A similar type was found by Hugh-Jones in 1955 in Jamaica. Consett investigated conditions in Natal and established that the disease was common among Indians living there but rare in Europeans and Bantu Africans. The Indians' diabetes was said to be the same mild type as in Ceylon and Jamaica, and as such divergent from the European and North American type. As a reason for the high frequency of diabetes in the Indians of South Africa, Consett largely gives environmental factors, chiefly the enormous consumption of certain plants as food. These plants are not eaten by the negroes. It would therefore be interesting to make an investigation in Trinidad where the two races, Indians and negroes, also live in the same external conditions.

There are then many important problems concerning diabetes mellitus which still await solution. This is partly connected with the fact that diabetes is still a collective name for a number of different metabolic disturbances, alimentary glycosuria (sugar excretion in the urine following the consumption of very large quantities of sugar), the non-malignant so-called senile diabetes, the typical diabetes in middle-aged individuals, and a severe juvenile form. As long as these forms of glycosuria are classed together, it is difficult to get exact answers to all questions.

Diabetes insipidus

As I said above, it is very possible that Galen knew of cases of this rare disease, in which constant thirst and enormous quantities of urine are such predominating symptoms that they cannot be overlooked. The disease was distinguished from the usual diabetes mellitus by Willis in the seventeenth century. Its hereditary character was discovered by Lacombe in 1841. With such an obviously hereditary disease as diabetes insipidus, research into geographical conditions is only possible in a relatively stable population with

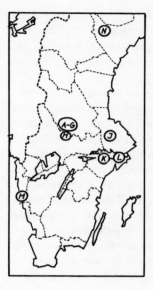

Diabetes insipidus in Sweden 1945–54, after H. Forssman. In the families examined, A–H show sex-linked heredity and good results with pituitrin treatment. The J family shows sex-linked heredity but no effect from pituitrin and the same is said to be the case with the uncertain family N. The families K, L, and M show autosomal dominant heredity and good results from pituitrin treatment.

good records, going far back in time. The disease occurs in two forms, the nephrogenic form due to a kidney anomaly and which is not affected by pituitrin, a substance from the posterior hypophyseal lobe, and a form sensitive to pituitrin in which damage can be localised to the hypothalamus.

In Sweden, H. Forssman had done research into both these forms and their incidence, heredity, symptoms and treatment. There are in Sweden at least seven large families with diabetes insipidus, but their origins are different and they have no evident blood ties. In three families in central Sweden and on the west coast it is a case of autosomal dominant genes and treatment with pituitrin has been successful. In two families in Dalarna it is a case of sex-linked genes, and here too treatment produced good results. Finally there are two families with sex-linked heredity, but with these the pituitrin treatment is ineffective. A form which is sex-linked and reacts to pituitrin has recently been described in Japan.

Other hormone disturbances

Protracted undernourishment, probably in association with continuing avitaminosis, causes hormone disturbances, especially of a

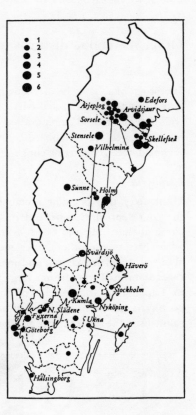

Distribution of porphyria in Sweden after J. Waldenström (1937). The size of the dots indicates the number of cases found at the time. The lines show family relationships.

hypophysial genital nature. During the Second World War in Germany there were a noticeable number of cases of adiposity in young girls, whose menstruation had ceased at the same time. Students of the pathology of African negroes, like Davies (1952) and Carothers (1953), have discussed the influence of chronic undernourishment in the sexual sphere. Davies mentions how extremely common gynecomastia (woman's breast) is in grossly undernourished men, and considers that a general lack of sexual balance with a tendency to homosexuality is evident there. Margaret Mead found somewhat similar conditions in the Far East, where Malayans and others not infrequently exhibited feminine types, though without association with homosexuality.

Other metabolic disturbances

Amyloidosis

Investigations have been made in Israel into a newly described hereditary disease, familial Mediterranean fever, and the frequently consequent amyloid degeneration of the kidneys. Out of 262 patients in Israel, 250 were Sephardic Jews but only 6 Ashkenazic. There is considered to be here a congenital metabolic disturbance.

Porphyria

Until 1937 this peculiar metabolic disturbance was very rare on the continent of Europe and in South Africa, whereas in Sweden alone at that time 150 cases were known. Today, thanks to Engel, Waldenström and others, over 200 cases are registered; in Denmark about 30 cases are known and in Norway about 10. Of the Swedish cases about half stem from a large family called Laestadius who came to Lapland in the middle of the seventeenth century. Cases of porphyria have also occurred in two Lapp families who grazed their reindeer in the same region, so a family relationship can be suspected.

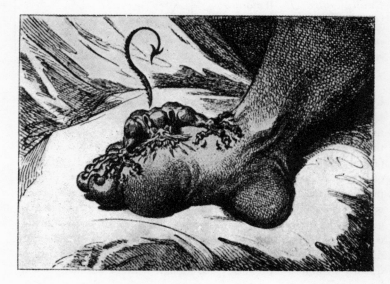

Attack of gout. Cartoon by J. Gillray, 1799.

Other families, with no provable family relationships to the above, live on the coast of Norrland, in central Sweden and on the west coast.

Gout, diathesis urica, chiragra, podagra

Real gout, which is sometimes associated with arteriosclerosis, diabetes and adiposity, is a metabolic disease characterised by a disturbance in the uric acid metabolism, a pathological increase in the uric acid in the blood, attacks of acute pain in the joints and deposits mainly of urates in the joint cartilage and in certain other places. With pains in the wrists, gout is often called chiragra and, with symptoms in the basal joint of the big toe, podagra—an expression which is also used to cover the whole disease.

This is a highly hereditary disease which in about half the cases also shows an association with other metabolic disturbances, among others, kidney stones. Besides heredity, way of life also plays a large part, especially immoderation in food and drink. An old Latin-German verse runs:

> *Vinum der Vater,*
> *Coena die Mutter,*
> *Venus die Hebamm*
> *machen das podagram.*

(Wine is the father, food is the mother, Venus the midwife, who make podagra.) The old name *arthritis divitum*, rich man's gout, has much truth in it. *Arthritis pauperum*, poor man's gout, was ordinary rheumatoid arthritis.

Gout is without doubt a very ancient disease. Joint diseases were described by Hippocrates and many other Greek and Roman doctors, including Aretaeus. Erasistratus is said to have treated Ptolemy for gout in Alexandria. Arab and mediaeval authors also describe joint affections, but it is not possible to distinguish clearly what could have been gout from other painful joint complaints. At the time of Rome's decline Seneca mentions that women had gout as often as men, because of their dissolute way of life, and Galen considers that the disease had increased for the same reason.

The oldest unmistakable record that gout existed thousands of years ago is found in the remains of an elderly man from early Christian times, who was buried on the island of Philae on the Nile. The joints of the feet, knees, arms and hands show typical changes and in addition he had so-called senile arthrosis. Towards the end of the Middle Ages, Paracelsus described cases in all probability of real gout, as did later the great English doctor Sydenham, who suffered from the disease himself for nearly forty years. His classic work *Tractatus de podagra et hydrope* (Treatise on gout and dropsy) came out in 1683 and contains his own case history. Finke mentions that 'Newton, during the whole of the time he was writing his *Optics* abstained completely from meat and lived only on vegetables'. Broadly speaking, gout was much more common a few hundred years ago than now, which must surely be linked with our present more natural way of life.

Previously, England and Holland were the special homes of gout. The very experienced pathologist Rössle says that he has never seen a single case in Basle, but many in Jena and Berlin, where wine and beer consumption is considerable. In Scandinavia the disease is

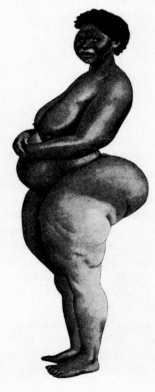

'Hottentot Venus', a Koranna woman of about 20, with a high degree of fat deposit, especially evident on the buttocks (steatopygia).

rare nowadays, and I myself have seen only about ten typical cases in 15,000 autopsies. The disease seems to be rare in the tropics, perhaps because of a more vegetarian diet.

Adiposity

This disturbance of balance has been known since time immemorial and in certain cultures is regarded as a sign of wealth and beauty. Thick deposits of fat on the hips, thighs and buttocks are said to be to a certain extent a racial characteristic in women, for example the steatopygia in certain Negro peoples. The first 'Hottentot Venus' was shown in Paris in 1814. Despite all that has been written on adiposity and obesity, opinions are still very divergent as regards the internal mechanism and as to whether endocrine, constitutional, hereditary or psychical factors are most important or simply faulty diet. The facts are that certain families consist mainly of thin individuals and that in others fat men and women predominate. The question anyway falls outside the realm of historico-geographical pathology. That the Mediterranean races are inclined to obesity is considered to be due to an earlier mixing with Negro blood.

4 Diseases of the Blood-forming Organs

The blood groups, variations in the form of the blood corpuscles, different forms of haemoglobin

It is not possible here to go into the large and interesting field of the different blood groups, their occurrence and relative frequency within the ABO-system, or into the incidence of the Rhesus factor and its importance to genetics, anthropology and pathology (see also

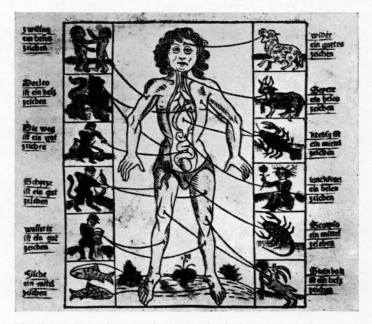

Bleeding and purging were important hygienic and medical measures, and the first medical script to be printed was a bleeding and purging calendar for the year 1457, printed in Mainz at the end of 1456 in the famous 36-line biblical type. The instructions for suitable blood-letting days shown here are of a somewhat later date, about 1485. A very interesting history of blood-letting, which falls quite outside our terms of reference, has been written by R. Fåhraeus, and others.

pp. 7 and 13). Nor can a survey be given here of the geographical incidence of divergent forms of red blood corpuscle, e.g. sickle-shaped and elliptical forms (drepanocytes and elliptocytes), or of other forms of haemoglobin and their geographical incidence.

Hitherto no one has found any serological characteristics in the blood which occur regularly in one human race but not in the others. A gene called Fy has been established which is very common in Negroes but extremely rare in whites in the USA and England. An antigen called Diego is considered to be an exclusively Mongolian gene (*Science*, 1961). It is lacking, however, in Indian tribes living on the periphery, e.g. the Patagonians, but is found in those which are considered to have arrived later. Some serologists and anthropologists have tried to improve on the old race classifications and have listed the following major racial groups:

1. Earlier Europeans.
2. Europeans.
3. Africans.
4. Asiatics.
5. Americans.
6. Australians.

It is, however, not certain if this classification will become definite. Among other things there remains to be investigated the connection between the Diego-positive, relatively late, immigrant American, 'old inhabitants', whose tribes show large differences between each other and their nearest neighbours and relations in north-east Asia, and the Diego-negative 'marginal' Indians. Diego has never been shown in people of pure white descent.

Pernicious anaemia

Authors of the past like the German Lebert and the Englishman Addison were the forerunners of Biermer who was the true discoverer of this common and important form of anaemia, which was formerly incurable and deserved its name of pernicious, death-bringing. The disease is of definite geographical interest as its frequency varies greatly from country to country, or perhaps one should say from one climatic zone to another. At a geo-pathological conference in Stockholm in 1937, the international report gave the following figures:

Cases of pernicious anaemia per 100,000 inhabitants (1936) (after de Langen and Askanazy)		Pernicious anaemia as a percentage of all autopsies (1936)	
Sweden	9·18	Warsaw (prosector)	1·39
Canada	9·1	Stockholm	0·9
England	8·9	Toronto	0·85
USA (north)	6·9	Greifswald	0·83
Switzerland (1926)	6·5	Berlin	0·66
Norway	5·5	Göttingen	0·45
Holland	4·4	Geneva	0·45
Switzerland (1935)	4·1	Lausanne	0·44
Italy	2·3	Vienna	0·44
Japan	0·6	Hamburg	0·43
Ceylon	0·3	Berne	0·42
Haiti	0·2	Königsberg	0·35
Java	0·0	Warsaw (Paskiewicz Inst.)	0·34
		Munich	0·33
		Chicago	0·27
		Freiburg i. B.	0·24
		Heidelberg	0·16
		Chile	0·12
		Japan	0·086

All these figures should be judged with some caution, as, for example, the apparent difference between the two reports from Switzerland in 1926 and 1935 can hardly correspond to the actual conditions, but is due to technical differences. In addition, improved clinical diagnosis has obviously increased the number of cases of pernicious anaemia, while today's effective therapy has brought the formerly very high mortality down to a minimum.

In Sweden, where diagnosis of pernicious anaemia is fairly uniform in all hospitals and clinics, an investigation I made on the basis of hospital reports from 1951–53 showed certain clear differences in the frequency of pernicious anaemia which could hardly be due to different diagnosis or different facilities for blood-tests for the inhabitants in the various regions. The figures are, as can be seen, on a completely different and much higher level than those published in 1937. This is probably entirely due to more exact diagnosis by which much earlier and milder cases can now be recognised as pernicious anaemia. If one excludes Gotland, then the tables show a very interesting decrease in the frequency from north to south, a fact which corresponds with the conditions stated earlier.

The three northernmost counties and Dalarna	approx. 350 cases in 100,000
Five neighbouring counties in central Sweden	approx. 308 cases in 100,000
Stockholm	approx. 241·5 cases in 100,000
Five neighbouring counties in south Sweden	approx. 221 cases in 100,000
Gotland	approx. 171 cases in 100,000

Kolstad's investigations in a limited area, a county in southern Norway, showed quite large differences between the districts. In one parish in 1935–53 over twenty new cases were diagnosed annually, in others ten to fifteen, and in yet others only five. The reasons for these large variations are not known, but hereditary conditions and differences in environment might be considered.

WHO gives statistical reports on the mortality in pernicious anaemia for the years 1950–56. These should have a certain limited value.

	per 100,000
Ireland	4·3
Scotland	3·4
England	2·3
Denmark	1·8
Italy	1·3
W. Germany	1·2
Norway	1·1
Holland	0·9
France	0·7

Non-European countries:

Australia	2·0
Canada	1·4
USA	1·1
Japan	0·5

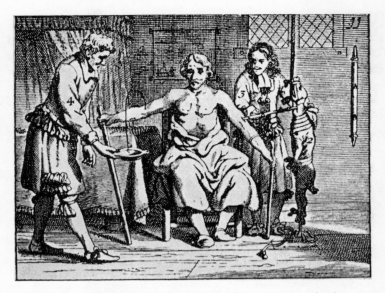

The history of blood transfusion falls outside our terms of reference, but can perhaps be briefly mentioned. After theoretical discussions, experiments were made on animals and humans, and the Frenchman Jean Denis carried out the first one of its kind in 1666. Lack of technical knowledge and complete ignorance of the composition of the blood made the results so discouraging that the method did not come into use until very much later. The above shows the transfer of blood from a dog. Late seventeenth century.

Bothriocephalus anaemia, anaemia perniciosiformis bothriocephalica

This severe anaemia, which has been known for about eighty years and which occasionally develops in carriers of the broad tapeworm, *Bothriocephalus latus*, occurs in all countries in which this tapeworm is common. This form of anaemia is found particularly in Finland and this is of course mainly associated with the wide distribution of the broad tapeworm as a result of eating semi-raw fish. This form of anaemia is also well known in the northernmost parts of Sweden. Not all worm carriers sicken, by any means, which is probably due to constitutional circumstances, to the worm's position in the intestine and to the number of worms. The number of cases of worm anaemia in Helsinki at the end of the nineteenth and beginning of the twentieth century was greater than the number of the then diagnosed cases of pernicious anaemia. Then the relative frequency of worm anaemia declined considerably, but in the mid-1930s there were still, according to Saltzman, two cases of worm anaemia for every five of pernicious anaemia. The role of constitutional factors is shown in that women sicken more often than men, and partly in that worm anaemia occasionally appears in the same families as pernicious anaemia. According to Nyberg, who made a thorough study of worm anaemia in 1960, its cause is essentially that the worm deprives its carrier of a large part of the vitamin B_{12} necessary to blood-formation, and as this vitamin 'holds a key position in numerous metabolic processes', the worm must be considered to be a much more serious enemy to its carrier than is generally supposed. Thanks to improvements in hygienic conditions and also chiefly to better information on the danger of worms, in recent years cases of worm anaemia have become rarer in both Finland and Sweden.

Hypochromic anaemia

Anaemic states have been known since the golden age of classical medicine in Greece, Rome and Arabia. The expression chlorosis, indicating the pale facial colour with a greenish tint, was first introduced at the beginning of the nineteenth century, particularly to characterise the anaemia and fatigue of young girls of the time. If one reads the medical literature of the end of the last century, one gets the impression that chlorosis was regarded as a true endemic condition, particularly in the northern countries like Sweden and Norway, but also in Canada and the USA.

The incidence of hypochromic and achylic anaemia in different parts of the world is still insufficiently known. Lundholm's investigations into this disease-complex and its occurrence in Jämtland in northern Sweden have established that it has a clear hereditary character and that consequently constitutional factors are here too of great significance. He found, for instance, that siblings of patients suffered from hypochromic anaemia to an extent of 12·4 per cent of those examined, or about ten times more than in ordinary hospital material. It was almost entirely women who had this form of anaemia.

Hereditary haemolytic anaemia

The hereditary form of jaundice caused by abnormal destruction of the red blood corpuscles was probably first observed by Minkowski in 1900. The disease is caused by a hereditary abnormality in the normal breaking-down of the used red blood corpuscles. The hereditary circumstances have been particularly studied by Meulengracht who has shown, among other things, that in such families an average of half of the children fall ill and that healthy children have healthy descendants.

This disease is extremely rare in China and exists there only in certain national minorities (Bernard, 1959).

Mediterranean anaemia, thalassaemia, Cooley's anaemia

This hereditary blood disturbance was first studied in the Mediterranean, where it is chiefly found in Italians and Greeks and their descendants. Continued investigations have, however, shown that it occurs in many other places, for instance among Jews in Kurdistan, in southern China, Tonkin, Thailand, South East Asia, Java and the Philippines. There is a centre of the disease in the Congo. Outside this relatively connected zone, there are scattered smaller centres and single cases, in Germany, France and England, among North American Negroes, in Mexico and South America. By far

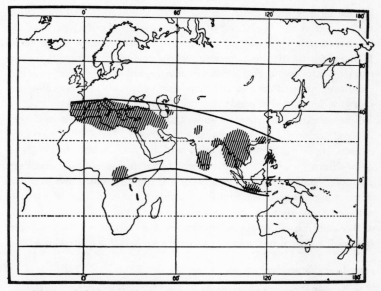

Incidence of thalassaemia in the eastern hemisphere where the centres for the disease's genes seem to lie within a broad belt including parts of Europe, Africa and Asia (after McKnight and McKnight).

212

the densest concentration of cases is found in Italy south of the mouth of the River Po, near Ferrara, Padua and Ravenna, but Sicily and Sardinia also have many cases. The disease occurs in two forms, a severer form with quite high mortality, and a milder form, often without symptoms.

There has been much speculation as regards the peculiar geographical distribution of this disease. As it evidently involves hereditary factors, an explanation for the smaller centres and scattered cases has been sought either in prehistoric migrations or in continued occurrence of the mutations.

Drepanocytosis, sickle cell anaemia

This anomaly, which is sometimes associated with anaemia, occurs mainly among the Negroes of Africa and North America, but is also known in Greece, in the region of Lake Kopias, in Arabia and India. Many Negro tribes have no fewer than 4 per cent heterozygotes. This anomaly is commonest in East Africa but is also seen quite often in West Africa. Negro tribes with and without drepanocytosis live side by side but do not mix sexually with each other. It has been

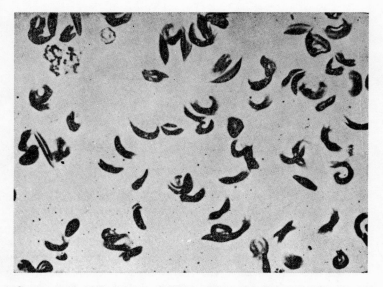

Smear of blood from an individual with sickle-shaped red blood corpuscles, drepanocytes.

213

discussed whether the anomaly came from India across Arabia, or vice versa and spread in an easterly direction. Roper and others have shown that heterozygotes (with drepanocytes) are more resistant to malaria than normal individuals and that the resistance is directed towards *Plasmodium falciparum* (see p. 138).

So-called 'brush skull' (Letterer), which occurs in various forms of severe chronic anaemia and which can be regarded as an attempt by the organism to compensate for chronic lack of blood, will be dealt with later (on p. 262).

Hereditary bleeding disease, haemophilia and thrombopathia

It cannot be stated with certainty how long true haemophilia, hereditary bleeder's disease, has been known. According to Rothschild certain commandments in the Talmud concerning the circumcision of boys whose brothers have died after the operation indicate

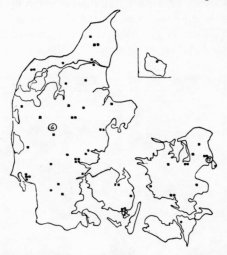

Distribution of haemophilia, bleeder's disease, in Denmark in 1943, when Andreassen investigated 67 Danish families with 81 bleeders.

that the risk was understood or the symptoms of the disease known. There is even mention of three sisters, whose firstborn sons had bled to death after circumcision, and this points to a certain insight into the hereditary character of the disease. Jewish and Arab doctors seem to have known of bleeding to death from sores and mucous membranes from the third century, whereas such conditions are not mentioned by the classical Greek and Roman doctors. One comes across sixteenth-, seventeenth- and eighteenth-century reports on mediaeval literature of bleeding which would correspond to haemophilia, but it was not until the end of the eighteenth century that family histories of bleeding in the male members were recorded. The first to show clearly the hereditary course of the disease is said to have been the American doctor, Otto, at the beginning of the nineteenth century, and the name haemophilia was introduced by Schönlein in 1828.

A number of other haemorrhagic diseases, predispositions to bleeding, have been distinguished over the years from haemophilia in a narrower sense with its characteristic heredity. It is not possible here to go into the geography of the different forms, mainly because definite data are not yet available.

In Sweden in 1944 Sköld found sixty families with true hereditary haemophilia and he has gone through their genealogies. The disease is said to be most common in Småland. In Norway in 1947–49 Imerslund carried out geographical and genealogical investigations into familial haemorrhagic diseases (thrombopathias).

To these diseases belong the hereditary thrombopathias which exist in several families on the island of Åland. They were originally demonstrated by von Willebrand and can affect both sexes. This form of bleeder has recently been the subject of further genealogical and geographical investigations by Eriksson (1960) which analysed in particular the seventh generation back and also the largest (1,300 people). The source is presumably the small isolated island of Sottunga, where no fewer than 20 per cent of the population have the disease. On Åland with its 22,000 inhabitants and geographical isolation, practically every person has several hereditary predispositions to diseases which do not necessarily occur at all. A propositus who was examined, Hildegard, with severe but not lethal haemophilia, had in the seventh generation only thirty-nine ancestors instead of sixty-four, i.e. a loss through intermarriage of nearly 40 per cent. This is a case of a non-sex-linked heredity with dominant hereditary course.

So-called 'Christmas disease', which is more or less similar to true haemophilia and affects only men, belongs here, and also Owren's parahaemophilia (1947) and Glanzmann's hereditary thrombasthenia, as well as a couple of other haemorrhagic diatheses.

Hereditary infantile agranulocytosis

A newly discovered hereditary form of agranulocytosis (lack of white blood corpuscles) in children, found by Kostmann, has hitherto been shown only in a geographically isolated place in northernmost Sweden, north of the Gulf of Bothnia. This is a case of primary inferiority in the red bone marrow with sharply reduced formation of white blood corpuscles. Children who are not treated die. The cause seems to be a simple recessive autosomal mutant gene.

Infectious horse anaemia

Finally, a few words on an infectious anaemia which occurs in the horse family and shows a very clear geographical distribution. In all hitherto investigated countries, it has a stationary distribution and can therefore be called an enzootic. This is clearly a case of an infectious disease, the agent of which is not known, but there probably are as yet unknown factors involved. It is not likely that mosquitoes act as transmitters, but it is possible that the chemical or physical properties of the earth's surface play a certain part (Dobberstein and Hemmert-Halswick). The disease has a wide distribution in Germany, also in former East Prussia and Silesia, in north-east France, northern Switzerland and the northern part of the Scandinavian peninsula, especially west Norrland and Jämtland. It is also known in south-east Europe, northern Japan and large parts of the United States and Canada.

5 Diseases of the Circulatory System

Vascular diseases

Arteriosclerosis

Arteriosclerosis means a thickening and stiffening of the walls of the arteries. The more recent term atherosclerosis (Marchand) does not indicate the localisation of the lesion, but describes both the processes which constitute the morbid change: *athera*, the porridge-like consistency in the fatty parts of the artery wall in advanced cases, and *sclerosis*, the hardening. These anatomical terms correspond to grave general nutritional disorder, especially in the cholesterol metabolism. Incipient and slight arterial lesions give no clinical symptoms; therefore geographical investigations of the disease must be founded almost exclusively upon autopsies.

This arterial change generally appears with increasing age, but should not be called an age-disturbance in itself, rather a metabolic disease. It can occur early in life but can equally be almost completely absent at a great age. The most important localisations are the aorta, the arteries of the heart, brain and kidneys, and the peripheral arteries, especially in the legs, but it can also occur throughout the body's arteries.

The disease is found in mummies of the ancient civilisations—the best known examples are Egyptian, and among them that of the Pharaoh Menephtah, son and heir to Rameses II, has been thoroughly examined. Some consider that he was the Pharaoh who drove the Jews out of Egypt and who, according to Exodus, was drowned in the Red Sea. This is however, contradicted in that the mummy shows a very old man with severe arteriosclerosis and calcification of the vessels. Ruffer found arteriosclerosis in Coptic mummies of the first century A.D. It has also been found in mummies from pre-Hispanic Peru, but never to such an advanced degree as in those of Egypt. The explanation for this could lie in that the Peruvian Indians followed a different diet, more vegetarian and less fatty than that of the wealthy Egyptians we have been able to examine—poor Egyptians were generally not embalmed and only their skeletons remain. The Egyptians probably also lived to a much greater age than the Indians and this must also be taken into account when attempting to explain the differences.

As far as the distribution and intensity of arteriosclerosis are concerned, in different parts of the world, in different races, populations, social and economic classes, and also as regards the influence of food on the development of vascular changes, comprehensive investigations have been carried out during recent decades. There is, of course, no lack of earlier investigations, but their limitations and lack of important data, such as division into age-groups and sexes, lessen their value in the present discussions on the conditions surrounding the occurrence of arteriosclerosis. Investigations by Ito in 1930 should be mentioned as he came to the almost certainly correct conclusion that atherosclerotic changes occur somewhat later in life in Japanese than in Europeans.

In 1934 arteriosclerosis was discussed at an international conference in Utrecht. Studies from all over the world had been brought to the conference, but unfortunately the material was mostly inadequate and details of age and sex often incomplete. In the case of more primitive people and illiterates, to a great extent one had to rely on more or less subjective assessments of age as most information on age was lacking.

Studies of the frequency and intensity of arteriosclerosis in Sweden were carried out for this conference by H. Sjövall, by Wihman and Björnvall and by Lundquist, in accordance with a programme planned by E. Sjövall and F. Henschen. It aimed at finding out whether any differences could be shown in the incidence of the disease in the different parts of our long country, with its different climatic conditions and large variations in peoples and diet. The investigation relied entirely on autopsies, for arteriosclerosis, especially in its lower grades, can in fact only be studied in autopsy material. The investigation was carried out partly in Lund, where the material largely consisted of people from fertile southern Skåne; partly in Stockholm with its urban population; and partly up in Umeå, where the surrounding country with its population living largely on a milk and vegetable diet and fish was reflected in the autopsy material. It was then shown that the frequency and forms of arteriosclerosis were almost identical in Lund and Stockholm (changes in the abdominal aorta of elderly and often quite fat women from the

Skåne countryside possibly being greater than in Stockholm, and arteriosclerosis in the vessels of the heart, or coronary sclerosis, being perhaps more noticeable in older male Stockholmers than in the Lund material). In contrast, a clear difference was established between the Umeå material and that from central and southern Sweden. In the inhabitants of Västerbotten, largely thin people, arteriosclerosis was generally less severe, and the incidence of the most severe types of change was virtually non-existent in the rest of the material. The whole process had evidently developed later in life and more slowly, very rarely reaching the high grades which were to be seen in cases from Lund and Stockholm. The interesting thing is that this clear difference between material from Västerbotten and that from more southerly areas has lately vanished. This is from experience of ordinary autopsy results as well as my own impressions during two periods as locum in Umeå. Prosperity has allowed people to eat and put on weight as much in upper Norrland as in other parts of the country and therefore to develop just as severe arterial changes as elsewhere.

Numerous more recent investigations into arteriosclerosis in the aorta and the arteries of the heart, which have been carried out with the necessary discrimination, present a good picture of the incidence

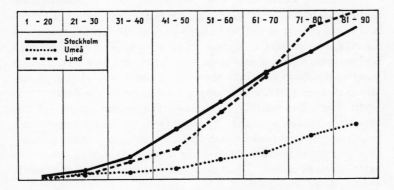

The relative frequency and intensity of arteriosclerosis in autopsy material from Lund, Stockholm and Umeå in 1934. The rise in arteriosclerosis per decade of life is seen to be steeper in Stockholm than in Lund during both the important decades from the ages of 41 to 60. By contrast the disease increased in Lund during the last two decades of life. The Umeå material shows a strong contrast with its relatively rare and considerably milder arteriosclerosis. See also text.

of the disease within different races and populations as well as those environmental factors which are thought to influence the development and intensity of the process. About the endogenous (internal) factors which undoubtedly play at least as important a role in this metabolic disturbance, little is known apart from the generally known fact that predisposition to the disease is hereditary.

A presupposition in all scientific investigations of arteriosclerosis is access to large quantities of autopsy material together with reliable data on the age of the dead person and, when it is a question of mixed racial populations, his race, in which case a specialised population like the Jews should also be taken into account, as has happened in New York, for instance. First the aorta is examined as it gives a valuable picture of the intensity of the change; but on the other hand it tells little of the clinical importance of any particular case. One has even reached the paradoxical statement: aorta change is not a disease but a disfiguration. Much more important from a clinical point of view is atherosclerosis in the arteries of the heart, with or without damage to the heart muscles, and also in the arteries of the brain. I shall return to changes in the smallest arteries or arterioles, when I discuss hypertension, high blood pressure.

In those parts of Western Europe where in peace-time people live on abundant calorie-rich fatty foodstuffs, in the Scandinavian countries, Holland, West Germany, the Netherlands, most of France and Great Britain as well as in large parts of the United States and Canada, one finds the highest frequency, earliest manifestations and severest forms of atherosclerosis. There are, however, modern investigations which seem to show that manual work plays a protective part, even with the consumption of calorie-rich and fatty foodstuffs. Gsell has recently investigated the inhabitants of a Swiss mountain village who live on such food but nevertheless show relatively low lipoid values in the blood, scarcely any arteriosclerosis and a general freedom from heart and brain complaints of an arteriosclerotic nature. They grow old and continue at hard work, even at an advanced age.

Statistically speaking, atherosclerosis declines swiftly—and presumably individually too—when supplies of food become shorter and especially when there are restrictions on the consumption of animal fats (the importance of vegetable fats is still under discussion). The first to point this out is said to have been the pathologist Aschoff who found that the disease declined in Germany during the shortage years after the First World War. Similar experiences were found in Germany, Finland, Sweden and Norway during and after the Second World War. Compulsorily limited diet and especially the decrease in consumption of fat had a very evident and favourable effect on the health of the people; atherosclerosis declined, perhaps not so much in the sense that already developed changes diminished—which does also occur—but in that the disease neither developed so early nor reached such severe forms, perhaps principally in the coronary arteries of the heart, in which myocardial infarct resulting from coronary occlusion consequently became less common.

This was shown in my academic lecture in 1946, in which the decline in atherosclerosis was also demonstrated in a decline in the mortality curve. It can be said without exaggeration that the Swedish people had never in their history been so healthy nor mortality so low as during those crisis years when people generally complained that they could never eat their fill. When the crisis was over and people could eat as much as they wanted, could manage and afford, then an increased mortality occurred, i.e. those who thanks to the restrictions on foodstuffs involuntarily had had their lives lengthened by a year or two, then died as a result of a swift return to their old food habits. It is also of considerable interest that both the arteriosclerosis and the mortality graphs showed a minor decline on an earlier occasion, namely during the economic crisis at the beginning of the 1930s, when the Swedish people had to tighten their belts somewhat, to the advantage of their health. Vartiainen (1947) came to the same conclusion in Finland where the crisis was much more severe, so did Malmros in Sweden (1950) and Ström and Jensen in Norway in 1951. It is barely necessary to say that too severe restrictions on foodstuffs accompanied by vitamin deficiency are directly harmful.

Relative intensity of arteriosclerosis registered at autopsies in Helsinki before and after the war and the years of crisis, divided into the different decades of life. White columns 1933–38, black columns 1940–46. (After Vartiainen and Kanerva, 1947.)

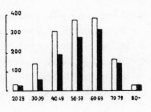

A parallel to this decrease in the intensity of atherosclerosis caused by times of crisis is shown in a study by Wynder and others of changes in the coronary vessels with damage to the heart among males of the Seventh Day Adventists in the USA, whose members do not smoke or drink and exercise moderation in respect of animal foodstuffs. In men belonging to the sect, coronary sclerosis occurred, statistically speaking, at a greater age than in other men, and it was also milder, especially in men under sixty. Perhaps the investigation should have been complemented by one into their physical constitution to see whether the men of the sect were not overwhelmingly asthenic, i.e. relatively weak and thin.

The large poor areas of southern Europe show a contrast to conditions in the above affluent countries. There the inhabitants to a great extent live on a vegetable and fish diet, and atherosclerosis is not so pronounced. Unfortunately large-scale studies based on autopsy results are lacking.

Even more marked is the difference between the all too well nourished parts of Europe and North America on the one hand and the greater part of the rest of the world on the other. This is shown clearly by comprehensive comparative studies which have been carried out recently. The explanation of these differences, as far as one can judge, is principally found in variations in food and way of life and probably also in psychophysical reactions, though not directly in anthropological differences. Several of these investigations deserve further reference.

Epstein and others investigated conditions among workers in the clothing industry in New York in which Jews and Italians were active. The Jewish workers had heart symptoms about twice as often as the Italians, while aorta changes showed no difference. Presumably the food of both categories was quite different in its composition. Larsen found in Hawaii much more coronary sclerosis among 'caucasians' than among 'orientals', i.e. East Asians. Large-scale comparative studies of atherosclerosis in the aorta and the arteries of the heart and brain have been made by Hirst and others, covering the USA, Jamaica, Japan and South India. In Los Angeles coronary sclerosis was more severe before the age of 60 than in India and Japan where coronary sclerosis and thrombosis were considerably rarer. Investigations in South Africa show, according to Siew, that severe atheromatosis of the coronary arteries is very common in Europeans but very rare in Bantus. A comparison between New Orleans and Guatemala City in Central America, made by Fejada and Gores, showed milder and later-developed atherosclerosis in the latter. US Negroes had about twice as severe atheromatosis in the coronary arteries as Negroes in Haiti, and similarly the average heart weight in American Negroes was higher (328 gm) than in Haiti's Negroes (269 gm). These differences might well be explained by the different diets, the US diet being the better with more animal protein and, in particular, more fats than that of the Haiti negroes, with its overwhelmingly vegetable content. Glotzer very rarely found coronary thrombosis in the poor Negroes of New York. An investigation into atherosclerosis in the aorta and coronary thrombosis in diabetic Negroes and whites showed, according to Anderson and others, no clear difference between the two races. In Singapore the occurrence of atheromatosis in the vessels of the heart has been studied in Chinese and Indians living side by side in the same city but in different cultural and dietetic circumstances. It was found that changes in the coronary arteries were much more common in Indians. The Indians in California 'never', according to Gilbert, have atherosclerosis with thrombosis in the coronary arteries. By contrast it was impossible to find obvious differences in Mexico with its considerable racial mixture and minimal differences in way of life, especially as the average age of individuals examined was no more than about 40.

Finally, a study by Sacks in Cape Town should be mentioned, based on 1,251 not especially selected autopsies. Male Bantus, consisting only of poor negroes with a meagre diet, had less coronary sclerosis between 40 and 59 than whites. A comparison touching on conditions after 60 showed that very few Bantus live that long. The difference was not so pronounced between poor whites and Indians. Sacks considers, correctly, that if the investigation had also included well-to-do whites the differences would have certainly been much greater.

According to Davies, who has a great deal of experience, atherosclerosis is unusual and coronary thrombosis extremely rare in the Africans of Uganda. Vandeputte investigated conditions among the negroes of the Congo and found that atherosclerosis occurred just as early in them as in whites, but that severer forms with calcification and thrombosis were rarer than in Europeans. On the other hand Mawpure Vovor considers that coronary thrombosis was by no means a rarity in the Negroes he examined.

One of the few studies from India was published in 1962 by Murthy and his colleagues. It is based on 260 medico-legal autopsies and shows clearly that 'the more advanced changes are less pronounced in this Indian material than in the white inhabitants of the USA and South Africa.'

WHO has published data on the mortality in coronary thrombosis and related diseases. The highest mortality is in the USA, followed by Finland, Norway and Japan. According to the same source, mortality from coronary sclerosis during recent years is in Israel 88·3–130·3, in Japan 41·2–46·3 and in Ceylon 29·2–23·6, all per 100,000 inhabitants. These figures given by WHO should be regarded with caution, as reliable comparisons between countries with so many and great dissimilarities as regards clinical and pathological-anatomical material are at present scarcely possible.

From the above, however, it appears that the differences between different countries and populations are considerable. The present plan for international research has a large target—to show, through a common, uniform and strictly carried-out programme, how great these differences are and which factors are their basis, i.e. what part race, food, work, blood-pressure and other agents play in the incidence of arteriosclerosis, one of the most important diseases of today.

Heart diseases

Both the coronary arteries and their different branches have few and small connections—the so-called end arteries. The study by Pepler and Mayer of conditions in Bantu Negroes and in whites is therefore of very great interest. They have found better developed connections, anastomoses, in Bantus than in whites. If this proves to be true, it is an important racial difference. This difference is said to have nothing to do with hypertrophy and atherosclerosis.

Heart hypertrophy

A physiological adaptation of the heart to permanent heavy work has been known for a long time, not only in humans but also in animals. Hirsch tells of hypertrophy in populations who always do heavy work, as opposed to sedentary townspeople. S. E. Henschen found in 1898 that the Lapps in general have larger hearts, in relation to size of body, than southern Swedes. Esguerra Gomez has studied heart hypertrophy in Indians who do heavy work at great heights. Davies and Ball, in comparisons between the heart weights of Africans in Uganda and Europeans, have found slight hypertrophy in a third of the Africans examined, moderate hypertrophy in a third and severe (40–180 per cent) in another third. No definite cause could be established, but this too is certainly an example of adaptation in a people who live in primitive conditions. Stieve found a heavier heart in grouse that live up in the snowy regions of the Norwegian mountains than in birds which live in sheltered scrub vegetation where pressure on the blood circulation is less.

Endocarditis and myocarditis, inflammation processes in the inner membrane of the heart and muscles, are of geographical interest only in exceptional cases. In Venezuela Jaffe and, later, Gould found a chronic myocarditis with heart weakness in up to 20 per cent of autopsy cases. For a long time the reason was not clear, but Gould's investigations, which include most of the Latin-American states, indicate that it might possibly be a question of a chronic endemic form of Chagas disease (p. 136). Davies has found a somewhat similar chronic endomyocarditis of an obscure nature in Uganda; these changes have also been observed in other places in East and West Africa and in former Rhodesia.

Hypertension, 'high blood-pressure'

The causes of high blood pressure and its different forms are among the problems which are still being discussed in the medical world. It is therefore not yet possible to answer all the questions which arise when one considers the incidence of hypertension diseases in different races and population groups, and especially when individuals of one geographical or racial group move to an environment which is in all respects alien to them. As far as the white race is concerned, it is considered that urbanisation and in particular life in large cities expose the individual to a 'chronic psychosomatic overloading' (Büchner), which is an important cause of the occurrence and frequency of genuine hypertension, and also of death. It is thought that Chinese, in so far as one can generalise, seldom have hypertension in their own country but that after a period of time in the USA they quite often develop high blood pressure. Murrill found in Puerto Rico that there were generally no differences between coloureds and whites. According to Davies, hypertension in its different forms is quite rare in Negroes in Africa but common in Negroes in the USA. Similar findings are reached by Moser (1960). Negroes from Liberia have low blood pressure, lower than Negroes in other parts of Africa, the West Indies and in the USA. Hypertension seems to develop more easily in them than in orientals and whites. Moser also gives urbanisation, civilisation, hostilities, worries and irreconcilabilities between different racial groups as reasons for a rise in blood pressure. It is therefore uncertain whether such a thing as racial predisposition to hypertension exists, as has been suggested in some quarters. Darby's investigations into blood-pressure conditions in Ethiopia show low blood pressure throughout, in men of between 25 and 44 117/72, in women somewhat lower. Only 1 per cent of the men in this age-group showed a higher level than 140/90, and 2·5 per cent of those over 45 had such levels. Broadly speaking, the same applied to women. No pregnant or breast-feeding woman showed hypertension levels. Ehrström's and Abs's studies of conditions among Eskimoes, whose average age, on account of infectious diseases and accidents, is very low, 20–27, seem to show that low blood pressure in young individuals often rises to high figures, 200–240, in those somewhat older. There is not thought to be any connection between their fat- and protein-rich diet and their hypertension, and everything indicates that the Eskimoes thrive best if they are allowed to live in peace with their own primitive régime.

Diseases of the veins

Varicose veins in the leg are a complaint which has been known since ancient times and is also found represented in Greek art. With blood clot formation or thrombosis in the veins, usually those of the extremities, a part or the whole of the thrombus, which can be 50 cm long, can come loose from the vessel wall, forming an embolism, is carried in the bloodstream and lodges almost always in the pulmonary arteries. Such thromboembolism is often fatal.

In times of forced restriction of food supplies, thromboembolisms seemed to decline and then to rise again when access to food became easier. Rössle found this in Germany after the First World War. Adelsten, Jensen and Hamperl came to the same conclusion. In

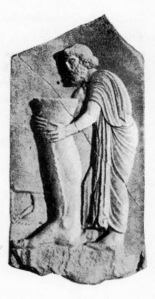

Votive tablet from the Asklepeion in Athens. The relief shows a leg with varicose veins. From Holländer, Plastik und Medizin.

times of severe restrictions and undernourishment, cases of pulmonary embolism were relatively few, but when the restrictions were lifted and many people again became fat, the number of thromboembolisms rose. Comparisons between the frequency of thromboembolisms in Skåne in two separate periods, 1927–28 and 1957–58, showed, according to Kaij, no obvious differences, but neither did these two periods show differences as regards the state of nourishment.

It is interesting that thromboembolisms are rare among more primitive peoples such as African negroes and the natives of India. Mawpure Vovor saw only 10 cases in 50,000 surgical and obstetric operations, of which 254 were cases of Caesarean section and 43,472 deliveries. The rarity of thromboembolisms in the Negro peoples of Africa shows that this disturbance is a disease characteristic of modern civilisation, a consequence of far too rich diet, obesity, a sedentary life and neuro-vegetative instability.

According to Halse and Quennet and to Mawpure Vovor, tropical inflammatory migrating thrombophlebitis, which has a wholly different, unknown cause and development, should be sharply distinguished from simple thromboembolism.

227

Telangiectasia haemorrhagica hereditaria, Rendu-Osler's disease

This disease is hereditary in both sexes and appears in an expansion and weakness in the walls of the small surface veins and capillaries, which cause bleeding. The disease is today known and described in many countries. A particularly instructive family tree includes the descendants in six generations of a Mormon pioneer who passed on the disease to numerous offspring by his four wives.

6 Diseases of the Respiratory System

Upper respiratory channels

Chronic inflammation and tumours of the sinuses of the nose and in the air-containing cells in the mastoid processes, the prominent bone processes behind and above the ears, are known from ancient Egyptian burial grounds, owing to changes in the bone, the result of severe disease. An example from the Italian Renaissance is mentioned on p. 263.

The bronchial tubes and lungs

The old-established names for inflammation of the lungs, pneumonia and peripneumonia, are found in the *Hippocratic Collection* and in non-medical writers such as Plutarch, but it is probably uncertain which lung diseases are referred to.

Among lung changes of geographical interest, lung emphysema, chronic distension of the smallest bronchii and lung alveoli, should be mentioned. It is found particularly in the Peruvian Andes in Indians, including women, who do heavy work at a height of perhaps 4,000 metres. These Indians, who suffer from emphysema, with their short growth and enormously large thoraxes, can be seen in Lima in a special institute for the examination of individuals who work at great heights.

A group of lung diseases of geographical and social interest are the pneumoconioses, lung-dust diseases, of which there are a large number of different forms, depending on what kind of dust is breathed in. The most common form is the generally quite harmless anthracosis, carbonisation of the lungs from coal dust, which is found in less severe forms in virtually all inhabitants of large cities, but especially in certain occupations such as coal-loaders. The most important form is silicosis, silicium lung, which has already been discussed under occupational diseases on pp. 181–2 and is put here for the sake of completeness.

All these pneumoconioses are often found in combination with lung tuberculosis, and it can be difficult to distinguish between coniotic and tuberculous indurations, scars in the lungs.

7 Diseases of the Digestive System

The teeth

The teeth and jaws, owing to their resistance to decay, are good objects of palaeopathological research. Changes in the teeth have been shown in the oldest remains of human beings, particularly abrasion from the hard food of the time which probably also contained small particles of stone from primitive grindstones. In ancient Egypt, especially in the south towards Nubia, many of the skulls from 6,500 years ago show severe abrasion of the teeth with exposed pulp and occasionally as a result severe inflammation in the tooth alveolars and adjacent parts of the jaws. In mummies of the upper classes and the Pharaohs, severe abrasions in the teeth are also occasionally seen, particularly in that of the ninety-year-old Rameses II whose teeth are otherwise good. Similar conditions are quite often found in skulls of the European Stone Age, as well as in later ones of the pre-Christian and Christian eras and on into recent centuries. Severely worn teeth are also occasionally found in pre-Columbian American skulls.

Another change in the teeth, known from very early times, is tooth stone formation which can reach very advanced stages, especially in the Orient, probably partly because of the old custom of chewing betel nuts. Herodotus and Pliny tell of oriental rulers and warriors who are said to have had a connecting plate of bone instead of teeth; it is possible that these might have been particularly severe formations of tooth stones (Thourén).

Caries has often and correctly been called a disease of civilisation. In primitive people at the hunting stage this tooth disease is rare, but with the transition to settling, farming and eating cooked, treated foodstuffs, it becomes more common. This can already be seen in the ancient civilisations of Egypt, Assyria and Babylon, where in certain population strata and during certain periods of history caries was almost as common as it is in many civilised countries today. Similar conditions prevailed in Etruria, Palestine, India and China.

Earlier archaeological accounts of tooth caries in skulls must always be treated with caution. More recent investigations into a number of authors, especially that of Sognnaes, have shown how difficult it is in fact to distinguish between genuine caries which has arisen during life from caries-like changes which occur after death and are mainly caused by the acid earth in which the teeth have lain. Sognnaes' investigations are based on 290 teeth with caries-like changes from Palaeolithic Palestine, pre-Dynastic Egypt, prehistoric Greece, mediaeval Norway and pre-Columbian America.

Palaeolithic human teeth are usually free of caries, but in earliest Neolithic times changes began to appear. According to Mummery, 2·2 per cent of the Neolithic long-skulled English races show caries, while in the contemporary short-skulled races as many as 22·8 per cent had caries, a fact which could be explained by differences in the composition of food (presuming that these are cases of true intravital caries). In ancient Egypt, according to Sudhoff, caries was rare, but somewhat later in the Old Kingdom, about 3000 B.C., caries in the upper classes became almost as frequent as among civilised people today. In contrast, teeth from the burial grounds of the poor were almost free of caries, but were very worn, probably because of the sand in the food caused by grinding. During the Ptolemaic period and in Byzantium the caries frequency rises, especially in older individuals.

Similar conditions are met in Europe. In the skulls of French Neolithic cave-dwellers only 1–1·2 per cent show caries. Holmer and Maunsbach, who in 1956 examined 4,187 teeth from the Swedish Stone Age, found no more than 49 teeth with caries (1·17 per cent).

In the great number of skulls from different parts of Europe, caries is found to a varying extent—between 15 and 33 per cent. A considerable proportion of skulls in pre-Columbian America also show caries. It is interesting that caries was markedly more common in the civilised cultures of Mexico and Peru than among the wild Indians in Louisiana and Arkansas in the USA, where it was very rare.

Only a couple of generations ago there were primitive people with a very low caries frequency. They included people who were scarcely touched by civilisation, such as the Eskimo and certain Lapp tribes, the people of north-east India and the remaining indigenous peoples of New Zealand and the Fiji Islands. On the other hand there were at that time other so-called primitive peoples, Polynesians, Australians, Tasmanians, south-east Indians, Kaffirs and East and West Africans, showing caries in over 40 per cent, but the geographical and demographical differences here were very great.

An investigation into tooth disease in the far north of Sweden, carried out by Westin, Holtz and Lindström in 1929–31, showed that women had much more caries than men. In the age group 16–45, their caries frequency was double that of the men—later on in life the difference was less pronounced and at least 95 per cent of both sexes had caries. Otherwise the caries frequency varied from one isolated district to another. One parish, Stensele, for some unknown reason (food, few sweetmeats, fluoride in the water?) had remarkably little caries. In Finland the recent war years brought with them a very interesting and marked decrease in caries in children (there was an acute shortage of sugar).

In the fight against caries, for healthy teeth, a very active substance has been found in fluoride. It is still too early to state to what extent the naturally varying fluoride content in drinking water and food appears in the geography of caries, but it does not seem improbable that the fluoride content is one of the active factors.

Periodontitis, alveolar pyorrhoea

Here too one must beware of confusion with post-mortem changes which destroy the tooth alveolar walls. Moodie says that the giant reptiles, fossil mastodontic rhinoceroses and primitive three-toed horses of the Chalk age already show jaw changes, which he compares with alveolar pyorrhoea. According to Schwalbe and Virchow, alveolar pyorrhoea was to be found in archaic skulls from Upper Egypt, occasionally with signs of septic processes round the teeth. Sudhoff mentions a young woman of 800 B.C. who had lost all her teeth and showed atrophy of the alveolar walls. A similar severe condition was found in King Magnus Ladulås (d. 1290), who during his life lost all the teeth in his upper jaw as a result of periodontitis and had only a few tooth roots left. Such changes have been described from pre-Columbian Central and South America as well as in European material from antiquity, the Middle Ages and the Renaissance.

The stomach and intestines

Ulcus ventriculi et duodeni, gastric and duodenal ulcer

This disease which is nowadays so common seems to have been first described at the beginning of the nineteenth century by Vetter

(1803), but the first classic account was not given until 1821 by Cruveilhier. The disease is almost certainly a very old one, but formerly was probably much less common than now. Gastric ulcer shows large geographical variations in frequency but adequate exact parallel investigations are still lacking. The true frequency can only be found in a great deal of autopsy material in which all the stages of the disease, from the small erosion up to the minute, almost invisible scar, are registered.

Most authors who have dealt with statistics on stomach ulcers consider that the disease has gradually become more common and that men nowadays are affected more often than women, who once predominated. It should be noted, however, that this higher figure for men in many places is not very pronounced, for instance in Stockholm, where in 1943 Falconer found ulcers and scars in 18·14 per cent of the men and 17·86 per cent of the women. Again, in Hamburg in 1941 Klein found it in 19–22 per cent of men and 13–15 per cent of women. In Japan after the last war the disease was three to five times as common in men as in women (Kurokava and Masuda, 1957). Ulcers became much commoner there than before and now, by comparison with twenty-two other countries and as regards division into ages, the frequency is unusually high in all age groups. Fairly analogous experiences are found in other countries which suffered through the war.

Certain observations point to the presence of a racial (or environmental?) predisposition. This is what Straub and Schornagel found:

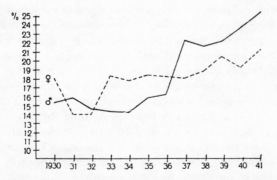

Stomach ulcer frequency in autopsy material in Stockholm from 1930–41, after B. Falconer (1943). Note the rising frequency and that nowadays men have stomach ulcers more often than women.

Chinese Indonesians had ulcers fifteen times as often as the Javanese. In several tropical and sub-tropical countries of Asia and Africa, ulcers are noticeably often localised in the duodenum, while the stomach is free. Payet found 80–90 per cent of ulcers localised in the duodenum. As far as the pathogenics of the disease are concerned, the significance of psychosomatic disturbances should be mentioned, and this applies not only to Europe and the USA, but also to the negro inhabitants of Central Africa (Davies).

Watkinson has shown large geographical differences in the frequency of ulcers in Great Britain, often greater in the north than in the south and almost throughout considerably more in men than in women. In the USA coloureds until quite recently had stomach ulcers much less often than whites, but now the frequency in coloureds is rising, presumably in association with the rise in their standard of living and in added psychological pressures.

There is a definite relationship between predisposition to stomach ulcers and the blood groups. If a person belongs to blood group O, he has about a 35 per cent greater chance of having ulcers than if he belongs to any other groups (Aird and others). This has also been recently noted in Shanghai (Dao Chin and others, 1958) where it was found that 41·23 per cent of individuals with ulcers belonged to blood group O, while in the control group of those free of stomach troubles only 32 per cent belonged to this blood group. However, a similar clear correlation could not be shown by Speiser in Vienna.

Ulcerative colitis and regional enteritis (inflammation of the large intestine with ulcers and regional inflammation of the small intestine) are two forms of intestinal affections which, together with transitional forms, have recently attracted considerable attention; their causes are largely unknown. It has been shown that they seem to have a certain geographical and demographical incidence. Melrose found that ulcerative colitis in England has a clear statistical tendency to decline in frequency from south to north; it is clearly less common in northern towns than in those of the south. In five Scottish towns the frequency is 6·9 per 10,000, in London 15·5 per 10,000. In the United States it is said to be the other way round— less common in the south than in the north.

Another peculiar demographic condition is considered to have been found in an examination of US veterans by Acheson. These intestinal diseases were four times more common among Jewish veterans than among the rest; even if the cases were divided into geographical regions, Jewish soldiers still showed a clear majority in all regions except one. There is no known satisfactory explanation for this, but it is thought that perhaps neuro-vegetative disturbances might be a cause.

Appendicitis

Periods with restricted supplies of finer foodstuffs and greater consumption of coarse bulky food seem to diminish the frequency of appendicitis. Purely vegetarian diet which changes the bacterial flora of the intestine is almost certainly not insignificant. Hamperl found a decline in the frequency of appendicitis in north Russia which in 1918 suffered severely from food shortages after the Revolution. In south Russia, which suffered less, the frequency of appendicitis did not noticeably decrease.

According to American reports, appendicitis is six times as common in whites as it is in coloureds. It is probably very uncertain whether this figure applies to true appendicitis, rather than to cases which have been operated on after clinical diagnosis of appendicitis behind which, as is well known, lie widely different functional and anatomical conditions, amongst others true appendicitis itself. In Stockholm an investigation I carried out showed that only about one-quarter of the appendices that were taken out after diagnosis of appendicitis were in fact cases of true appendicitis.

Anal fistula is quite an interesting disease from a historical point of view and was known and treated by the surgeons of India and ancient Greece. When the gourmand Louis XIV, *le Roi Soleil*, contracted one, interest in anal fistula became especially noticeable. A vast number of doctors and surgeons were consulted and different, usually totally irrational remedies were tried, first on his loyal subjects and then on the king. Finally the king's chief surgeon, Félix, undertook a small operation with a little knife he had himself made with a knob-shaped tip and this led to an immediate cure. It is not surprising that the operation then became almost fashionable. It was probably a troublesome and painful complaint for the king and affected his temper and capacity to govern, and his long rule has even been divided into two periods—before and after the fistula operation.

Anal fistula appears quite frequently in patients with lung tuberculosis and can then be of a tuberculous nature. In the mid-nineteenth
century it was thought that lung tuberculosis increased if the anal
fistula healed and things went so far that an anal fistula was produced
in the tuberculous person to let the diseased matter, *'materia
peccans'*, have the necessary outlet, a curious revival of the ancient
humoral pathology.

Haemorrhoids, piles, which often give rise to bleeding from the
anus, were formerly the object of great interest in the period of
blood-letting, and haemorrhoid bleeding was considered important
to the whole economy and health of the organism. Haemorrhoids
can be said to be a disease of civilisation, like varicose veins in the
legs. It is said that neither of these forms of dilatation of the veins
exists in Negroes living in primitive conditions.

The liver

The three great human races are mainly distinguished by a number
of external differences—at least these differences are the easiest to
demonstrate. In addition, with more detailed examination, other
very interesting differences can be shown, for example in the
macroscopic and microscopic construction of the brain. Certain
functional differences have also been established, especially in the
secretory system. It has not been, however, possible to find specific
differences in the biochemical activities of the liver.

Cirrhosis of the liver, different forms of liver atrophy

At the first conference of geographical pathology in Geneva in 1931,
the main theme was cirrhosis of the liver, its causal conditions and
geographical distribution. At that time, the general opinion was
that alcoholism was the most important cause of cirrhosis and in
many countries it was also possible to establish a parallel between
alcohol consumption and cirrhosis of the liver, as well as an increase
in cirrhosis if alcohol was not restricted or became considerably
cheaper. Wegelin, for instance, found just such a direct connection
in Berne, where cirrhosis had increased in the years 1910–30 at the
same time as an increase in drinking caused by the lowering of the
price of spirits. In eastern Switzerland, where cider and beer are the

most common drinks, cirrhosis of the liver was said to be substantially rarer than in central and western Switzerland. The well-known clinician Staehelin also maintained that in Switzerland alcohol was the most important cause of cirrhosis of the liver. On the other hand it was stated that cirrhosis was rare in Copenhagen and Skåne although a great deal of spirits were drunk there, and many people at the conference doubted that alcohol was the predominant cause of cirrhosis.

Atrophic cirrhosis of the liver is now regarded as the final stage of a number of different injuries to the liver, among which alcohol plays an important part. Several serious nutritional disturbances and inflammatory changes in the biliary passages are also of great importance. It has gradually become clearer that in a large number of cases injuries to the liver of a virus nature give rise to cirrhosis. Finally there remain a number of cases in which its cause is unknown. The figures which are given here do not clarify the causes and development of cirrhosis. All recent research indicates that the different pathogenic forms of cirrhosis of the liver are nowadays represented in very different circumstances in different countries. Cirrhosis is, for instance, not uncommon in Muslim countries where the abuse of alcohol hardly exists, so other causes, for example virus hepatitis, must be important. In Japan, as Amano and Yamamoto have recently shown, most of the cases of cirrhosis are the result of virus hepatitis and not even as much as 10 per cent are caused by alcohol. In Jamaica, where cirrhosis of the liver is found in no less than 4·9 per cent of autopsies, 90 per cent of the cirrhosis cases were divided into three groups of roughly the same size: (1) post-necrotic cirrhosis, following vital infection (30 per cent); (2) through changes in the hepatic arteries (28·5 per cent); (3) through obstruction of the veins of the liver (30 per cent). As a reason for this was given the consumption of large quantities of bush-tea, in particular *Crotalara fulva*. Cirrhosis after injuries to the biliary passages was found in only 1·3 per cent. In contrast, in Egypt no less than 71 per cent of cirrhosis cases are said to be due to bilharzia eggs (Hashem). In certain parts of India and in Djakarta, there is in children of 1–3 years of age a so-called infantile biliary cirrhosis, the nature of which is as yet not really known. This might possibly be due to some food deficiency, but toxic and infective factors cannot be excluded. Roulet points out how often African Negroes show liver injuries. In many cases this is probably the result of a deficiency in food, especially a shortage of protein.

237

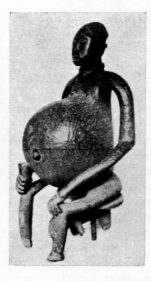

Wooden statuette from the northern Cameroons representing an African with advanced ascites or fluid in the peritoneal cavity, probably from cirrhosis of the liver. Ethnographical Museum, Berlin.

On the other hand, the importance of alcohol is upheld by Davidson and Popper in the USA and by Gros, who investigated the conditions in the wine-growing districts of Germany. Cases of cirrhosis following hepatitis and associated with dystrophy, nutritional disturbances, do occur, but 260 autopsies of cirrhosis from Mainz show that abuse of alcohol comes far ahead of other causes. Formerly the role of alcohol was overstressed, Gros says, and then hepatitis and dystrophy were overstressed in the same way. It is evident that the different causes show marked geographical variation in their significance.

As far as one can judge, it will be a long time before a uniform, international and universally acceptable classification of cirrhosis of the liver is possible.

According to the report from WHO on the years 1950–56, certain European countries such as Denmark, Finland, Iceland, Norway and Sweden show a moderate rise in deaths due to cirrhosis of the liver, and there were similar conditions in Holland and the British Isles. West Germany showed a sharp rise, from 9·2 per 1,000 to 12·4, West Berlin from 15·9 to 28·7 and France from 16·3 to the high figure of 32·5, all in the year 1956. Unfortunately it is an open question as to how far these figures are comparable and to what extent one can attribute the rise of cirrhosis to the increased

238

consumption of alcohol, which seems to be an international phenomenon.

In North America deaths from cirrhosis have also risen somewhat, in Canada from 4·5 per 1,000 to 5·2, and in the USA, among whites from 9·5 to 10·5 and among coloureds from 6·5 to 7·5. In South Africa the number of deaths from cirrhosis of the liver increased a little and here too whites showed more cirrhosis than coloureds, and Asiatics slightly more than Negroes. A similar increase in deaths from cirrhosis also occurred in Japan, from 6·8 to 9·2.

Gallstones, cholelithiasis

Very little is known about the occurrence of gallstones in ancient Egypt. Only a very few cases are known from mummies as their viscera were destroyed in embalming. Earlier reports on the frequency of gallstones in Europe are almost completely lacking, but according to von Haller they were a common complaint in the eighteenth century in Göttingen, Swabia, Hungary and England. According to Bollinger, during the latter part of the nineteenth century gallstones were considerably more common in Basle than in Munich.

In St Erik's hospital in Stockholm all the gallstones found in autopsies in the years 1930–46 were registered and it was shown that the frequency fell somewhat during the economic crisis of the early thirties and even more so during the restrictions of foodstuffs during the war period. Before and after this period almost 25 per cent of all

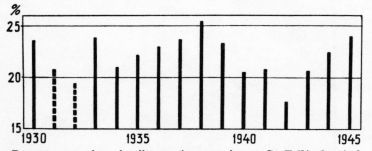

Percentage number of gallstones in autopsies at St Erik's hospital, Stockholm, 1930–45. The low figures from 1931–32 are uncertain, but could correspond to the then prevalent economic crisis. The significant fall in the cases of gallstones during the period of crisis, with a minimum in 1942, is very noticeable. (After F. Henschen, 1946.)

Stockholmers had gallstones; during it the frequency fell to 17 per cent.

Among non-European countries, Thailand should be mentioned, as there in 1960 Stitnimankorn in 3,283 cases of autopsy material found 46 cases (1·4 per cent) of gallstones. In Japan the gallstone frequency varies from place to place but it remains between 3·05 and 6·8 per cent, according to Kido in 1930.

A similar investigation is reported by Enderlin in 1958 from Zürich, where among 4,100 autopsies he found 1,000 cases with gallstones or gallstone operation, i.e. about the same percentage as in Stockholm. Every fourth woman and every tenth man had gallstones.

Gallstones do not necessarily produce morbid symptoms. The majority of the men and women who at autopsies are found to have concretions in the gall bladder, almost certainly never had any idea that they had gallstones.

8 Diseases of the Urinary System

Urolithiasis, stone formation, concretions in the urinary passages

The formation of solid bodies, concretions in the kidney-pelvis, urethra and bladder, has almost certainly been a very common disease in all periods of history. However, only a few cases are known from ancient Egypt—a boy from pre-Dynastic times is supposed to be the oldest. Both Elliot Smith and Shattock mention a few cases. The reason for this apparent rarity is no doubt the embalmer's technique of removing the organs at embalming. As urinary stones were a common complaint, the lithotomist's art was developed to perfection in the surgery of the time and it flourished in ancient China, in India and Europe. The term lithiasis stems from the *Hippocratic Collection*. Arab doctors mention urinary stones. A mediaeval legend about the Emperor Henry II (*c.* A.D. 1000) and his stones is very well known; the operation which was performed on him has been rendered into sculpture by Tilman Riemenschneider in the cathedral in Bamberg, though it is considered by many more likely to represent a castration.

Exact information about the frequency of urinary concretions is lacking, but it is known that they were an extremely common complaint in Holland two or three hundred years ago. In Amsterdam there is a large collection of them, some beautifully set in metal. Urinary stone, according to C. P. Thunberg, was also a common complaint in eighteenth-century Bengal. One has the impression that urinary stone, especially in children, has become less common during the last century. Finke's reports from England of the end of the eighteenth century seem to indicate a varying frequency from town to town, which in itself does not seem improbable. In Norwich 1 in every 55 operations was for urinary calculus, in Newcastle 1 in 287 and in Manchester only 1 in 557. Lilian Jonsson has made calculations on the occurrence of urinary calculi in Stockholm both in old times and 40–20 years ago, which seem to show a falling frequency. In children, mostly boys, the number fell from 0·084 per cent to 0·016 per cent, and in adults during the same period from

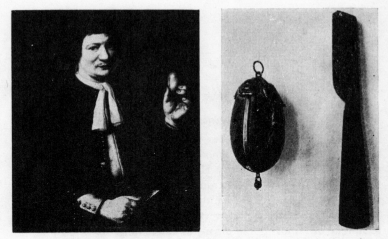

A seventeenth-century Dutch stone-carver shows with satisfaction the urinary stone which he has removed from himself. In his right hand he holds his knife. The picture to the right shows the beautifully set stone and his knife. In Amsterdam there is a large collection of urinary stones often decorativly set and inscribed.

0·77 per cent to 0·19 per cent of cases of disease. Men made up between 90 and 95 per cent of the cases in adults.

It is difficult to find definite figures for the frequency of kidney stones. If one relied entirely on the numbers of operations then one would think the number of cases had risen considerably, but this is probably more apparent than real. A compilation of the number of kidney stone operations in Sweden shows a considerable rise; however, it certainly cannot be taken as evidence of a real increase, mostly rather of an increased frequency in the operation. The figures show annual average numbers of operations.

1911–14	1915–18	1919–22	1923–26	1926–30	1931–34	1935–38
5·55	6·55	11·37	16·30	26.41	44·14	64·83

In Germany, Austria, France, Switzerland and Lithuania, Praetorius, Grossmann, Blum, Bibus and others all have found an increase, but in Holland, the home of urinary calculi, they have become rarer. In Dalmatia Racic found them mainly among the poorer classes. McCarrison has investigated the high incidence in poor people in India. In large parts of the Near East, it is a very common complaint which is to a certain extent associated with ordinary inflammations of the bladder and also avitaminosis. The chemical composition of the concrements varies from country to country, probably according to different foodstuffs. In Egypt there is to a large extent a special factor, namely the very common bilharzia infection in the bladder wall which has already been dealt with on pp. 153–4.

9 Diseases of the Reproductive System

Abnormalities

The forms of bisexuality or hermaphroditism, in which the female form, face and breasts are associated with male external organs, are of great cultural, artistic and medico-historical interest. Bisexual themes are widespread in the myths and rituals of the past. In the East it was once thought that there originally existed an androgyne, i.e. a double-sexed deity, as a symbol of potential fertility and that this androgyne then split in two, man and woman. In the ancient Egyptian myths Isis says: 'There is no god who can do what I have done, nor a goddess. I made myself into a man, although I was a woman.' In the ancient Jewish scripts and in Plato there are also glimpses of such bisexual beings. In the art of Egypt, India and especially of Greece and Rome there are numerous representations of hermaphrodites. It is impossible here to go further into the question of how far these bisexual creatures derive from ancient representations and true observations of individuals of mixed external sexual types, or to what extent they are purely imaginative creations by the artists. As with many other cases of abnormalities, Janus's head for instance, there are probably representations inspired by real human abnormalities. A hermaphrodite such as the beautiful bronze statuette from Mirecourt, now in Epinal, can be produced as evidence. It has a woman's breasts but the external sex organs show realistic hypospadias, i.e. a very small penis with a channel-like urethra in the under surface. As an example of bisexuality being shown in animals also, one can mention the great dragon in the St Göran group in Storkyrka in Stockholm, Berndt Notke's masterpiece. It is a hermaphrodite, as also are Chinese dragons which the art-historian Carl Neumann told me are said to be bisexual, while European dragons are said to be male.

Male reproductive organs

WHO in 1959 gave a report on deaths from prostatic hypertrophy, enlargement of the prostate gland, but the tables do not permit any conclusions about the true frequency of the disease. A compilation of deaths from prostatic hypertrophy among blacks and whites in the United States is of much greater interest. According to this, coloureds in 1957 showed a mortality of 40·5 in 100,000 and whites only 25·2. One must, however, approach these figures with discretion. They do not necessarily show a racial difference and could well indicate that whites seek treatment for prostate enlargement earlier and more commonly than do coloureds. Before prostatectomy, the removal of the organ, became an ordinary operation with minimal mortality, 'urine-block' or 'stone' was a very usual disease as well as a common cause of death. In many cases of 'stone' the disease was of course not prostate hypertrophy, but urinary calculus, which has already been dealt with on pp. 241–2.

Female reproductive organs

WHO in 1959 gave a table of mortality during the years 1955–57 from complications in pregnancy, delivery and during climacteric. The sharply varying figures to a certain extent correspond to the care of women in these three categories. The figures show a maximum in Ceylon of 370·8 per 1,000 and figures of about 300 in Mauritius, Colombia and Trinidad. Low figures, 48·2–41·2, are found in Denmark, England and Scotland, and the lowest in Sweden (36·4) and among US white women (27·6).

Seizures, eclampsia, in association with delivery, and their causes were discussed at the conference of geographical pathology in Paris in 1960. As far as the frequency was concerned, it was evident that these morbid states show both historical and geographical, or rather ethnographical frequency. This can be for different reasons. During the latter part of the First World War, cases of eclampsia decreased in Germany and then rose again to the old level after the war. This, according to Hinselmann, is associated with restricted and poor diet. According to Hauch and Lehman, the variations are more likely due to the low frequency of primigravidae which increased after the war. Remmelts and De Snoo are also of the opinion that in the first place it was the composition of the material with numerous primigravidae which made the frequency of eclampsia rise; dietetic conditions also contributed. Some researchers considered that there were no differences in the incidence associated with climate and race, while others stressed the significance of demographic circumstances such as the race and age of the women. Anyhow a considerable decline in pre-eclampsia and eclampsia was noted. Before the Second World War the frequency was estimated at 2–3·5 per thousand, but after the war it was said that the frequency could only be expressed in fractions of 10,000.

Pike and Dickins have investigated blood-group conditions in pregnancy toxaemia, pre-eclampsia, and consider it is shown that the disease is statistically most common in women of group O.

10 Diseases of the Muscular and Skeletal System, Deformities

Skeleton and joints

The great significance of bone and joint changes in palaeo-pathological research has already been dealt with in the Introduction. When all the soft tissues of the body have long vanished, the skeleton and teeth may still remain and give us a certain, although often very limited, idea of the diseases of that time. The skeletal system reacts to only a few diseases in such a characteristic way as to enable definite diagnostic conclusions to be drawn from the prehistoric or historical material at hand. Many bone changes are also difficult to interpret if one does not also have the soft tissue changes; in addition there are post-mortem changes with the release of the minerals of the skeleton in a wet and acid environment, as well as damage by insects and worms.

Under favourable circumstances skeletal and dental remains can, with the help of modern techniques, be profitably used and give gratifying results, as Hammerlund-Essler has shown. Even research into blood groups can lead to definite conclusions through the examination of old bone material, even if only minimal quantities

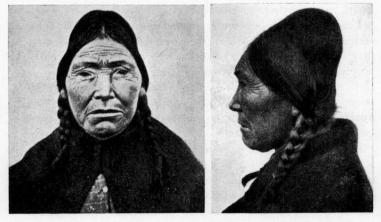

Eskimo woman with unusual deformity of the skull. From American expedition to Arctic North America.

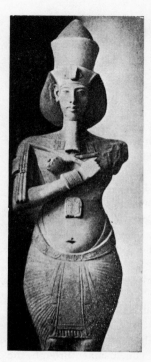

*The great statue of Akhen-
aton in the Egyptian
Museum in Cairo. Note
the narrow waist, broad
hips and long narrow face,
which in profile has a
projecting jaw.*

of haemoglobin are preserved in the bone marrow, as Madeleine
Smith has recently demonstrated.

I can here only briefly touch on the numerous artificially achieved
skeletal changes, which are in themselves very interesting, whether
they are deformities, trephinations, scarifications, burn marks, or
purely traumatic injuries from cuts, stabs, crushing or accidents.
Deformities of the skull by suitable treatment of the soft pliable
cranium in childhood have occurred in both the ancient and modern
world. In Riddarholm church in Stockholm there are a Swedish
queen, probably from Frisland, and her daughter, who, according to
Fürst, had their skulls treated in accordance with mediaeval fashions.

In this connection perhaps a few words can be devoted to the
strange head and body shape of the Pharaoh Akhenaton and to the
shape of his daughters' heads. As far as the Pharaoh himself is
concerned, his head at least was probably of the shape which
contemporary sculptors and caricature drawings portray: a long
narrow drawn-out skull and more or less female features. His famous

248

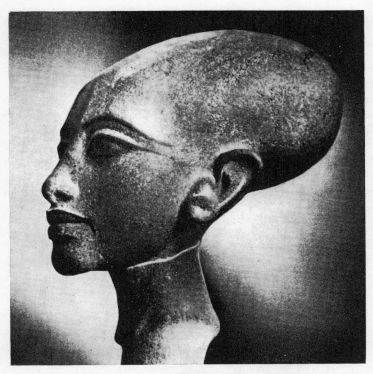

Egyptian princess, one of the daughters of Akhenaton, with a strange, flat, projecting head. It is not known whether the shape of the head was hereditary, whether it came from artificial moulding during childhood, or was simply an expression of the fashion in art at the time.

colossal statues show a narrow body and waist but broad female hips. It has been surmised that he was in fact a woman (Lefebure, 1890) or a eunuch (Mariette, 1855). His peculiar skull has even been interpreted as evidence that he was acromegalic and others speak of 'hypogonadism', 'clinical intersex', or 'hypopituitary eunuchoidism'. Feminine features have also been seen in his psychical behaviour; he was not aggressive and lacked the instinct of self-preservation. In addition his religious fanaticism and the building of a new city are said to indicate more of feminine emotionalism than mature masculinity. The mummy which is thought to be Akhenaton's is said to be severely damaged by water seeping down through a crack in the roof of the tomb, which makes it precarious to draw definite anatomical conclusions. Similarly Elliot Smith considers Akhenaton is a case of hypogonadism with delayed bone development, as the bone development is said to correspond to 23–26 years of age, but his historical age should be 37–40. The strange shape of head in his daughters, which is somewhat similar to his own, could be inherited or the result of deliberate compression of the skull, or else quite simply an expression of the sculptural fashions of the time.

Another artificial deformity is the ancient Chinese custom of binding women's feet from early childhood, forcing them into a pointed position with the toes bent under the sole of the foot. Many poets have praised these tiny feet which have been compared to

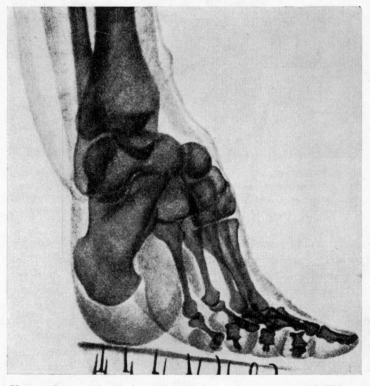

X-ray photograph of the deformed foot of a 32-year-old Chinese woman with the toes bent back under the sole of the foot (after Hans Virchow).

golden lotus flowers or golden lilies (Fang and Yu Fy, 1960).

Trephinations of the vault of the skull are essentially rare finds in ancient and mediaeval burial grounds, of both the Old and New World. Occasionally more than one hole is found in the skull; some have evidently not been done with rotating instruments, for they are squarer in shape, while others are beautifully rounded. Many cases are operations performed after or just before death; in others the patient must have lived on for a shorter or longer period, probably at least several months, judging from the scarred healing of the bone edges. In one Peruvian pre-Hispanic skull it is believed that a piece of bone had been inserted into a cranial defect, probably of a traumatic or inflammatory nature. It is not possible

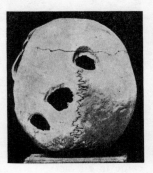

Vault of skull from a pre-Columbian Peruvian with three partly healed trephinations.

to go here into the 'indications' for these operations—whether they were done for predominantly medical or for ritualistic or magical reasons. Anyhow, such various artificial skeletal changes form an interesting field for research in which medicine, ethnography and archaeology co-operate with great success.

Deformities

Deformities of the external form have played a large part in the mythology and art of the past. Many fantastic mythical figures can be traced to direct observation and imitation of deformities in humans and animals. The Greek Cyclops myth and the double head of Janus have many parallels in human teratology, the study of deformities. The double eagle in the Habsburg imperial coat-of-arms probably had its origin in a case of so-called duplicitas anterior, i.e. a bird monster with two heads. In the Nordic sagas trolls are often represented as dwarfs.

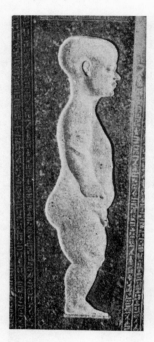

Pouoinhetef, an achondio-plastic dwarf, employed by Djiherpto, an important courier to Pharaoh Nec-tanebo II, 350 B.C.

The frequency of deformities in new-born infants seems to be the same in all races. In over 2,000 African infants, 5·4 per cent had deformities of some kind, mostly polydactylism and fistulas round the ear passage, but rarely deformities in the central nervous system (Simkiss and Love).

Deformities of the chondrodysplasia type (achondroplasis, etc.) were remarked very early on. The popular Egyptian god Bes, with his great head and short limbs, has been interpreted by researchers such as Dawson as a representation of chondrodystrophy, and by others as a man originally from a pygmy tribe in the interior of Africa. The oldest known skull showing chondrodystrophy dates from the eighteenth Dynasty in Egypt and belonged to a 20–25-year-old woman (Seligmann and Keith). Mettenleitner has described a chondrodystrophic skeleton, probably from the Merovingian period. It is not possible to mention all the portraits of dwarfs, mostly achondroplastic, which are found in the art of recent centuries, for instance in Velasquez. Grebe has recently dealt with this theme. All the grander courts, especially in Spain and Italy, but also occasion-

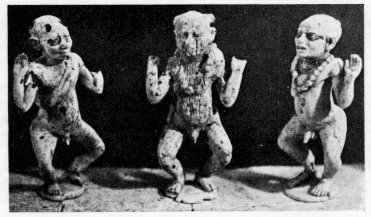

Three dancing dwarfs or perhaps pygmies imported from Central Africa to amuse important Egyptians.

ally the Swedish court, had dwarfs in attendance. In Mantua, in the Gonzaga family's ducal palace, there is a whole suite of small rooms and staircases with low steps for the dwarfs.

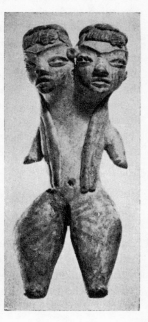

Deformity with symmetrical cleft of cephalic extremity, duplicitas anterior. Ancient Mexican sculpture, 10·5 cm high.

253

Chondrodysplasias are hereditary diseases but the difficulties in tracing their heredity have been very great as such deformed people do not often bring children into the world. In Denmark and southern Sweden the genetic and geographical conditions have been investigated by Mörch. Chondrodysplasia, according to him, is the result of a mutation, the frequency of which can be estimated at about 10 per 100,000 new-born infants and about 2 per 100,000 adults. In geographical isolation a collection of cases can occur. Related but not identical hereditary skeletal anomalies have been described in Norway by Bennevie in 1915, and in Sweden by Silfverskiöld in 1925, Ribbing in 1937 and Böök in 1950. During an anthropological expedition to Cyprus in 1952, I visited, among other places, a Turkish village in which there were numerous chondrohypoplastic people among the approximately 1,400 inhabitants.

Another hereditary bone disease which also has geographical interest is osteogenesis imperfecta, inherited brittleness of bones, which was first described in 1788 by the Swedish army doctor O. J. Ekman in seven individuals belonging to four generations in Dannemora in Uppland. Smårs has shown on a map the incidence of cases in Sweden, which are to a considerable extent distributed according to density of population. In 1957 the frequency for the whole population was about 4 per 100,000.

In this connection perhaps one can mention a bone change, the nature of which is still very unclear, Kaschin-Beck's disease. It manifests itself in a shortening of the long bones and a swelling of the joints, especially in the hands and feet, and it is endemic in Korea, Manchuria and Siberia. Morbidity varies considerably and in some places over 10 per cent of the population may be affected. It is commonest in low-lying delta country and its cause is suspected to be a chronic intoxication, possibly from mould fungi (Nomoto, 1958).

Anomalies in the skull and its bone formation, and in the spinal column

Abnormal skull shapes of all known types are familiar from the burial grounds of Egypt and among many other peoples. Among historic personalities with strange skull forms one can name Pericles, who because of his conical skull was called 'onion-head' by the Athenians and whose portrait busts always show a tall helmet; Erasmus, who to hide the shape of his ugly, abnormally short head, always wore a stuffed biretta on the back of his head; and Emanuel

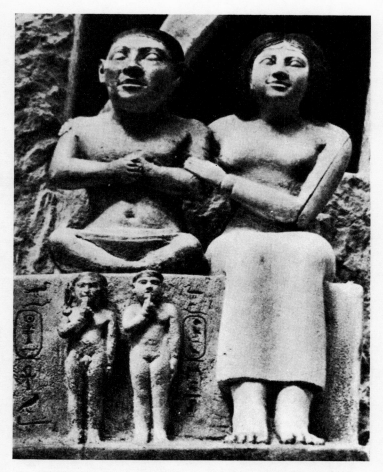

The famous family group of Seneb with his wife and two children. Seneb is generally characterised as an achondioplastic dwarf, but his head is not of that type; it is more like a case of micromelia, short arms and legs. The group was found walled in and well hidden so that posterity should not be able to see Seneb's deformed limbs. There is something very touching about the group with the wife's tender gesture and the attractive children.

Swedenborg whose abnormally long and narrow skull was completely hidden under a curly wig. Supernumerary skull bones, 'Inca bones' and 'ossa wormsiana' (ossa suturiala), have also often

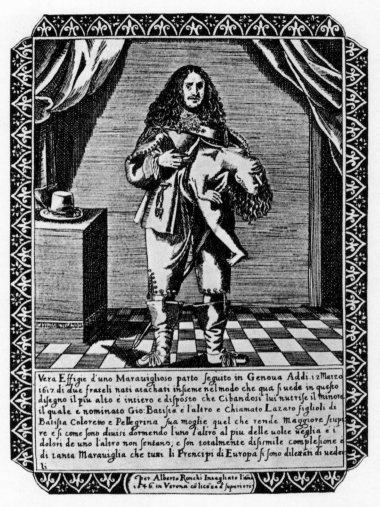

Vera Effigie d'uno Marauiglioso parto seguito in Genoua Addi.12Marzo 1617 di due frateli nati atachati insieme nel modo che qua si uede in questo disegno il piu alto e intiero e disposto che Cibandosi lui nutrise il minore il quale e nominato Gio:Batista e l'altro e chiamato Lazaro figlioli di Batista Coloreto e Pellegrina sua moglie quel che rende Maggiore stupore e si come sono diuisi dormendo l'uno l'altro al piu delle uolte ueglia e i dolori de uno l'altro non sentano, e son totalmente disimile complesione e di tanta Marauiglia che tutti li Prencipi di Europa si sono dilettati di uederli

Per Alberto Ronchi Insaghato l'an.
1646 in Verona cõ licenza d superiori

Asymmetrical double deformity with an apparently normal half (autosite) and a severely reduced half joined to the autosite at the line between the chest and upper part of the abdomen (parasite), a sterno-pagus parasiticus. This monster, which caused an enormous sensation in the seventeenth century, was born in Genoa where the autosite was christened Giovanni Battista and the parasite Lazaro. The autosite went to Holy Communion but the parasite was refused it as it could not speak. The picture is from Verona, 1646.

256

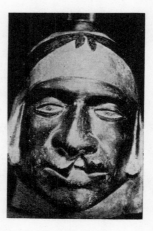

Cleft lip, 'hare-lip' or cheiloschisis. Peruvian ceramic from the Mochica civilisation.

been described. In Peru, Inca bones occur in about 5 per cent of all skulls and in the West Indies they are almost twice as common, in some groups the frequency rising as high as 20–23 per cent. The persisting 'metopic suture', in the centre line of the forehead, is also of interest and in most cases soon disappears. In ordinary cases its frequency is 1–4 per cent but in isolated places can rise to 30 per cent (Gejvall).

Congenital bone defects have been described in a number of cases,

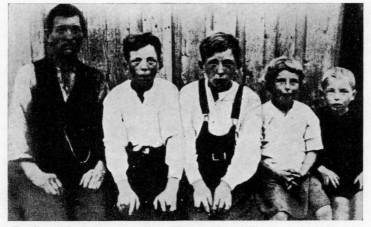

Family with finger anomalies. Three such families were examined by Bonnevie in 1919 and all three originated from the same parish in south Norway.

257

usually of brain rupture, encephalocoele, or so-called dermoid cyst lying partly inside and partly outside the cranium, or meningioma from the brain membrane. These have been found in ancient Egypt and in an Alaskan Eskimo. An Egyptian archaeologist found a mummy of an anencephalus, a deformed human embryo without a brain, buried among the ape mummies in Heliopolis. Finally it should be mentioned that among the skulls of America's prehistoric Indians, several cases have been found of a very rare anomaly, atresia (absence) of the external ear passage.

Cases of cleft lip, jaw and palate (cheilo-, gnatho- and palato-schisis) occurred in ancient Egypt and Peru, and this deformity was known and portrayed in ceramics.

A number of different deformities of the spinal column which need not be specified here are known from Pharaonic Egypt and ancient Peru, as are also congenital hip luxations.

Deformities of the hands and feet, fingers and toes, mainly supernumerary or 'webbed', are quite common, and mostly are cases of congenital inherited characteristics. A number of Danish and Swedish researchers have studied these anomalies which often occur in isolated places.

In palaeontological and anthropological literature one often finds accounts of variations in the thickness, density and weight of the skull, which are unusual and which are occasionally stated to be pathological or characteristic of certain races. According to Martin, Herodotus states that Persians were said to have especially thin skulls and Egyptians especially thick ones. Thin skulls are also said to be typical of Etruscans and Polynesians. Cushing and Eisenhardt mentioned the unusual thickness of the Negro skull. It has not really been established that different races have different skull thicknesses and similar generalisations can naturally only be confirmed if a sufficiently large amount of material is investigated and also categorised by sex and age, which is very rarely the case. The thickness and weight of the skull depends on a number of different kinds of factors, endocrine factors probably being decisive. Of the different types of skull-thickening which the American S. Moore described, frontal hyperostosis, first described by Morgagni, is incomparably the most important and interesting. It occurs virtually only in women after the menopause (Henschen). The cranium of the elderly woman in the Oseberg ship in Oslo, possibly the famous Queen Åsa, has this bone change.

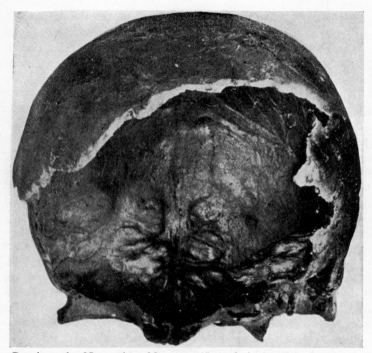

Cranium of a Norwegian old woman (Iron Age), found in the Oseberg ship. The cranium, the back of which is missing, is seen from behind and shows a symmetrical nodular new bone formation on the inside of the frontal bone, a typical Morgagni's hyperostosis. Much points to this being the skull of Queen Åsa. (After Henschen, 1949.)

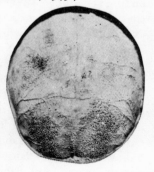

Interior of cranium with thousands of small holes, so-called cribra cranii. (early nineteenth century, Stockholm), probably a manifestation of chronic nutritional disturbance (after Henschen, 1960).

An American, Angel, has studied porosity and sclerosis in prehistoric and more recent skulls. He is of the opinion that variations in the porosity of the skull are connected with nutrition and social structure. In ancient Greek skulls of about 2000 B.C., porosity is said to be a common change, and also in those from the period of decline that followed the era of prosperity. Such changes should perhaps be regarded with caution; against Angel's explanation is the fact that the skull is only to a very limited extent associated with alimentary (hunger) osteopathia (see below). One has more reason to suspect that the porous skulls in question have been exposed to decalcification in acid soil over the centuries.

A strange skull change, pitted atrophy, which is occasionally found, has been observed particularly in crania from the Middle Kingdom by the famous Egyptologist Elliot Smith. He has connected this with the wearing of heavy wigs; the matter cannot be discussed here, but nevertheless his theory seems very unlikely.

Hydrocephalic crania have been described from different prehistoric and historical periods. According to Grimm, the earliest dates from the late Stone Age and belongs to a five- or six-year-old child. Even at this early time, it seems that sick children were cared for. A number of similar skulls are known from Egyptian burial grounds from archaic to Roman times. Similar skulls from elsewhere have also been described. Gejvall investigated two cases from the mediaeval churchyard on the island of Frös.

In this context perhaps a few words should be said on the peculiar changes which go by the name of cribra cranii et orbitalia and which have long been considered to be characteristic of certain races and geographical regions. Their appearance has already been touched on (p. 175). Mongolians and Negroes are said to show such cribra to a considerably larger extent than Europeans. Møller-Christensen's excavations of two mediaeval Danish monasteries, Æbelholt in northern Själland, and Næstved in southern Själland, of the same period, in almost the same region and with the same population, have shown clear differences in the incidence of these cribra. In the northern monastery which was an ordinary cloister and probably quite prosperous, cribra were rare whereas in the southern monastery, which was a leprosarium and partly lived on alms, the changes were considerably more common. This seems to me to indicate that skull changes have something to do with nutritional circumstances and probably with the morbidity too. A circumstance which also points in this direction is that these skull changes can again be found in skulls from ancient times in the pathological museum in the Karolinska Institute, Stockholm, but were not once observed in the 2,000 crania, the interiors of which were carefully examined over a period of two years in the 1940s.

The bone and joint change described by P. Marie, which goes by the name of hypertrophic pulmonary osteoarthropathy, is occasionally seen in chronic heart and lung diseases and is principally manifest in the long bones and the fingers. It can easily be confused with syphilis. In the examination of the skeletal remains of King Magnus Ladulås in Riddarholm church, where he was buried in 1290, Fürst in 1920 found similar very pronounced changes which provoked a scientific discussion. At the time of the king's death syphilis had not yet occurred in Europe and both E. Sjövall and L. Aschoff were able to exclude it with good grounds. But it is known

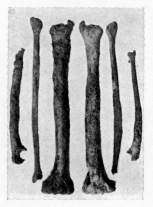

The long bones from the skeleton of King Magnus Ladulås from his tomb in Riddarholm church, showing severe chronic changes in the bone surface, probably as a result of a chronic heart or lung disease from which the king seems to have suffered. Magnus died in 1290.

from the Chronicle of Erik that the king for many years suffered from a chronic disease which certainly did not prevent him carrying out his duties in an excellent manner.

Tyrgils Knutsson wrote:

> As he felt that his sickness was so
> severe, that he could not escape death,
> then he chose before he died
> a wise man, faithful and loyal,
> to rule over the kingdom.

Alimentary osteopathia (hunger osteopathy), which occurs in severe undernourishment, according to Klotzbucher and Daliche, principally affects the spine and ribs, less often the upper and even more seldom the lower extremities. The skull seems to be least affected; in cases examined, only in 6 per cent. This is said to be a case of an avitaminosis D in association with a lack of calcium, phosphorus and protein. The name hunger osteopathy, according to Knorr, is rather unfortunate as one never sees such skeletal

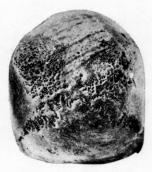

Prehistoric cranium with strange porosity, reminiscent of 'brush skull' in certain forms of anaemia (from Adachi, Porosität des Schädeldaches, *1904).*

changes before the age of 45 and it is said to be in fact more a case of presenile and senile skeletal changes. The as yet not completely explained problem of alimentary osteopathia has been mentioned here because such skeletal changes are probably to be expected if one could examine skeletons from the great population groups in Asia and Africa who live under miserable nutritional conditions.

Rhachitic skeletal changes are, as far as one can judge, extremely rare in archaeological material, both in Egypt and in America. Nevertheless, it is possible that a few typical cases have been found in Scandinavia (Fürst; Gejvall). In one of the cases from northern Sweden the molar teeth were also characteristically changed.

Spongy hyperostosis of the skull, 'brush-skull'

This strange skeletal change which occurs in certain anaemias (p. 214) also has palaeopathological interest. Hrdlicka found it in ancient Peruvian skulls from the coast but not in the inhabitants of the Andes, and Williams, who examined 176 pre-Hispanic Peruvian crania, also found it in both children and adults. It is said to be especially common in Yucatan, Mexico, where Hooton found no fewer than 14 cases in 21 child skulls; also in New Mexico and Arizona, USA. Pre-Columbian skulls from other parts of the USA showed the same peculiar change.

Disuse atrophy of the skeleton is seen after early paralysis of the muscles, especially with 'polio' in children. Rolleston found a shortening of the left arm in a Stone Age skeleton but whether this was a case of polio is not known. In Egyptian mummies atrophies of one leg have been repeatedly observed, after polio as far as can be judged, and Michell found a similar case in a mummy more than 5,000 years old. Pharaoh Siptah had an atrophy and 'pointed foot' which was almost certainly a result of polio in childhood. A very beautiful portrayal of an early 'polio-atrophy' of the leg can be found on a stone relief carving in Copenhagen which shows the Eighteenth Dynasty priest Ruma supported by a stave as he offers sacrifices to the gods (p. 45). In a case described by El Batrawi, from archaic times, the bones of both legs were thin but not particularly shortened. This case has been interpreted as double-sided paralysis of the legs (paraplegia). Ribera painted what is probably a case of poliomyelitis with residual atrophy and contraction in the right arm and leg (p. 47).

Inflammatory bone changes of a septic nature are found in very early human remains, though not very extensively. When considering changes in such old skeletal remains, one must in any case be extremely cautious, as post-mortem processes of different kinds are often similar. An example of a septic process from a relatively late date is the well-known cranium of Lionello d'Este which shows a severe relapsing mastoiditis from the middle ear, inflammation of the mastoid process behind the ear.

Joint and spinal changes of a non-inflammatory nature, arthroses and spondyloses

Boudouin calls these changes 'the oldest diseases in the world', a remark which is probably true if one adds 'that are known'. The facts are, however, that the giant reptiles of the Chalk Age showed joint and spinal changes which are exactly similar to those which afflict older people today and cause them so much trouble. Animals from much later geological periods also sometimes show these changes.

Human beings have suffered from arthroses and spondyloses since the earliest Stone Age, and examples occur from the upper and lower Pleistocene periods. Skeletons from the oldest eras of Egypt, Nubia, China, Scandinavia and North and South America give us a wealth of similar skeletal changes, but they are not always easy to interpret.

The difficulty lies in deciding whether they are cases of joint and spinal injuries mainly due to wear and tear, or whether they are to a certain extent, perhaps even quite often, due to what is nowadays called rheumatoid arthritis. The Egyptologists Elliot Smith and Dawson consider that their Egyptian and Nubian skeleton collections mainly show 'rheumatoid' changes; they believe too that a special Egyptian complaint is involved which affected quite young individuals. Whether their interpretation is correct must be left at that. The same diagnostic difficulties apply to joint and spinal changes in American Indians.

Arthroses and spondyloses are also common in skeletons from considerably later periods than that of the Pharaohs. Gejvall has shown how common they were in his studies of a large amount of material from the mediaeval churchyard on Frösö. It is probable that the heavy mechanical labour these Jämtlanders had to do from quite an early age contributed to the incidence of the changes.

Changes in the joints of the jaw have often been found in skeletons of pre-Columbian North American Indians, but it is difficult to say whether they had been of an inflammatory or degenerative nature.

Muscular diseases

Several muscular diseases have shown themselves to be hereditary, but in a population which is not markedly stable from generation to generation, they are of no particular geographical interest. An example of a muscular disease of a hereditary character with a limited geographical distribution is dystrophia myotonica. Its frequency in Denmark is estimated at 2·5 cases per 100,000 inhabitants and in Switzerland it is about twice that, 4·9 per 100,000. In a recently published study, Rolander and Floderus have shown that the disease occurs in Norrbotten county with a frequency of at least 37 cases per 100,000 inhabitants, and that it is principally localised in the south-eastern region (Boden, Luleå, Kalix and Haparanda).

11 Diseases of the Skin

Different artificially caused skin changes, such as tattooing and deliberately acquired, severe, thick scars or keloids, I ignore here, although they are of great cultural, historical and psychological interest. The only one I will mention is the so-called 'Weichsel pigtail', *plica polonica*, a mass of matted hair, dirt, sweat, lice and other matter at the back of the head, which was once commonly worn in Poland. Finke, who seems to think it a case of disease, writes 'that it affects the poor more than the rich, nor does a high degree of cleanliness protect one from it'!

Hereditary skin anomalies and diseases occur in all parts of the world. If they occur in geographically isolated areas, then they become of great interest.

Albinism is found in all races. In white populations it is rare— one case per 10–20,000 individuals. Albinism is known as dominant heredity in certain negro tribes. In 1960 Björnberg reported on albinism in the Cuna Indians in Panama and Colombia, where it is

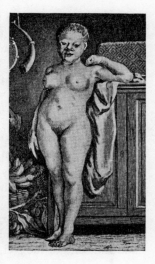

White Negro girl of about 18 from the West Indies. Her parents were imported from the then Gold Coast and, like her brothers and sisters, were black. Drawn from life by Buffon in 1777 and published the same year in his Histoire Naturelle.

265

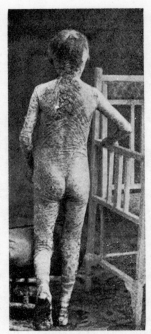

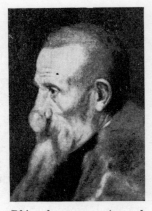

Rhinophyma or 'pound-nose', chronic inflammation of the skin and glands of the tip of the nose, which is often portrayed in art. Painting by an unknown artist, Stockholm.

Case of ichthyosis or scaly skin, exhibited as 'Elephant Girl Suzy' at fairs (1961).

said to be common as 1 in 200–300. These albinos are called 'moon-children' or 'moon-eyed', their skin is white to pink, often freckled, and the hair on their heads and bodies is white to straw-coloured. The lack of pigmentation in their eyes leads to photophobia, light-shyness, and the children have to stay indoors in daytime. It is possible that Columbus saw them on his fourth voyage. They correspond to Linnaeus's *'homo nocturnus'*.

An example of a strange hereditary skin anomaly is the Norwegian family with 'dappled skin'. Sundför investigated this in 1939. The family live in a very small area of central Norway and the disease takes the form of severely pigmented, usually symmetrical patches on the face and all over the body; in sunlight the patches turn very dark.

An interesting hereditary skin change is keratodermia palmaris et plantaris, a severe thickening of the horny skin of the palms of the hand and soles of the feet. According to Floderus, it is common in

266

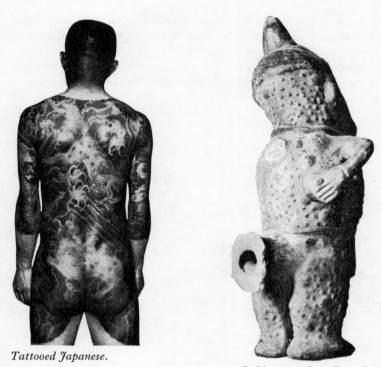

Tattooed Japanese.

Itching rash. Peruvian ceramic. (Leprosy? Pinto?)

Norrbotten in Sweden, where over 700 cases have so far been registered. There is said to be no similar concentration of this skin anomaly elsewhere. Another hereditary skin change, which in severe cases can lead to death, even in children, is ichthyosis, a thickening of the horny layers of the skin, like fish-scales. Groups of cases also occur in geographically isolated areas.

Psoriasis is in many cases one of the most easily recognisable skin diseases. It has, however, long been confused with other skin changes, especially leprosy, scabies and pellagra. These severe scaly and irritant skin diseases could once not be distinguished, in Assyria, Babylon, ancient Egypt, the Near East, India and China. The Hebrew word *zaraath*, the Indian word *vipadika* and the terms *lepros* and *psoriasis* used by Greek doctors really mean something other than scaly skin rash. Those who had psoriasis were simply

267

put together with the lepers and referred to as *'pauperes Christi'* (the paupers of Christ), who were forced to live in isolation with special warning signs of recognition.

According to G. Lomholt (*Psoriasis*, Copenhagen, 1963), psoriasis is more common in cold and temperate climates than in warmer zones, and is rare in the tropics.

12 Diseases of the Sensory Organs

Blind Peruvian Indian. Polychrome ceramic from the Mochica civilisation.

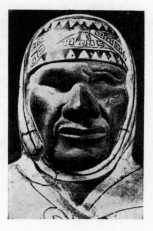

The eye

Blindness is a concept which means many things, according to the degree of sight. Nor does the word say anything about the causes. The number of blind people varies extensively from country to country, as do the most important causes of partial and vanished sight.

Among the different forms of blindness are several of great geographical interest, including hereditary amaurosis, recently described by Alström, which occurs in northernmost Sweden and has been known since the end of the sixteenth century. A form of hereditary sight degeneration due to the degeneration of the macula, the middle part of the retina, occurs in a parish in Dalarna. It has been possible to trace this back four and probably six generations (Barkman, 1961).

In the countries of the West the number of blind is estimated at about 1·5 per thousand. In Sweden a figure of 10,000 has been reached, corresponding to an equivalent frequency. In contrast there is India, where the estimated number of blind is as much as 2,000,000. As examples of how the causes of blindness vary from

269

country to country, the following facts are of interest. In England, according to Sorsby, the most important causes are cataract and senile changes in the macula; after these follow eye changes with severe myopia, short-sightedness and diabetes in the 50–69 age-group; finally a number of hereditary and congenital anomalies and certain forms of inflammations (iridocycltis, iritis).

In Ethiopia, Torgersruud calculates the following statistics for causes of blindness: ulcers in the cornea 27 per cent, syphilis 16 per cent, external injuries 14·6 per cent, trachoma 13·9 per cent, glaucoma 13·9 per cent, other causes, including smallpox, 14·6 per cent. Trachoma does not play the same role there as in Egypt. The number of blind in China and India is still very great. In India only a few years ago there were 1·5 million blind and 4·5 million partially sighted, mostly because of trachoma, smallpox, gonorrhoea, syphilis and other inflammations, as well as worm infestation. In China it is estimated that at that time there were approximately the same number of blind. In the rural districts of Bengal, Sen lists the eye changes which lead to blindness in the following order: cataract, glaucoma, keratitis, trachoma. In Hong Kong, Korea and Formosa lepromatous changes are particularly prominent, and also corneal injuries and eyelid changes of different kinds, especially following trachoma. According to Chitnis, the most important cause of blindness in India is smallpox, next come eye diseases in infants, especially trachoma, and then inadequate diet, hereditary and congenital defects, treatment by quacks and syphilis. Mann and Löschdorfer, who studied eye diseases in Papua and New Guinea, found trachoma in 53 per cent of all those examined. In one village where 378 eye patients were examined, no fewer than 85·7 per cent had trachoma. Quite the most important causes of blindness here were external injuries. As these peoples seldom reach old age, cataract played a very small part indeed.

Cataract has been known for a very long time. In India it is called 'the shining white pearl' and, according to Susruta, was treated surgically centuries B.C.

Colour blindness

Red-green colour blindness, which is sex-linked, occurs in Europe in about 8 per cent of men but is very rare in women, about 0·5 per cent. It occurs when the X-chromosomes have been damaged. It has been said that red-green blindness is much rarer

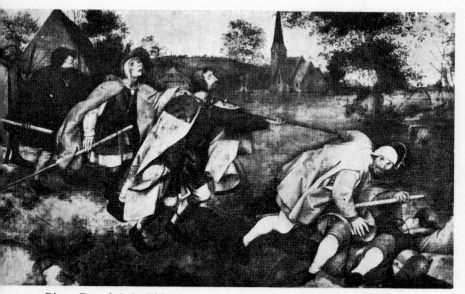

Pieter Breughel the Elder (1525–69), The Blind, *signed 1568. Museo Nazionale, Naples,*

in most of the other races. Several investigations have been carried out into the incidence of colour blindness in different races, partly, however, based on very little material. According to Yang Chun and others, a survey covering 13,071 Chinese showed an incidence of 5·22 per cent in men and 0·47 per cent in women. Another Chinese survey had given an incidence of 5 per cent and 0·8 per cent in women; only red-green blindness was investigated. An investigation in Australia showed 7·3 per cent of defective colour sight in white men and 0·61 per cent in white women; in coloureds 3·2 per cent and 0 per cent; and in indigenous Australians only 1·9 per cent and 0·031 per cent. So Australia's primitive races have better colour sight than Europeans. Certain Indian tribes and Todas are said to have even fewer colour blind and among Eskimoes only 0·8 per cent of the men are said to be colour blind.

Total colour blindness (achromatopsia, monochromasia), in which all perception of colour is absent, is extremely rare and its frequency in Europe is estimated in general to be 1 : 100,000 or even 1 : 400,000. In geographical isolation it can be considerably more common. On the little island of Fuur in Limfjor, Denmark, Holm and Lodberg in 1940 found no fewer than 23 cases among the island's 1,600 inhabitants, i.e. a frequency of more than 1·4 per cent. Immigration and emigration caused the frequency to fall in following generations. In the above-mentioned Chinese surveys, no case of total colour blindness was found.

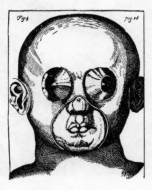

Treatment of squint or strabismus by a facial mask. Engraving from a work by Georg Bartisch (1535–1607), eye surgeon to the Elector of Saxony.

The ear

In congenital deaf-mutism, consanguinity, i.e. intermarriage between related carriers of the tendency, plays a large part, and can lead to groups of cases in geographically isolated areas. In north Sweden a short while ago there was a region with no fewer than 0·145 per cent deaf-mutes. The frequency in Stockholm at the same time was 0·049 per cent.

Liu-Juei-Hua and others have recently examined 560 children from both the Peking schools for the deaf (347 boys and 313 girls) and they found that about three-quarters suffered from deafness which they had contracted during their first four years. In 1·2 per cent there was congenital syphilis.

13 Nervous and Mental Disorders

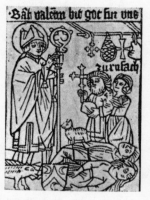

St Valentine of Rufach with two epileptics and two men praying. Woodcut from Alsace of c. 1480.

Only in very rare cases is it possible to mark the early occurrence of nervous and mental disorders. In palaeopathology (the science of diseases in ancient times) one can find examples of abnormalities in the brain and spinal cord such as anencephalus, encephocele, hydrocephalus and atrophies and paralysis after poliomyelitis, and these have already been dealt with. Facial paralysis was already known to doctors of the classical period. Galen mentions a case of loss of sensation in the hand after injury to the spine.

A disease with very old roots indeed is epilepsy—*morbus sacer*, the holy disease. There is no difference, wrote Hippocrates, between the 'holy disease' and any other. If people think it divine, then there are many holy diseases and not just this one. According to Wellman, however, this famous remark does not stem from Hippocrates and his pupils, but from Alcmaeon of the ancient Croton school. Many Greek and Roman authors wrote about epilepsy, as did Arab and European mediaeval doctors. Several of the greatest figures in history suffered from epilepsy, Mahomet being the best known, who, because of his many epileptic attacks, was considered by the people to stand near to Allah and to gain strength from him to prophesy. Exact information on the number of epileptics does not

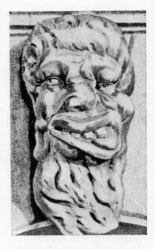

Mask from the church of S. Maria Formosa, Venice. The great neurologist Charcot explained that this was not an imaginary portrait but showed a hysterical spasm of the lips and tongue.

exist but in the United States it is estimated that there are about 800,000, i.e. 1 per 200. The history of focal epilepsy has been described by Fulton in 1959.

Knowledge of hysteria also goes back a long way in time. Passio hysterica was for a long time understood to be a disease emanating from the uterus, *hystera*. Indian and Arab doctors knew the symptoms of hysteria very well, but that it was in fact a nervous disorder was first shown by Piso in 1714.

The fundamentals for a comprehensive geography of nervous and mental disorders do not as yet exist. Reference can be made to

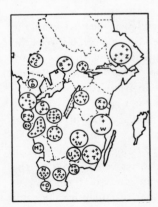

The 23 loci of juvenile amaurotic idiocy in Sweden in 1920s (after T. Sjögren). All the loci are country parishes, often quite isolated and with little movement in or out.

sample trials covering a small number of countries and diseases. The same applies to the incidence of mental defects, oligophrenia, in their different types and grades. As they are often cases of hereditary intelligence defects and nervous and mental disorders, countries with areas still geographically isolated devote themselves to research into the hereditary circumstances of these abnormalities, and in this the Scandinavian countries have been well to the fore. If these diseases occur in higher frequencies within geographically isolated areas and if with the help of archives and other records one can trace them far back to a certain limited area and family circle, then they naturally become of great geographical interest.

Myoclonus epilepsy can be cited as an example of a nervous disease occurring in a limited area. Lundborg carried out research into this disease at the end of the last century. In Sweden it was then known only on the Lister peninsula in western Blekinge. There, from the eighteenth century on, there was for economic reasons a considerable amount of consanguineous marriage, from which hereditary tendencies have become manifest. Lundborg was of the opinion that the morbid tendency had originally come to Blekinge from outside, but this is very uncertain. The disease is found in several European countries and I myself have seen cases from the region round what is now Leningrad. It has also been described by Janssen in a negro family in Ruanda-Urundi, where it is said it can be mapped geographically.

Another hereditary disease with a geographically limited locus is juvenile amaurotic idiocy, studied by T. Sjögren in 1931, which has twenty-three loci in southern Sweden, generally in remote districts with considerable consanguinity. Due to the present increased marital connections with the country as a whole, this recessive hereditary disease is rapidly declining. Sjögren also investigated the inherited form of dance-disease, Huntington's chorea, in two parishes in northern Sweden, and the numerous Swedish loci for hereditary motoric disturbances, hereditary ataxia. A form of hereditary tremors, which are very rare in Europe as a whole, was described by Velander in an isolated Swedish community in upper Norrland on the border of Lapland; it was further studied by Larsson and Sjögren in 1960. Mjönes in 1947 investigated the geographical distribution of paralysis agitans, a paralysis associated with tremors, and he found that 47 per cent of all cases lived within two small areas of the country. Finally, one should mention a

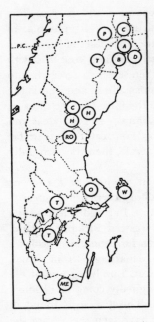

Loci of several Swedish hereditary diseases:
A. Agranulocytosis. B. Congenital blindness. C. Chondrodysplasia. D. Dystrophia myotonica. H. Huntington's chorea. ME. Myoclonus epilepsy. O. Osteogenesis imperfecta. P. Polydactylism. RO. Rendu-Osler's disease. T. Tremor hereditarius. W. von Willebrand's thrombopathia.

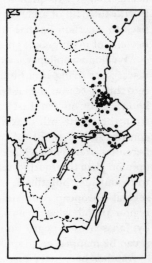

Hereditary distal myopathy. The place of birth of the first known case or transmitter of myopathy in 72 families (after Lisa Welander, 1951).

relatively recently discovered neuro-muscular disease to which Lisa Welander has given the name myopathia distalis tarda hereditaria. It is concentrated in a small area of central Sweden.

A recently discovered nervous disease, possibly of a hereditary degenerative nature, occurs in the eastern mountain districts of New Guinea. It is known as *kuru*, and is found mainly in the so-called Fore tribe and their neighbours, in all about 17,000 individuals (Klatzo; Gajdusek; Zigas). Mortality is high and the main symptom is ataxia. Severe microscopic changes are found in the cerebellum (little brain) and elsewhere. Fischer and Fischer very much doubt the hereditary character of the disease.

Among organic nervous diseases with no obvious prominent hereditary tendencies first and foremost comes sclerosis disseminata, multiple or disseminated sclerosis, which is characterised by

276

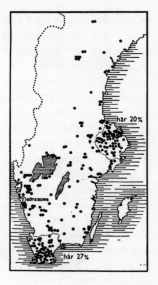

Incidence of paralysis agitans in Sweden (after Mjönes, 1949). 27 per cent all cases are in Skåne, 20 per cent in Uppland and neighbourhood.

numerous plaques in the brain and spinal cord with scar formation (gliosis). As with many other nervous diseases, geographical research is complicated by the difficulties which arise in early diagnosis. The number of registered cases in Europe is slowly rising, but whether this is due to a genuine increase of cases or, more likely, to improved diagnosis, is hard to say. A calculation of the frequency of the disease in Europe probably gives some kind of picture of its incidence, if an uncertain one. The highest figures per 100,000 are shown in Scotland and Northern Ireland with 3·0 and 3·1; Ireland shows 2·6, England only 1·8. High figures are found in France (2·9), in Austria, Switzerland and Denmark (2·2–2·0 per 100,000). Sweden shows 1·3–1·1. In North America, Canada shows no increase and low figures much as in Sweden, and the USA come lowest, with only 0·9 per 100,000. Here the division between the two races may be considered of some interest if one can assume that Negroes seek medical aid to the same extent as whites. In whites the number rose from 1,227 (1950) to 1,343 (1956), and in Negroes during the same period from 51 to 66. These figures do not correspond to the relative size of the two races but may possibly show that whites are affected by the disease more than twice as often. It is also possible that the disease is in fact rare in Negroes. The figures from Japan are markedly low: in 1950 57 cases, in 1956 54, which would correspond to only 0·1 per 100,000 inhabitants.

A study of the geographical distribution in Sweden was made in 1942 by Sällstrom who, however, could not show any clear geographical localisation tendencies. Since then other investigations have been undertaken in which attempts have been made to correlate the geographical, geological, climatic and hereditary factors.

In the USA Lichtenstein thinks that he can show that multiple sclerosis is more common in low temperatures and unstable atmospheric conditions, as in Canada and the northern USA, than in the southern part of North America, and he maintains that similar conditions can be shown in Italy and Turkey. A study of 1,782 US veterans gave fairly consistent results, if they were divided according to places of birth. The disease increased from south to north in all states regardless of the longitude, and also if Negroes were kept separate. Canada, however, showed higher figures than were expected. These reports on a higher frequency in temperate than in sub-tropical zones have since been confirmed from both America and Russia.

The significance of genetic factors has also been investigated. According to Curtius, a genetic factor can no longer be doubted, but the hereditary predisposition may suppress significant manifestations and in addition allergic conditions are said to contribute in the genetically determined constitution. Both McKey and Myrianthopoulos have, like two earlier researchers, tried to solve the problem of an eventual heredity by the twin method, i.e. they have investigated whether twins have multiple sclerosis more often then others, and they consider that a hereditary factor is shown. Finally Georgi and colleagues (1961), in investigations into the frequency of the disease in Switzerland and East Africa, think they can show that the disease is not of an infectious nature but is caused by an agent as yet unknown. A collection of cases within a certain family does not necessarily mean heredity but can be explained in other ways.

Mental disorders

Until quite recently there were available only few investigations and brief reports on the occurrence and forms of mental disorders in

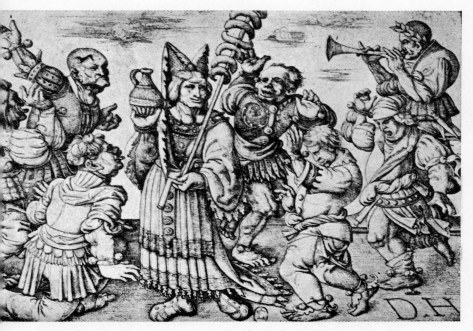

The Dance of the Lunatics, *early sixteenth-century engraving by Daniel Hopfer. Six lunatics dance to the music of a trumpeter wearing a laurel wreath, round an old woman with a wine jar and a long stick of sausages. The woman has a nodular goitre.*

different races, and the study of 'comparative psychiatry' founded by Kraepelin in 1904 has as yet not advanced very far. But with the knowledge we have today of the widely differing psychosomatic characteristics of different races and populations, we may justifiably presume that there are at least certain differences between the great races of Mongolians, Negroes and whites and also within different populations. It is a fact that variations in environmental conditions and what is called civilisation are of great significance in the forming of types of mental disorder and neurosis. As Yap so rightly states, there is no justification for judging, by orthodox European and North American psychological and psychiatric norms, neuroses and psychoses in alien races and populations who live under quite different forms of civilisation. Presumably, as Yap says, there are in certain cultural areas specific characteristic mental disorders which

279

are hereditarily, psychologically, culturally and sociologically pre-determined and which are also based on special climatic factors, nutritional conditions and the effect of drugs.

A work called *Culture and Mental Health* (1959), published by Opler, marks a step forward. In it, twenty-two anthropologists, sociologists, psychologists and psychiatrists attempt to give a picture of the effects that civilisation and the stresses which accompany it have on spiritual health. Standardisation of methods of work and comparable material are of course the prerequisites for obtaining comparative results by such studies. An example of the facts which are thought to have been established is a statement by Wittkower and Fried on the subject of 'transcultural psychiatry'. In general in primitive civilisations schizophrenics are calmer than in the West. The blunting of emotions and other signs of psychic decline have been described from Africa and India. Manic-depressive psychoses are rare in technically backward populations, but in contrast acute and chronic manic forms are relatively common. The specific syndromes which have been called koro, imu, latah, amok, Arctic hysteria, etc. are briefly mentioned on p. 197. A closer study of these problems, which are both interesting and difficult to treat, is here impossible, the more so as the literature on the subject is already very great and increasing rapidly.

In Denmark, Norway and Sweden there has been an attempt to define statistically the psychic health of the population over more or less limited areas, and, with some reservations, to draw conclusions about the population of the whole country. In Denmark Strömgren made such investigations in 1935–50 and to them can be added Svendsen's (1952) into psychical disorders in Denmark during the Second World War. In Sweden as long ago as 1932 T. Sjögren began a similar study of a north Swedish peasant population; he continued in 1948 with a study of genetic and psychiatric circumstances in a west Swedish population; and he has now, together with Larsson, completed an investigation into a large Swedish coastal population (1954). They have estimated the number of psychoses and oligophrenias (mental deficiency) in the total population of Sweden, showing both the number of cases found in 1945 and the estimated number for 1965. Naturally in many respects their figures cannot be definite but they are none the less of very great interest indeed. The table below shows the number of patients in thousands.

	1945			1965		
	Men	Women	Both sexes	Men	Women	Both sexes
Schizophrenia	21	18	39	24	20	44
Manic-depressive psychosis	8	14	22	10	17	27
Senile and pre-senile psychosis	3	6	9	5	8	13
Other forms of psychosis	10	10	20	12	12	24
All psychoses	42	48	90	51	57	108
Oligophrenia, over 10 years of age	20	15	35	22	17	39

In addition there are Essen-Möller's study of mental disorders in rural inhabitants in Sweden (1956), Hagnell's studies of neuroses in southern Sweden (1959) and an investigation carried out by Fölling, Mohr and Ruud into the form of mental deficiency known as oligophrenia phenylpyruvica (recessive hereditary mental deficiency with excretion of phenylpyruvic acid in the urine), which occurs, among other places, in Norway. It also is found in the British Isles where it is more common in Wales than in England.

Coming to psychical disorders in populations which are radically different from our own, only a few examples can be given here. Chinese who live in the USA are said to suffer from neuro-psychiatric disorders to a much greater extent than in China. In Java, melancholic depressions are much more common among immigrant Chinese than among indigenous Javans. Negroes who work far from their homes show similar psychical disorders, whereas they are rare in Negroes living in their original environment. In Kenya, as in Java, manic-depressive psychoses are said to be rare among the native inhabitants. On the other hand Hrdlicka states that Indians in South America have more psychoses than whites. Lima Nato has given interesting accounts of psychopaths in Pernambuco, now Recife. Ehrström has described mental disorders in certain Eskimo tribes.

Deleterious psychic effects are also found in workers who move from one European country to another. Poeck has described 'hypochondriac depressions' in Italian workers who have found employment in Germany but cannot adapt themselves to their new environment.

Modern life in Europe and North America almost certainly favours the occurrence of neuroses and other psychical disorders. The well-known American clinician Rowntree (1958) emphasises 'the ascendancy of nervous and mental disorders. Half of our 700,000 hospital beds are taken up by patients in this category. Judging from medical statistics we shall soon be a nation of neurotics.'

Collective mental disorders

An extremely interesting chapter in the history of mental disorders is the subject of collective psychosomatic manifestations, psychopathically based excesses in different forms. A good deal is known about the excesses of every conceivable kind which took place at cult ceremonies in honour of the gods of Assyria, ancient Egypt and Greece. The best known perhaps are the Dionysiac ceremonies with their ecstatic participants. In this context attacks of berserk rage, sustained by drugs, are also relevant. During the Middle Ages, outbreaks of mass religious mania became almost a folk-disease in Europe. Raving flagellants, men and women, marched unrestrainedly through many countries. In convents similar acute mass psychoses occasionally occurred. The fourteenth and fifteenth centuries saw occurrences of so-called St Vitus's Dance, which may have occasionally been a genuine chorea or dance-disease of the Sydenham or Huntington type. The Blockberg assemblies, which in Scandinavia had their equivalent in the Blåkulla assemblies, are all part of the epidemic incidence of psychopathy. These terrible witch-hunts went on all over Europe and continued right into the seventeenth and eighteenth centuries, a shameful blot on the history of Europe. In Sweden, Dalarna was particularly notorious. As late as 1836 a 'witch' was so maltreated that she died, on the Hela peninsula outside Danzig (Casper).

Similar but considerably more peaceful collective psychical excesses occurred only a few generations ago in eastern parts of the United States with the 'Jumpers' and 'Barkers'. The 'Shaker' sect, too, a branch of the Quakers founded in England about 1700, moved to the USA where it flourished during the second half of the nineteenth century.

Other examples of individual or epidemic infections of a hysterical kind are the *minryachit*, known from China, Malaya, Burma, Siberia, the Philippines and even Africa. The demoniac possession which occurs in medicine men can also occur epidemically, as can yogism and the abnormal condition known as 'amok' in which various toxins can also be involved. Other abnormal conditions which deserve mention in this context are 'Arctic hysteria', severer forms of Lapp

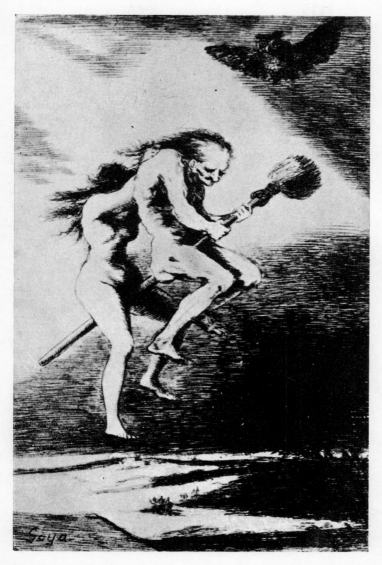

Engraving by Francisco Goya (1746–1828). A witch rides away with a young woman. Goya's text below reads 'Linda maestra' (roughly 'sweet mistress').

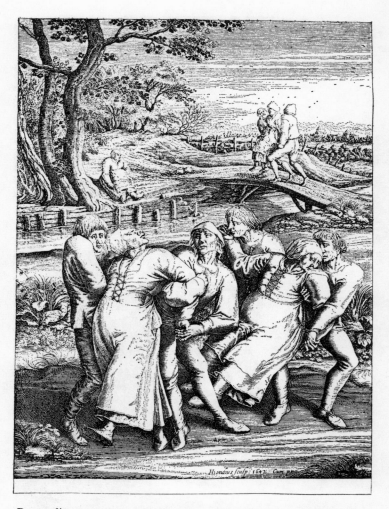

*Dance-disease, mass psychosis or hysteria. Etching by Hondius (1642)
after a painting by Breughel.*

disease, and 'Tropenkoller', koro, imu and latah. The 'Windigo
psychoses', of certain Canadian Indian tribes can manifest
themselves in murder and cannibalism (Wittkower and Fried,
1959).

284

Suicide

The frequency of suicide, both attempted and successful, varies both historically and geographically and will therefore be briefly dealt with here. The official figures must be treated with caution and in any case they are minimum figures. It is also obvious that such factors as race, culture and religion have a very great influence. Religion generally has a restraining influence. According to WHO, Turkey, Greece, Italy, Spain and Portugal show remarkably low figures, 3·8–8 per 100,000 inhabitants. Marked contrasts are shown by many countries in central and northern Europe, the highest number being in West Berlin with an average of 32·6 and a maximum of 34·2 per 100,000. Very high figures also came from Austria (23·9), Denmark (22·1), Finland (21·9), Hungary (21·7), and Switzerland. Especially low figures are shown by Ireland (2·4), Scotland, Holland and Norway. I shall come back to conditions in Sweden below.

Countries where different races or adherents of different religions live side by side are of especial interest. In Toronto during the years 1925–38, Frank found 4·5 suicides among Protestants, 5·6 among Jews and no fewer than 11 among Roman Catholics, all calculated per 100,000 inhabitants. In the USA as a whole in the years 1955–57 the equivalent of 10·5–11 per 100,000 committed suicide, but among US Negroes only the equivalent of 3·8–4. In the Union of South Africa whites showed a figure of 11·3–11·5, Asiatics 12·4–10·0 and Negroes only 2·3–2·8. Among non-European countries, Japan in 1955–57 had very high figures—25·2–23·9.

It is known from experience that urbanisation and city life, with many individuals living in isolation, raise the figures for suicide and attempted suicide. The same applies presumably to detribalisation in Africa, involving the dispersal of tribes with their ancient customs and sense of community.

In Sweden, with its relatively unified population which, however, lives under differing climatic and social conditions, with a few cities and densely populated areas such as Malmöhus county, and with large thinly populated rural areas, the official figures show quite large variations. The highest frequency occurs in Stockholm and Malmöhus county, both with 21·2 per 100,000. Jönköping county, where the Free Church movement is very pronounced, has low figures, as do Blekinge, which is considered a rather poor area, and the strictly High Church county of Göteborg and Bohus, all with 12–11·5 per 100,000 inhabitants. The lowest figures come from the great, thinly populated areas in the extreme north, the counties of Norrbotten and Västerbotten, with 8·0 and 6·7 per 100,000 inhabitants—figures which are in contrast to the high figure of 21.9 in neighbouring and equally thinly populated Finland.

14 Tumours

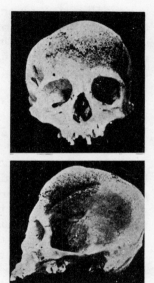

Peculiar porous bone over-growth on the cranium of a pre-Columbian Indian, due to a meningoma or tumour growing out from the dura mater of the brain. Several similar cases of bone overgrowth are known from North and South America, and from Egypt.

History

Tumours are found in early palaeontological material but naturally almost exclusively in the skeleton. They may be primary bone tumours, which are known in both the Old and the New World, or primary tumours in the soft tissues, particularly the prostate, mammary and thyroid glands. We know very little about primary tumours of the soft tissues in those remote times. One of the extremely rare cases is P. Møller's case of calcified tumour inside the thorax.

Of the primary bone tumours, multiple exostosis (growths on the bone) and non-malignant osteoma (bone tumours) are the best known. In some cases a severe blow or trauma lies behind the incidence of osteoma. Another form of bone overgrowth is quite often found with meningoma, tumours growing outwards from the dura mater of the brain which can affect the skull bone and occasionally give rise to very pronounced raised bone formations. Several such cases are known from pre-Columbian America, both North and South (MacCurdy; Moodie; Abbot and Courville; Cushing and Eisenhardt; Netsky and Lapressle). An example of a malignant bone tumour is a colossal osteosarcoma which MacCurdy has described in a pre-Hispanic Peruvian. Osteosarcomas in the femur and pelvis are also known from ancient Egypt, even occurring in the mummy of an ape, which had a large one in the armpit. Another primary tumour in the skeleton is multiple myeloma growing from the bone marrow, a small number of cases of which are known from both the Old and the New World.

Metastatic, secondary tumours from ancient Egypt are also known, especially in the cranium (Elliot Smith), and Møller and Møller-Christensen have described a case in a young woman from mediaeval Denmark.

Representations of tumours also occur in art. There is a well-known Greek statue, a votive image, which is considered to portray a tumour in the mammary gland. From Peru there is a ceramic representation of what is thought to be an eye tumour. One finds accounts of malignant tumours and their treatment in ancient Egyptian and Indian texts. In the Ebers papyrus, according to Sigerist, cancer is a tumour which is not to be touched. On the other hand it is known that the Egyptians used a caustic ointment for treatment of surface cancers—unguentum aegyptiacum, composed of arsenic and vinegar—which was still used in the sixteenth century. The Indian epic *Ramayana*, of about 2000 B.C., mentions tumour treatment by a red-hot iron. Herodotus relates how Democedes, a Greek slave at the court of Darius the Great in Susa, is said to have cured Cyrus's daughter, Queen Atossa, of a cancer or abscess of the breast about 520 B.C.

The old name *karkinos* (cancer) was used, according to Galen, for certain tumours, especially cancer of the breast, because of the tumour's tendency to spread out like the claws of a crab. The word carcinoma comes from the Greek verb καρκινόω, to spread out, like for instance the roots of a tree or crab feet, and means in particular an open ulcerating tumour. Leonides of Alexandria defied Hippocrates' warning against operating on cancers and tried to operate on a breast cancer with a knife and red-hot iron. Galen,

Cranium of pre-Columbian Peruvian with a large bone-forming sarcoma or malignant tumour of a non-epithelial nature (after MacCurdie).

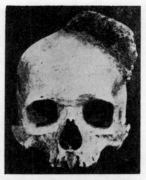

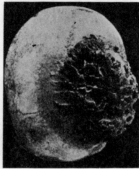

Pre-Columbian Peruvian cranium with artificial deformity and large irregular defect which was once interpreted as a trephination but is more likely due to destruction of the bone caused by a tumour. National Museum, Buenos Aires.

who was doctor to the Roman Emperors Marcus Aurelius and Commodus, also left a contribution to the study of tumours. According to Sigerist, there is no mention of cancer in mediaeval medical literature. Clemmesen records that the first description of a group of cancer cases as an occupational disease dates from the beginning of the sixteenth century when Agricola and Paracelsus, who were both interested in mineralogy, described what they called '*mala metallorum*' (evils of metals), now known as '*Schneeberger Lungenkrebs*', naturally without realising that it was a case of a specific form of lung cancer associated with radioactive mine dust, which was not properly understood until the present century (1926).

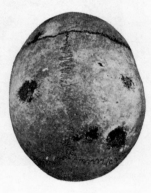

Vault of the skull of a mediaeval woman aged about 30, found in Aebelholt Cloister in Själland. It shows five irregular holes which are probably due to destruction of the bone through cancer metastasis, secondary cancer from a tumour in some organ, or multiple myeloma, a rare bone-marrow tumour. Closer diagnosis is not possible.

It is not necessary here to consider the more recent developments in the study of cancer since the accounts of Virchow and others in the middle of the last century, or the latest progress due to the perfecting of the light and electron microscope.

Geography and demography

It would be hazardous to attempt to give a brief, comprehensive and, as far as possible, dependable account of the geographical incidence of tumours and their frequency in different demographic categories. The difficulties are associated with incomplete statistics, with widely differing competence in doctors and hospitals, with varying willingness of populations to seek medical aid, and with variations in scientific diagnoses and nomenclature. Thus reports from different countries are often incommensurate and unsuitable for the purposes of a comparative study. As early as 1886 Hirsch

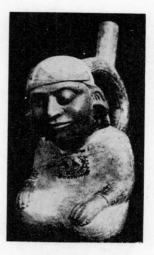

Indian with tumour or some other affection of the left eye. Peruvian terracotta, Mochica civilisation.

quite rightly complained about the lack of reliable mortality statistics on tumours.

It was for a long time believed that tumours were 'diseases of civilisation' and that primitive peoples were largely free of this scourge of civilised man. To a certain extent this is absolutely true, but these so-called 'primitive peoples'' relative freedom from tumours is largely due to the fact that their average life-span is so short that the individual seldom lives to the age when most cancer cases arise.

A tumour panorama covering the whole of the world will long remain an unfulfilled dream, since for every country, even for every region, considerable prerequisites must be fulfilled if reliable international statistics are to be achieved:

1. An adequate number of observations on every specific form of tumour, preferably collected over a short, carefully defined period of time by experienced clinicians and pathologists and analysed in accordance with modern methods.

2. Information on the sex index: i.e. the relative numbers of men and women; separate reports for the two sexes; division into age-groups—something which has been impossible in large areas of the world where illiterates seldom know their age.

3. Information on whether large cities are involved, or suburbs, or smaller towns, or more or less densely populated areas; further information on local conditions—division into occupations, form

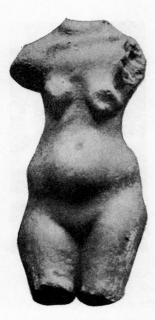

Torso with contracted cancer in left breast. Evangelical School Museum, Smyrna.

and extent of industries with possible pollution of air and water.

4. Information on social conditions, nutrition, deficiency diseases, habits, good and bad (tobacco and alcohol).

5. Information on whether different races live together, and on adherence to different religions, if this applies.

6. Information on the origin of the material, whether autopsies, biopsies, material from a well-equipped hospital, from private doctors or based on non-medical reports.

7. Information on whether morbidity or mortality figures are given; whether the cases are treated or untreated, and in the former case, whether the treatment is surgical, therapeutic or of any other kind.

Geo-demographic information gains considerably in value and interest if information on historical changes in the tumour panorama can also be given. Every tumour is a disease in itself, and the causal complex of tumours can only be found if information on as many different factors as possible is available and taken into consideration.

In a short and comprehensive account of the geographical incidence of tumours, one can choose two ways of approach. One can describe the whole tumour panorama of each individual country or region and then compare the different countries with each other, or one can deal with each particular form of tumour separately and compare its frequency in different countries. With either approach one quite naturally comes across the pathogenesis or conditions of incidence of the form of tumour. In order to condense this account as much as possible, there are below a number of tables on which anyone can, without too much effort, reflect and draw his own conclusions.

Total number of malignant tumours in certain countries according to WHO, 1950 and 1957. Mortality per 100,000 inhabitants.

	1950	1957		1950	1957
EUROPE			AFRICA		
Spain	98·2	102	Union of South Africa		
Italy	113·5	135·8	Asiatics	35·4	37·3
Iceland	132·9	144·3	Negroes	66·1	79·7
Finland	138·4	152·6	Whites	119·3	130·7
Holland	146·9	158·6			
Norway	158·4	160	ASIA		
Ireland	141·9	167	Japan	77·4	91·3
Sweden	154·6	167·8	Israel	77	93·9
France	173·1	189·5			
West Germany	186·4	192·1	NORTH AMERICA		
Denmark	177	196·3	US negroes	108·1	113·9
Belgium	207·5	208·6	Canada	127·7	129·8
Scotland	193·8	208·7	US whites	143·5	154
England	194·5	194·5			
Austria	—	246·2	AUSTRALASIA		
			Australia	127·5	131·5
			New Zealand	—	149·6

From this table it is evident that mortality from cancer seems to vary in different countries. The considerable variations depend to a certain extent on the widely differing average length of life but are also largely due to great variations in exactness and completeness: this is also shown in the steep rise in many countries from 1950 to 1957. The very high figure for Austria can be explained by the considerable urbanisation (Vienna predominating) and it is exceeded only by West Berlin whose figure, 295·9, is not included in the table.

These mortality figures, however, give an incomplete and partially false picture of the frequency of malignant tumours, and a truer picture would be given if the figures for tumour morbidity were available, for many malignant tumours can now be cured with modern treatment. It is virtually pointless to carry out research into the causes of tumours, when information on age, sex, place of residence (town or country), occupation, etc., is lacking. Not until such differentiation is made can a cancer register offer the degree of usefulness one should demand.

In this respect Denmark has taken a lead. There are also now similar registers of morbidity and mortality in several other countries, Finland, Norway, Sweden and the USA. Several African and Asian countries have produced good but incomplete reports.

As examples of a useful systematic collation of the frequency of several different forms of tumour in men and women in Denmark and, by comparison, in the USA, there follow two sets of tables in which all the information is adjusted according to age (Clemmesen, 1956). The figures give the frequency of tumours per 100,000 inhabitants.

(– and – – mean decrease and large decrease.

+ and + + mean increase and large increase.)

Denmark 1948–52   *USA 1947*

MEN	Copen-hagen	Provincial towns	Rural districts	10 cities Whites	Coloureds
Mouth and throat	8·4 –	7·6 –	10·1	21·1	10·9
Digestive organs	110·3 –	100·2 –	84·1 –	110·5	96·9
Oesophagus	8 –	5·1 –	3·8 –	8·3	9·7
Stomach	37 – –	43·4 – –	41·8 – –	34·1	39·6
Large intestine	22·8	19·3	14	26·2	13·9
Rectum	25·2	22·5	17·4	22·1	12·7
Liver	5·4	3·4	2	4·9	5·3
Respiratory organs					
Larynx and trachea	3·6 +	2·2 +	1	7·7	5·9
Lungs	43·6 + +	14·3 + +	8·3 + +	29·5	25·4
Prostate	22·2 + +	17 + +	15 + +	34·8	49·9
Bladder	15·3 + +	7·7	5·6 +	18·6	7
Skin (incl. melanoma)	24 + +	26·7 + +	23·2 + +	56·1	4·5
Leukaemia	8·4	7	6·6	9·1	8·6
All malignant tumours	284·8 + +	227·7 + +	185·7 + +	338·3	252·6

WOMEN

Mouth and throat	3·7	7·6	2·6	6·3	5·3
Digestive organs	72·8 –	70·7 – –	69·4 – –	79·8	68
Oesophagus	1·6 –	2·4	2·1 –	1·9	2·2
Stomach	23·6 –	26·7 – –	29·8 – –	18·3	22·8
Large intestine	21 +	17·8 –	16·4	27·8	16·2
Rectum	13·9 –	12·2	11·2	15·2	13·6
Liver	3 –	3 –	3·4 –	4·2	2·7
Respiratory organs					
Larynx and trachea	0·3	0·1	0·2	0·6	0·6
Lungs	6·1 +	3·3 +	2·7	6·5	5·8
Breast	57·4	49·3	40·9 +	72·6	53·9
Womb:					
Neck	38·4	34·9 +	20·2 + +	38·8	70·4
Body	14·4 +	10·9	7·9	10·3	11·2
Ovaries	15·3	12·3	10·8	14·7	9·9
Bladder	4·3	2·4	2·1	8	7·9
Skin (incl. melanoma)	16·9 +	16·5 +	14·4	39·5	6
Leukaemia	6 +	5	4·5	6·3	2·9
All malignant tumours	272·5 +	241·5 –	208·6 –	333·4	293

Here follow two more tables, for men and women, covering the cancer morbidity (frequency of the disease) in New York State, in which differences can be seen between town and country and between the two sexes.

Cancer frequency per 100,000, New York State (excl. N.Y. City), 1949–51

MEN Age adjusted	Metropolitan counties		Non-metropolitan counties	
	Towns	Country	Towns	Country
All localisations	267·2	226·1	257·7	202·3
Mouth and throat	15·8	12·2	16·1	14
Digestive organs	90	75·4	79·5	62·5
Oesophagus	7·1	4·8	5·1	2·8
Stomach	24·1	20·8	22·4	20·4
Large and small intestine	24·4	18·8	23·1	17·1
Rectum	19·3	15·6	15·8	12·4
Others (liver, biliary passages and pancreas)	15·1	15·4	13·1	9·8
Respiratory organs	40·3	31·7	30·7	22
Lungs and bronchi	29·2	23·9	20·8	15·2

MEN Age adjusted	Metropolitan counties		Non-metropolitan counties	
	Towns	Country	Towns	Country
Prostate	27·9	22·6	30·9	25·3
Bladder	13·6	13	13·6	9·5
Skin	32·1	29·3	42·6	35·5
Leukaemia	9·6	8·4	6·8	5·1

WOMEN Age adjusted				
All localisations	245·9 –	217·2 –	256 +	222·2 +
Mouth and throat	3·8 – –	2·6 – –	4·1 – –	3·3 – –
Digestive organs	62·7 – –	58·4 – –	63·3 – –	53·7 – –
Oesophagus	0·9 – –	1·4 – –	1·4 – –	1·1 – –
Stomach	12·1 – –	11·3 – –	10·5 – –	9·2 – –
Large and small intestine	25	22·2 + +	27·7 +	22·5 + +
Rectum	11·9 –	10·3 –	12·1 –	9·1 –
Others (liver, biliary passages, pancreas)	12·8 –	13·2 –	11·6 –	11·2 –
Respiratory organs	5 – –	4·7 – –	5·3 – –	3·6 – –
Lungs and bronchi	3·2 – –	3·5 – –	3·2 – –	2·4 – –
Breast	58·1	50·3	55·4	49·3
Female reproductive organs	55·1	48·3	67·4	59·8
Neck	24·6	20·7	32·4	27·3
Body	14·9	12·4	18·6	17·4
Bladder	4·4 – –	3·6 – –	4·6 – –	3·8 – –
Skin	23·4 – –	19·6 – –	25·2 – –	22·3 – –
Leukaemia	6 –	5·8 –	5·4 –	4·9

There follow figures from Finland, Japan and Sweden which illustrate the differences between their structure in composition of the population, average length of life, food, climate, social conditions and economic circumstances.

Saxen, Finland, 1954. Cancer mortality per 100,000 inhabitants and as percentages of total cancer mortality

	MEN		WOMEN	
	per 100,000	% of cancer deaths	per 100,000	% of cancer deaths
Total mortality in cancer	164·6	100	141·1	100·0
Mouth and throat	3·4	2·1	0·9	0·7
Digestive organs	82·4	50·1	75·8	53·7
Oesophagus	7·5	4·5	7·9	5·6
Stomach	56·3	34·2	46·4	32·9
Large intestine	4·3	2·6	5·5	3·9
Rectum	4·5	2·7	4·3	3
Liver and biliary passages	2·1	1·3	2·9	2
Pancreas	4·4	2·7	3·6	2·6
Respiratory organs	42·4	25·8	4·1	2·9
Lungs only	36·9	22·4	2·9	2·6
Breast			13	9·2
Female reproductive organs			22·4	15·9
Neck			6·5	4·6
Body			4·9	3·5
Prostate	6·8	4·2		

Japan, 1956. Cancer mortality per 100,000 inhabitants and as percentages of total cancer mortality

	MEN		WOMEN	
	per 100,000	% of all cancer forms	per 100,000	% of all cancer forms
Total cancer mortality	98·4	100	83·3	100
Mouth and throat	0·9	0·9	0·5	0·6
Digestive organs	78·4	79·7	51	61·2
Oesophagus	5·1	5·2	2·1	2·2
Stomach	53·3	54·2	32·9	39·4
Large intestine	1·7	1·8	2·1	2·5
Rectum	3·2	3·3	2·8	3·4
Biliary passages and liver	1	1	1	1·2
Pancreas	1·6	1·6	1·3	1·5
Respiratory organs	7·5	7·7	3·4	4
Breast			3·4	4
Uterus (with chorioepithelioma)			16	19·3
Male reproductive organs	1·1	1·1		
Excretory organs	1·7	1·7	1·1	1·3
Skin	0·7	0·7	0·6	0·7
Blood-forming organs	4·5	4·6	2·9	3·5

Sweden, 1958. New cases of cancer per 100,000 inhabitants and as percentages of all new cases of cancer

	MEN		WOMEN	
	per 100,000	% of all new cases	per 100,000	% of all new cases
All newly discovered cases (8,924 men 10,400 women)	241	100	280	100
Mouth and throat	8	3·2	5	1·6
Oesophagus	3	1·3	2	0·6
Stomach	41	17·1	25	8·8
Large intestine	20	8·1	20	7·3
Rectum	16	6·7	10	3·7
Liver and biliary passages	4	2·3	5	2·3
Pancreas	8	3·4	7	2·5
Lungs	20	8	7	2·3
Breast	1	0·2	67	24
Neck of womb	—	—	24	8·6
Body of womb	—	—	17	6·1
Ovaries	—	—	21	7·4
Prostate	40	16·7	—	—
Kidneys	10	4·1	6	2·2
Bladder	10	4·3	5	1·8
Skin (with melanoma)	10	4·5	8	2·8
Leukaemia	9	3·8	7	2·4

The cancer register for 1959, which has now been published, shows a slight, barely noticeable rise in new cases from 19,324 for 1958 to 20,220 for 1959. But cancer of the stomach has decreased in men from 17·1 per cent to 16·2 per cent of all cancer cases. It is also evident from the latest publication that the number of new cancer cases per 10,000 inhabitants is lowest in Jämtland, Härjedalen and Dalarna, highest in Stockholm, Uppsala, Malmöhus, Göteborgs and Bohus county, and in Gotland, with a maximum in Stockholm city of over 34 new cases per 10,000 inhabitants.

The above tables give some picture of the incidence of malignant tumours in men and women and in various organs in different countries.

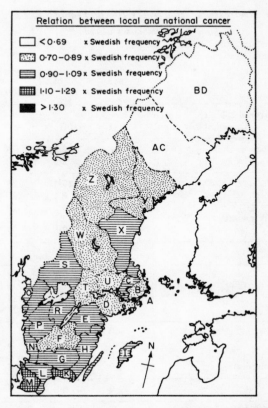

The map shows the relative frequency of all cancers in the different counties of Sweden and in Stockholm. The approximate frequency figure for the whole country is 261 per 100,000 inhabitants (241 for men, 280 for women). In both the northernmost counties, the frequency is only about two-thirds of the national frequency. In the dotted counties the frequency is well below the average. The horizontally striped counties show the equivalent of national frequency. High frequencies are shown in Blekinge and Malmöhus counties. Stockholm city shows the highest frequency. (After Cancer incidence in Sweden, 1958.)

There are, however, important questions which can only to a small extent be posed and answered by tables. They include whether racial predisposition and heredity exist in cancer, and the questions of age predisposition, of the significance of diet and deficiency diseases, of place of residence, its geology, its industries and consequent pollution of air and water, of the significance of occupation and profession, of the part played by external injuries and of habits in general.

Systematic study of the frequency of tumours is completely lacking in many countries, but observations and comparisons can still be of considerable interest. W. Fischer, who has studied the pathology of China (1958), says that bronchial cancer is common among men, that cancer of the gullet is more common than in Germany, that by contrast stomach cancer is about as common as in Germany, and that cancer of the liver is not, as had earlier been thought, the most common form.

Dungal has recently (1961) published an investigation into the frequency of lung cancer in Iceland, in which he states that the air in Reykjavik has been unusually clean since they began to use water from the hot springs for heating nearly twenty years ago. Cigarette smoking has increased considerably there and at the same time the lung cancer frequency has risen. According to Dungal the frequency of stomach cancer is extremely high in Iceland, and he associates this with the high consumption of smoked trout and mutton with a much higher than normal content of cancer-causing substances.

The position in countries where the population consists of several races who do not mix with each other is also of interest, despite incomplete information. Mardsen (1958) stated that in Malaya, where the population is composed of 49 per cent Malays, 38 per cent Chinese and 12 per cent Indians, lung cancer is more common in Chinese than in Malayans although both are heavy smokers. Throat, gullet and liver cancers are common in Chinese, cancer of the mouth common in Indians and lymphogranulomatosis rare in Chinese and Malayans. From Mozambique, Prates (1958) reported that both skin and breast cancers are more common in whites than in coloureds and that primary liver cancer is said to be more common there in the coloured population than in other parts of Africa. Cancer of the cervix of the womb, as opposed to cancer of the womb, is more common in Negroes than in whites. Lung cancer is rare.

Further information on the frequency of certain cancer forms can be mentioned. In the case of the two most important forms of cancer of the womb, cervix cancer and corpus cancer, it has been known for some time that Jewesses in both New York and Palestine have very little cervix cancer. The same is true of nuns. This subject will be dealt with further on p. 309. Cervix cancer is more common in towns than in the country, and is more frequently found in the southern than in the northern States, and more often among the poor than the better-off.

There are large fundamental studies by Davies, Higgins and Oettle and by Steiner of primary liver cancers in Africa. Contrary to what was formerly presumed, infestation by trematoda (sucker worms) in the liver is not of great significance, nor is it clear whether liver cancer always develops from a liver cirrhosis. In some places liver cancer is even more common than cirrhosis. The frequency of liver cancer varies geographically and its distribution coincides with that of virus hepatitis. It is therefore probable that liver damage from hepatitis starts the process, presumably reinforced by wretched diet, which was earlier thought to be a significant cause of the frequency of liver cancer in Africa.

Research into the geography and demography of the different forms of cancer is undoubtedly of great importance to the study of their hereditary and general causal conditions.

Possible racial significance

One would at first be inclined to ascribe a specific, perhaps large significance to race. But analysis shows that hardly anything definite is known about any eventual racial predisposition. The different races, by which I mean the genuine great races, mongolians, negroes and whites, live for the most part under such different external conditions, their length of life differs so greatly, their food too, that all these environmental factors more or less associated with race, become inter-determinative in the statistical calculation of cancer frequency.

If one uses the everyday meaning of race and looks for instance at circumstances in the Ukraine where thirty years ago the population was composed of Jews, Ukrainians and Russians, then there was there an obviously large difference, which is shown in the table opposite.

However, it is probable that the different cancer frequencies of the different population groups are not an indication of varying predisposition but mainly of the varying spiritual vitality and education levels of the three population groups. Among other things the table perhaps shows that Jews sought medical and hospital aid most often and Russians least often. Studies from other quarters,

Cancer in	Men	Women
Jews	89·7	86·9
Ukrainians	59·1	64·8
Russians	49·6	60·3

for instance from Tunis, Algeria and Morocco, mostly indicate that the population groups, whites, Jews and Moors, have about the same predisposition to cancer. In the case of coloureds and whites in the USA there are some definite differences as regards cancer frequency, but whether these differences are more apparent than real only further investigations can show; it is clear, however, that whites have considerably more skin tumours than coloureds.

Again, thirty years ago Dutch doctors made a thorough study of cancer frequency in the Javanese and Chinese of the East Indies. It was shown that mortality in these population groups was just about as high as in the inhabitants of Holland—if one considers parallel age groups. In the Javanese mortality was high at an early age, in contrast to which in the Chinese mortality increased with years approximately as in Europeans.

In many of the malignant forms of tumour it has recently been possible to show a clear, if generally only small, hereditary predisposition, but whether it is expressed in a geographically uneven distribution of cases, with hereditarily determined groups of one form of cancer in a particular region, is not known.

Sex differences need not be discussed further as they should be sufficiently clear from the tables.

Is the cancer frequency rising?

The rise with age of the frequency of cancer is a matter of great theoretical interest. Cancer is undoubtedly in general a disease of older age-groups. This is shown in graphs from all countries.

The reason for the increasing risk of cancer the longer one lives has not been entirely clarified. Formerly it was thought that the cells and tissues of the ageing organism were more predisposed to tumours, but the rising cancer frequency is probably a result of exposure over the years to different irritants which, when they have been active sufficiently long, cause cancer—perhaps even in individuals who lack an essential predisposition. It should, however, be stated that this cancer frequency rising for each year of life does not apply to all forms. Cancer in the female uterus reaches its maximum between 42 and 64 years of age, the maximum of the relatively rare testicle tumours falls between 40 and 50, and tumours of the nervous system in both sexes reach their maximum between 50 and 70 years of age. At advanced ages, after about 80, the cancer frequency falls considerably.

The significance of diet and deficiency diseases for the incidence of cancer is in some cases clear. As might be expected, cancers of the digestive organs and liver are particularly involved. With cancer of the gullet and stomach, considerable overweight in men is in all probability not a direct indication of sex predisposition, but due to the quantity and quality of diet and drink (tobacco? spirits?). The varying frequency of cancer in the pylorus can, as I said before, be considered socially determined to a certain extent. This has been

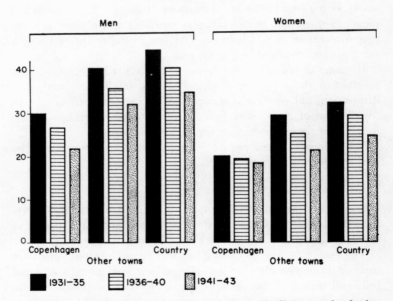

Deaths from stomach cancer as a percentage of all cancer deaths in Denmark. The frequency of stomach cancer seems to decline during the three periods which the investigation covers. (After Clemmesen.)

shown in comparisons between rural workers and city-dwellers in both Great Britain and Denmark, in studies of the incidence of gastric cancer within different social groups. On the other hand the frequency of cancer below the pylorus, i.e. in the large intestine and rectum, is said to be equally high in all occupations and social classes. The declining frequency of cancer of the stomach, which is true of many places—Denmark, the USA (according to Potter; Haenzel; and others) and also Sweden—is probably also associated with improved diet and a better 'stomach milieu', as I call it. The same applies to the fact that, according to surveys in such cities as Oslo and New Haven, USA, gastric cancer is more common in lower-income districts. In the case of liver cancer, Davies and other researchers, as I said before, have shown the significance of deficient diet which characterises certain parts of Africa.

The table overleaf, published by Potter, shows how in the USA certain forms of cancer increase while others decrease, and is of great interest. The figures are adjusted according to age.

The comparative frequency of different forms of cancer is by no means constant. For reasons one can only partly outline, one form gradually becomes more common in relation to others, which perhaps are on the decrease.

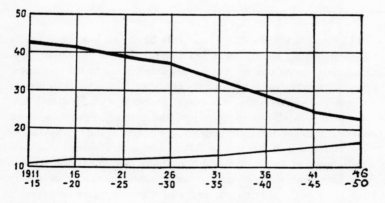

Deaths from stomach cancer (thick line) and from cancer of the large intestine (thin line) in Stockholm from 1911 to 1950, expressed as a percentage of all deaths from cancer (according to the official statistics).

		1933	1944	% Annual variation
	All cancers			
Men		106·8	116·9	+ 0·76
Women		125·3	122·7	− 0·38
	Cancers with falling tendency			
Men	mouth	6	4·2	− 3·8
	stomach	28·3	22·3	− 2·1
Women	mouth	1·3	0·9	− 3·4
	stomach	19·8	13·5	− 3·8
	Cancers with no clear tendency			
Men	oesophagus	3	3·2	0
Women	oesophagus	0·8	0·8	0
	rectum	5·2	5·5	0
	Cancers with rising tendency			
Men	pharynx	1·3	1·9	+ 4·9
	intestine	10·7	13·5	+ 2·1
	rectum	6·4	7·6	+ 1·6
	lung	4	8·1	+ 5·8
	'other respiratory'	0·6	3·9	+20·1
Women	pharynx	0·3	0·5	+ 5·6
	intestine	13·6	15·9	+ 1
	lung	2·2	3	+ 2·1
	'other respiratory'	0·2	0·8	+15·5

The significance of locality can easily be shown but the difficulty comes in seeing clearly what lies behind. It was shown in 1959 that in Norway, if one adjusts the primary figures to age and town/country, then the cancer frequency is highest in the two counties of Finnmark and Akershus and lowest in Sogn and Fjordane. For Sweden it was shown in 1960 that the primary figures, without adjustment to age and town/country, are lowest in the two northern-most counties and highest in Malmöhus and Blekinge counties, which, however, are exceeded by Stockholm city. It has been known for a long time that cancer is more common in towns, especially large cities with polluted air, and also that it is more common in industrial communities than in dormitory towns. Any real evidence to show that the geology of the soil and the composition of non-purified subsoil water has some essential significance for the frequency of cancer has not been forthcoming, although experiments have been made in this direction, especially in Holland.

Air pollution has gradually been shown to be of great importance to certain tumours, especially lung cancer, which is much more common in larger towns than in small ones, and relatively rare in the clean countryside; it is also in some areas ten times more common in men than in women. It is not yet entirely clear which substances are the primary causes, but it is certain that cigarette smoke is one of the most important. The pollution of the air has brought with it an important sanitary problem, which has already been dealt with on p. 176–7.

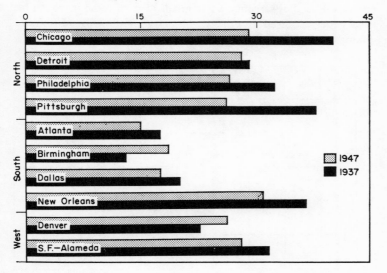

Incidence of stomach cancer in ten cities in the USA, in 1937 and 1947. The number of new cases per 100,000 inhabitants is shown. Stomach cancer frequency has declined in all cities except two, Birmingham and Denver. The reason for this is not known. (After Boles and Baum, 1955.)

It is known from experience that particular forms of cancer can occur in certain industries and occupations. The oldest known is the lung cancer in Schneeberg, Erzgebirge, mentioned elsewhere. The classic example otherwise is so-called chimney-sweep cancer in England, first described by Pott in 1775. The chemical irritation of the combustion products of coal produces cancer, especially in the

307

wrinkled skin of the scrotum. In the years 1880–92, 242 chimney sweeps died in London, 49 (22 per cent) of this form of cancer. During the period 1900–02 mortality had fallen a little, to 13 per cent. Other cancer forms associated with industry are skin cancer in brown-coal (lignite), tar and brick workers in Holland and Germany, paraffin cancer in Scotland and Germany, cotton spinners' cancer (from splashes of machine oil) in England, and skin cancer in petroleum refineries in France, Germany and Galicia. Radium poisoning as a cause of tumours is also known. In a factory in New Jersey where a large number of women workers were occupied in the manufacture of luminous watch dials, a considerable number of employees died of sarcoma, a malignant form of tumour, which had clearly been caused by the involuntary swallowing of minimal quantities of radium salt.

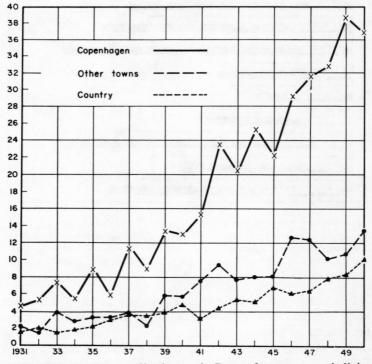

Rising lung cancer mortality in men in Denmark per 100,000 individuals, 1931–50 (after Clemmesen and Nielsen, 1954).

Liver, bladder and rectum cancers caused by sucker worms should also be included with forms of cancer occurring within limited geographical areas. They have been described in Africa, particularly Egypt (bilharzia), and the Far East.

Finally there are some forms of cancer, geographically more or less limited, which are associated with certain habits or customs. Among them is the widespread habit of chewing betel nuts in the Orient in which the mechanical and chemical irritation can lead to cancer of the mouth and lips; also so-called kangri or kashmir cancer, which men on the cold high plateau of Kashmir acquire from the burns on the stomach and thighs made by their portable glazed jars which they fill with red-hot charcoal, *kangri*, and wear round their waists in winter. The women do not wear these and have neither burns nor cancer. Many other examples of such cancers caused by external irritants could be given.

There are examples, too, of religious precepts and simple hygienic precautions giving protection against cancer, however incredible that may sound. It has been established for quite a long time that Jewesses who marry circumcised men, Jews and non-Jews, very seldom have cancer of the neck of the womb, cervix uteri, an otherwise very common form of cancer which in Sweden also is showing signs of increasing. This is associated with the Jewish law and custom of forbidding intercourse during menstruation and with circumcision, after which the fatty substance which is excreted in the foreskin, smegma, cannot collect and decompose in the absence of personal hygiene. This freedom from cervix cancer is also found in women who have become nuns in youth. Experience shows that decomposed smegma can lead to cancer of the penis, especially in China according to some reports.

Outlook for the Future

A question, perhaps not falling directly in the field of historico-geographical pathology but here worth answering briefly, in so far as that is possible, is one which is occasionally put with a certain anxiety: shall we succeed in eradicating most of the infectious diseases, among them tuberculosis, leprosy and syphilis, only to fall victims in the future to a much greater incidence of cardio-vascular diseases and malignant tumours? The answer is both yes and no.

As far as arteriosclerosis is concerned, with all its manifestations in the vessels of the heart, brain and legs, it undoubtedly lies within our power to keep this disease to some extent in check, even if we cannot completely overcome it. This I hope is evident from what I have said on the recent history of arteriosclerosis and its incidence within different population groups.

In the case of cancer, the situation is somewhat different. It cannot be denied that certain forms of cancer are increasing; this is largely due to the fact that the average life-span is becoming longer, so that many people now have cancer which they would not have had if they had died younger. But the increase in lung cancer, for example, as has been said, is directly associated with the increase in the pollution of the air we breathe, whether it comes from the tobacco which we or our companions smoke, from industry or from the combustion engines of motor traffic. On the other hand there is a definite indication that other forms, particularly one of the most important, cancer of the stomach, are decreasing, thanks to improved dietetic conditions and as a result of improvement of the 'stomach milieu' in which the cancer develops. The forms of cancer which are largely associated with unsuitable environment we can probably prevent. As for cancers of whose causes we still know very little, we must look, perhaps sooner than one dare hope, to discoveries which will clarify these too, and which will let us prevent and fight them more effectively than we know how to at present.

Added to this there is the rapid improvement in diagnosis,

through which we can recognise an early cancer both sooner and with more certainty, and the much improved methods of treatment in so many fields. All this means that one has no grounds for being pessimistic about medicine's future ability to win the battle against the two large groups of diseases which remain after the conquest of infectious diseases, cardio-vascular diseases and malignant tumours; here too medical research will advance successfully.

But one must not, however, forget that if we win the fight against infectious diseases, that will create a population which will rapidly lose the immunity the contraction of those diseases usually brings. One must therefore clearly understand that if one of these infectious diseases should for some reason suddenly reappear, for instance in bacteriological warfare, then the community must not stand unprotected. As with the perpetual threat of war, it is a matter of being prepared to meet force with force.

There are many who point to primitive peoples and their, broadly speaking, rare arteriosclerosis and low cancer frequency, but they ignore the fact that it is largely our high average life-span which is the reason for these two predominating in the list of diseases as causes of death. I am deliberately not speaking here of the terrible rise in accidents, especially road accidents, both directly fatal and those which cause lifelong invalidism with all its consequences to the individual and society. In the United States and in certain parts of Europe nearly half of all deaths of boys between the ages of five and nine are due to accidents, mostly road accidents.

We must not forget that the increased frequency of cardio-vascular diseases and tumours, as well as the numerous accidents on the roads and in industry, are indirect results of our much-prized material civilisation, and that in them we are harvesting the fruits, for good or evil, of the tree of knowledge which we ourselves have planted and of which we are so proud.

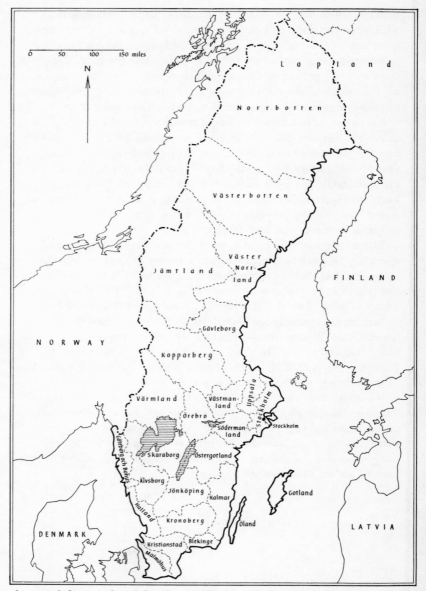

A map of the counties of Sweden, to illustrate the frequent references in the text.

A Select Bibliography

1 GENERAL

ACKERKNECHT, E. H. *Geschichte und Geographie der wichtigsten Krankheiten.* Stuttgart, 1963.

BROTHWELL, D. R. *Digging up bones.* Trustees of the British Museum, London, 1963.

CASTELLANI, A., and JACONO, I. *Manuale di clinica tropicale.* Turin, 1937.

DOERR, W. *et al. Gestaltwandel klassischer Krankheitsbilder.* Heidelberg, 1957.

DOLL, R. *Methods of geographical pathology.* Oxford, 1959.

HELLPACH, W. *Geopsyche.* 5th ed. Leipzig, 1939.

Hippocrates. With an English translation by W. H. S. Jones. 4 vols. London and New York, 1922–31.

HIRSCH, A. *Handbook of geographical and historical pathology.* 3 vols. London, 1883–86.

HUSS, M. *On Sweden's epidemic diseases.* (In Swedish.) Stockholm, 1859.

ILMONI, I. *Contribution to the history of diseases of the Scandinavian Countries.* (In Swedish.) 3 vols. Helsingfors, 1846–53.

Manson's Tropical diseases. Edited by Sir P. Manson-Bahr. 15th ed. London, 1960.

SIGERIST, H. E. *On the history of medicine.* Edited by F. Marti-Ibanez. New York, 1959.

SORRE, M. *Les fondements de la géographie humaine.* 3 vols. Paris, 1943–52.

WELLS, C. *Bones, bodies and disease.* London, 1964.

2 INFECTIOUS DISEASES

INTRODUCTORY

ANDERSON, G. W. *et al. Global epidemiology.* Baltimore, 1944.

DOMBROWSKI, H. J. 'Organismes vivants du paléozoique', *Presse Médicale,* **71**, 1963, 1147.

HENSCHEN, F. 'Anthropozoonoses', *Arch. Path.,* **59**, 1955, 517.

NICOLLE, C. *Naissance, vie et mort des maladies infectieuses.* Paris, 1930.
— *Le destin des maladies infectieuses.* Paris, 1937.
SIMMONS, J. S. *et al. Global Epidemiology. A geography of disease and sanitation.* 3 vols. London, 1944–50.

VIRUS DISEASES

BIETTI, G. B. *et al.* 'The current distribution of trachoma throughout the world', *Rev. Internat. Trachoma,* **39**, 1962, 113.
BRANDT, M. *Geopathologische Forschungen in der Sowjetunion.* Berlin, 1964.
COLLINS, S. D. 'Geography of poliomyelitis', *Publ. Health. Rep.,* **61**, 1946, 327.
DIXON, C. W. *Smallpox.* London, 1962.
DUBIN, I. N. *et al.* 'Statistical studies on cases of viral hepatitis. Armed Forces Inst. Pathology', *Schweiz. Zschr. Allg. Path. Bakt.,* **16**, 1953, 392.
FAVRE, M., and HELLERSTRÖM, S. 'The epidemiology, aetiology and prophylaxis of lymphogranuloma inguinale', *Acta Dermat.-Venereolog.,* **34**, Suppl. 30, 1954.
GALE, A. H. 'History of poliomyelitis in Great Britain', *Brit. Med. J.,* **1**, 1951, 511.
RENBOURN, E. T. 'The history of sweet and sweat rash from earliest times to the end of the 18th century', *J. Hist. Med.,* **14**, 1959, 202.
RHODES, A. J., and VAN ROYEN, C. E. *Textbook of virology.* Baltimore, 1962.
RIVERS, T. M., and HORSFALL, F. L. *Viral and rickettsial infections in man.* Philadelphia, 1959.
SYLVEST, E. *Bornholm disease.* (Danish, with English summary.) Copenhagen, 1933.
TOWNSEND, J. F. 'History of influenza epidemics', *Ann. Med. Hist.,* **5**, 1933, 553.
WAHLBERG, P. *et al.* 'Diphasic tick-borne meningo-encephalitis in the Åland islands', *Acta Med. Scandinav.,* **412**, 1964, 275.
WENNER, H. A. 'Psittacosis', *Advanc. Virus Res.,* **5**, 1958, 40.

RICKETTSIAL DISEASES

Bergey's Manual of determinative bacteriology. Baltimore, 1957.
BRANDT, M. 'Rickettsiosen in der Sowjetunion', *Referat, Osteuropa-Institut, Freie Universität Berlin,* **61**, 1964, 77.

KEIL, H. 'The louse in Greek antiquity, with comment on the diagnosis of the Athenian plague as recorded by Thukydides', *Bull. Hist. Med.*, **25**, 1951, 305.

LUOTO, L., and PICKENS, E. 'A résumé of recent research to define the Q-fever problem', *Americ. Journ. Hyg.*, **74**, 1961, 43.

RHODES, A. J., and VAN ROYEN, C. E. *Textbook of virology.* Baltimore, 1962.

RIVERS, T. M., and HORSFALL, F. L. *Viral and rickettsial infections in man.* Philadelphia, 1959.

BACTERIAL DISEASES

BOTHWELL, R. W. 'Epidemiology of human brucellosis in the United Kingdom', *Brit. J. Prevent. Social Med.*, **17**, 1963, 90.

BRANDT, M. *Geopathologische Forschungen in der Sowjetunion.* Osteuropa-Institut, Berlin, 1964.

DEFOE, D. *Journal of the Plague Year. London.* Library of World Literature, New York, 1960.

DEVIGNAT, R. *Répartition géographique des trois variétés de Pasteurella pestis.* Liége, 1952.

HECKER, J. F. C. *Der schwarze Tod im vierzehnten Jahrhundert.* Berlin, 1832.

JUSATZ, H. J. 'Tularämie in Europa 1926–1951', *Weltseuchenatlas*, **1**.

KAMAL, A. M. 'Endemicity and epidemicity of cholera', *WHO Bull.*, **28**, 1963, 277.

KELLETT, C. E. 'The early history of gas gangrene', *Ann. Med. Hist.*, **1**, 1939, 452.

KLEMM, DORIS M., and W. R. 'A history of anthrax', *J.A.W.M.A.*, **35**, 1959, 458.

MADSEN, S. 'Diphtheria in Denmark: from 23,695 cases to 1 case', *Dan. Med. Bull.*, **3**, 1956, 112.

Manson's Tropical Diseases. Edited by Sir P. H. Manson-Bahr. 15th ed. London, 1960.

OLIN, G. 'Une nouvelle épidémie de tularémie en Suède', *Bull. Off. Internat. Hyg. Publ.*, **30**, 1938, 2230.

— 'Studien über das Undulantfieber in Schweden', *Sv. Läk.-Sällsk. Handl.*, **61**, 1953, 1.

SEELIGER, H. P. R. 'Listeriosis, Epidemiology', *Karger's Gazette*, 1962, 2.

SIMMONS, J. S. *et al. Global Epidemiology.* London, 1944, vol. I.

TATE, W. J. 'The great plague in London 1665', *B.M.Q.*, **12**, 1961, 61.

TATENO, J. 'Tetanus', *Journ. Japan. Inf. Diseas.*, **36**, 1962, 194.

WHO Bull., **13**, 1955, 173. 'Typhoid—Paratyphoid'.

— **24**, 1961, 254. 'Gonorrhoea today'.

WHO Chronicle, **15**, 1961, 3. 'Past and present distribution of cholera'.

— **18**, 1961, 61. 'Diphtheria in the last forty years'.

TUBERCULOSIS

BARTELS, P. 'Tuberkulose (Wirbelkaries) in der jüngeren Steinzeit', *Arch. Anthropol. N.F.*, **6**, 1907, 243.

CHALKE, H. D. 'The impact of tuberculosis on history, literature, and art', *Med. Hist.*, **4**, 1962, 301.

DANIELS, M. 'Tuberculosis in Europe during and after second world war', *Brit. Med. J.*, **II**, 1949, 1065.

ELLIOT SMITH, G., and RUFFER, M. A. 'Pottsche Krankheit an einer ägyptischen Mumie aus der Zeit der 21. Dynastie', *Zur Histor. Biologie d. Krankheitserreger*, **H.3**, Giessen, 1910.

FRANCIS, J. *Tuberculosis in animals and man.* London, 1958.

HENSCHEN, F. 'Das Tuberkuloseproblem Schwedens', *Beitr. z. Klinik d. Tuberkulose*, **99**, 1943, 362.

SILVEIRA, J. 'Die Bekämpfung der Tuberkulose in Südamerika', *Beitr. Klinik d. Tuberkulose*, **127**, 1963, 35.

YELTON, S. E. 'Prewar distribution of tuberculosis throughout the world', *Publ. Health Rep.*, **61**, 1946, 487.

LEPROSY

COCHRANE, R. G. *Biblical leprosy.* Tyndale Press, 1961.

COCHRANE, R. G., DAVEY, T. F., MCROBERT, SIR G. *Leprosy in theory and practice.* Bristol, 1964.

DOULL, J. A. 'The epidemiology of leprosy: present status and problems', *Internat. J. Leprosy*, **30**, 1962, 48.

JOPLING, W. H. 'Leprosy and its management in Britain', *Lond. Clin. Med. J.*, **4**, 1963, 47.

MØLLER-CHRISTENSEN, V. *Ten lepers from Naestved in Denmark.* Copenhagen, 1953.

— *Bone changes in leprosy.* Copenhagen, 1961.

RICHARDS, P. 'Leprosy in Scandinavia. A discussion of its origins, its survival and its effect on Scandinavian life over the course of nine centuries', *Cantaurus*, **7**, 1960, 101.

SCHALLER, K. F. 'Seuchen im Wandel der Zeiten. Lepra und ihre Bekämpfung', *Zeitschr. Haut-Geschlechtkrankheiten*, **33**, 1962, 166.

SIMMONS, J. S. *et al. Global Epidemiology*. London, 1944, vol. I.

FUNGUS DISEASES ETC.

AJELLO, L. 'Geographic distribution and prevalence of the dermatophytes', *Ann. New York Acad. Scienc.*, **89**, 1960, 30.

BOCK, A. A. 'Epidemiological investigation of sarcoidosis. Discussion and summary', *Americ. Journ. Hyg.*, **74**, 1961, 189.

CONANT, N. F. *et al. Manual of clinical mycology*. Philadelphia and London, 1954.

EDWARDS, P. Q., and KIAER, J. H. 'Histoplasmosis. World-wide distribution', *Americ. J. Trop. Med.*, **5**, 1956, 235.

LÖFGREN, S. 'Conception of sarcoidosis' (in Spanish), *El Torax* (Montevideo), **10**, 1961, 1.

SPIROCHAETAL DISEASES

COCKBURN, T. A. 'Treponematoses', *WHO Bull.*, **24**, 1961, 221.

GUTHE, T., and WILLCOX, R. R. 'Treponematoses. A world problem', *WHO Chronicle*, **8**, 1954, 37.

HACKETT, C. J. *Bone lesions of yaws in Uganda*. Oxford, 1951.

— 'On the origin of human treponematoses', *WHO Bull.*, **29**, 1963, 7.

HAMLIN, H. 'The geography of treponematoses'. *Yale J. Biol. Med.*, **12**, 1939, 29.

HASSELMANN, C. M. 'Studien über die Histopathologie von Pinta, Frambösia und Syphilis', *Arch. Klin. Exp. Dermatol.*, **201**, 1955, 1.

HUARD, P. 'La syphilis vue par les médecins arabo-persiens, indiens et chino-japonais', *Hist. Méd.*, **6**, 1956, 9.

HUDSON, E. H. *Non-venereal syphilis. A sociological and medical study of bejel*. London, 1958.

ROMANO, A. 'The Candelaria cave in the Delicias valley' (in Spanish), *Tlatoani*, **2**, 1953, 5.

RIMPAU, W. 'Die Leptospirose als Problem der Geo-Epidemiologie', *Grenzgebiete d. Medizin*, **2**, 1949, 380.

STEWART, T. D., and SPOEHR, A. 'Evidence of the paleopathology of yaws'. *Bull. Hist. Med.*, **26**, 1952, 538.

STILLIAMS, A. W. 'The introduction and spread of syphilis in Europe', *J. Internat. Coll. Surg.*, **37**, 1962, 594.

TEMKIN, O. 'Zur Geschichte von "Moral und Syphilis"', *Arch. Geschichte Med.*, **19**, 1927, 331.

WILLIAMS, H. U. 'The American origin of syphilis', *Arch. Dermatol. Syphilis*, **16**, 1927, 683.

— 'The origin and antiquity of syphilis: the evidence from diseased bones', *Arch. Path.*, **13**, 1932, 783.

— 'Pathology of yaws, especially the relation to syphilis', *Am. J. Hyg.*, **25**, 1937, 477.

PROTOZOAL DISEASES

Amoebiasis, trypanosomiasis, leishmaniasis

BURROWS, R. B. 'Amebiasis in US and Canada', *Americ. J. Trop. Med.*, **10**, 1961, 172.

CORRADETTI, A. 'Italian foci of kala-azar and problem of leishmaniasis in southern Europe' (in Italian), *Rendic. Ist. Sup. Sanità*, **24**, 1961, 281.

MAILLOT, L. 'Distribution of Glossina and sleeping disease. Geographical races', *Bull. Soc. Path. Exot.*, **54**, 1961, 856.

MORRIS, R. C. *et al.* 'Kala-azar', *Americ. J. Med.*, **30**, 1961, 624.

PIETKARSKI, G. *Lehrbuch der Parasitologie.* Springer, 1954.

ROMANA, C. 'Epidemiological and geographic distribution of Chagas disease', *Bol. Ofic. Sanit. Panameric.*, **51**, 1961, 429.

WHO Chronicle, **17**, 1963, 43 and 443. 'Trypanosomiasis control in Africa'.

WILCOCKS, C. 'Leishmaniasis', *Trop. Diseas. Bull.*, **59**, 1962, 950.

WOODY, H. B. 'American trypanosomiasis. Chagas disease in USA', *J. Pediatr.*, **58**, 1961, 586.

Malaria, toxoplasmosis, balantidiasis, etc.

BEUTLER, E. *et al.* 'Sickle cell trait and resistance to malaria', *Brit. Med. J.*, **I**, 1955, 1189.

BREDE, H. D., and VAN NIEUWENHUYSEN, M. E. 'Balantidium coli', *S. Afric. Med. J.*, **36**, 1962, 937.

COATNEY, G. R. 'Simian malaria. Its importance to world-wide eradication of malaria', *J. Americ. Med. Ass.*, **184**, 1963, 876.

FLECK, D. G. 'Epidemiology of toxoplasmosis', *J. Hyg.* **61**, 1963, 61.

JONES, W. H. S. *Malaria, a neglected factor in the history of Greece and Rome.* With an introduction by R. Ross. Cambridge, 1907.

LANCISI, G. M. *De noxiis paludum effluviis eorumque remedio.* 1717.

MANSON-BAHR, R. 'The story of malaria: The drama and the actors', *Internat. Rev. Trop. Med.*, **2**, 1963, 329.

WHO Chronicle, **17**, 1963, 335. 'Malaria eradication in 1962'.

WRIGHT, W. H. 'Toxoplasmosis', *Americ. J. Clin. Pathol.*, **28**, 1957, 1.

WORM DISEASES

BRANDT, M. *Geopathologische Forschungen in der Sowjetunion.* Osteuropa-Institut, Berlin, 1964.

BUDDEN, F. H. 'Onchocerciasis', in J. H. Holmes, *Geographic ophthalmology.* Springfield, 1962.

DESCHIENS, R. 'Considérations épidémiologiques et sanitaires sur l'hydatidose humaine dans le bassin méditerranéen', *Bull. Soc. Path. Exot.*, **53**, 1960, 971.

FOG, H., and KONDI, A. 'Incidence of anemias, iron-deficiency and anchylostomiasis', *Ann. Trop. Med. Parasit.*, **55**, 1961, 25.

HIGGINSON, J., and DE MEILLON, B. 'Schistosomum haematobium infestation and hepatic disease in man'. *Arch. Path.*, **60**, 1955, 341.

MARKKANEN, T. 'Tapeworm anemia and economy of vitamins B in man', *Ann. Med. Int. Fenn.*, **51**, 1962, 229.

MACFARLANE, L. R. S. *Human protozoology and helminthology.* Edinburgh, 1960.

MEIER, K. 'Medina-Wurm', *Arch. Geschichte. Med.*, **30**, 1937, 69.

VON OEFELE, F. 'Studien über die altägyptische Parasitologie', *Arch. Parasitol.*, **5**, 1902, 499.

PIETKARSKI, G. *Lehrbuch der Parasitologie.* Springer, 1954.

VOGEL, H. 'Worms as cause of disease', *Triangle*, **3**, 1958, 174, 223.

ARTHROPODAN DISEASES

BATES, M. 'Human destiny influenced by insects' (in Spanish), *Rev. San. Hig. Publ.*, **30**, 1936, 506.

BURKS, J. W. *et al.* 'Norwegian scabies', *Arch. Dermatol.*, **74**, 1956, 131.

DUNGAL, N. 'Is leprosy transmitted by arthropods?', *Leprosy Review*, 1961.

DUNHAM, M. C. 'Swimmer's itch', *Maine. Med. J.*, **54**, 1963, 180.

FORD, J. 'The distribution of the vectors of African pathogenic trypanosomes', *WHO Bull.*, **28**, 1963, 653.

HOEPPLI, R. 'Early references to the occurrence of Tunga penetrans in tropical Africa', *Acta Trop.*, **20**, 1963, 143.

3 NON-INFECTIOUS DISEASES. DISEASES OF THE ORGANS

FAMINE, MALNUTRITION

BHATTACHARYYA, A. K., and CHANDURY, R. N. 'Aetiological investigations in kwashiorkor and marasmus II. Study in socio-economic aspects', *Bull. Calcutta Sch. Trop. Med.*, **10**, 1962, 100.

BENSON, P. F. *et al.* 'Rickets in immigrant children in London', *Brit. Med. J.*, **5340**, 1963, 1054.

COOKE, W. T. 'Malabsorption syndrome. Pathogenesis (Sprue)', *Amer. J. Clin. Nutr.*, **8**, 1960, 167.

HAMPERL, H. 'Beiträge zur geographischen Pathologie unter besonderer Berücksichtigung der Verhältnisse in Russland', *Ergebn. Path.*, **26**, 1932, 353.

HIGGINSON, J. *et al.* 'Siderosis in the Bantu in Southern Africa', *Amer. J. Path.*, **29**, 1953, 779.

JOOSTEN, J. H. 'Figures and the world's hunger', *Indian Med. J.*, **56**, 1962, 153.

Nature, **196**, 1962, 227. 'The challenge of hunger'.

RANGACHARI, V. 'Xerophthalmia and keratomalacia', In W. J. Holme, *Geographic ophthalmology.* Springfield, 1959.

ROSENSTEIN, L. M. 'Zur Psychopathologie des extremen Hungers', *Krankheitsforsch*, **3**, 1926, 118.

SMITH, D. A., and WOODRUFF, M. F. 'Deficiency diseases in Japanese prison camps', *Med. Res. Council Sprc. Rep. Ser.*, **274**, London, 1951.

WHO Chronicle, **17**, 1963, 161. 'Malnutrition and disease'.

POISONING AND OCCUPATIONAL DISEASES

DAVIES, P. 'Favism: a family study', *Quart. J. Med.*, **31**, 1962, 157.

DRINKER, P. 'Air pollution', *New Engl. J. Med.*, **264**, 1961, 754.

FRY, J. *et al.* 'Smog', *Lancet*, **II**, 1962, 132.

HALLIDAY, E. C., and KEMENY, E. 'Second report on air pollution measurements in the towns Pretoria, Johannesburg, Durban, East London', *Publ. Health Johannesburg*, **82**, 1962, 7.

HAYASHI, M. 'Acute radiation sickness and the amount of radiation.

Based on a study of material from the Hiroshima atomic explosion by the Okayama Med. Coll. team', *J. Jap. Med. Ass.*, **48**, 1962, 11.

IRUKAYAMA, K. *et al.* 'An organo-mercury compound extracted from sludge in the acetaldehyde plant of the Minamata factory', *Jap. J. Med. Progr.*, **49**, 1962, 536.

LAWTHER, P. W. 'Must we use the air in our cities as a sewer?', *Unesco Courier*, March 1959.

MILLS, C. A. 'Respiration and heart deaths in Los Angeles smogs', *Amer. J. Med. Sci.*, **239**, 1960, 307.

PRINDLE, R. A. 'Air pollution problems', *Amer. Rev. Respir. Diseas.*, **83**, 1961, 403.

ROTH, F. 'Über die Spätfolgen des chronischen Arsenismus der Moselwinzer', *Deutsch. Med. Wochenschr.*, **82**, 1957, 211.

SIGERIST, H. E. *On the history of medicine.* New York, 1959.

SINGH, A. *et al.* 'Skeletal changes in endemic fluorosis', *J. Bone Joint Surg.*, **44-B**, 1962, 806.

THACKRAH, C. T. *The effects of arts, trades, and professions of civic state and habits of living on health and longevity.* Leeds, 1832. (Quoted after Sigerist.)

WICKERSHEIMER, E. '"Ignis sacer" (Ergotism). The story of a name', *Ciba Sympos.*, **8**, 1960, 160.

ENDOCRINE AND OTHER METABOLIC DISTURBANCES

Thyroid Gland

GALLI-VALERIO, B. 'L'étiologie et l'épidémiologie de l'endémie thyréoidienne', *Kropfkonf*, **128**, 336.

HETTCHE, H. O. *Ätiologie, Pathogenese und Prophylaxe der Struma.* München, 1954.

— *Epidemiology of struma.* IVth Internat. Goitre Conf. London, 1960.

HÖJER, J. A. 'Untersuchungen über den endemischen Kropf in Schweden', *Zschr. Hyg.*, **110**, 1929, 239.

— 'Goitre studies' (in Swedish), *Svensk. Läk. Sällsk. Handl.*, **57**, 1931.

IVERSEN, K. *Temporary rise in the frequency of thyrotoxicosis in Denmark 1941–45.* Copenhagen, 1948.

JUSSILA, R. 'The general epidemiology of goitre in Finland' (in Swedish), *Nordisk Med.*, **57**, 1957, 807.

KELLY, F. C., and SNEDDEN, U. W. 'Prevalence and geographical distribution of endemic goiter', *WHO Monograph. Ser.*, **44**, 1960, 27.

KILPATRICK, R. *et al.* 'A survey of thyroid enlargement in two general practices in Great Britain', *Brit. Med. J.*, **5322**, 1963, 29.

MERKE, F. 'The history of endemic goitre and cretinism in the 13th–15th centuries', *Proc. Roy. Soc. Med.*, **53**, 1960, 993.

— 'Hat Paracelsus als erster über den Kretinismus berichtet und dessen Zusammenhangmit dem endemischen Kropf vermutet?', *Karger's Gaz.*, Sept. 1964.

PELTOLA, P. 'Goitrogenic effect of cow's milk from goiter district in Finland', *Acta Endocrinol.*, **34**, 1960, 121.

REISENHAUER, R. 'Die kartographische Darstellung der Struma', *Endokrinologie*, **40**, 1960, 27.

SÄLLSTRÖM, T. *Vorkommen und Verbreitung der Thyreotoxicose in Schweden.* Thesis. Stockholm, 1935.

STANBURY, J. B. *et al. Endemic goiter: The adaptation of man to iodine deficiency.* Cambridge, Mass., 1954.

WHO Chronicle, **14**, 1960, 339 and 345. 'Problems of endemic goitre'.

Diabetes mellitus

BARACH, J. H. 'Historical facts in diabetes', *Ann. Med. Hist.*, **10**, 1928, 387.

CAMPBELL, G. D. 'Some observations upon 4000 African and Asiatic diabetics collected in Durban between 1958 and 1962', *E. Afr. Med. J.*, **40**, 1963, 267.

D'ALONZO, C. A. 'Diabetes in an employed population', *Delaware Med. J.*, **34**, 1962, 284.

REMEIN, Q. R. 'Prevalence of diabetes in U.S.', *Ann. New York Acad. Sci.*, **82**, 1959, 229.

SCHERSTEN, B. 'Statistics of diabetes mellitus' (in Swedish), *Diabetes Conf. Hindås. Svensk. Läk.-Tidn.*, **58**, 1961, 2441.

WITTBRODT, H., and SANGE, G. 'Beitrag zur Frage der Diabeteshäufigkeit', *Deutsch. Gesundheitswesen*, **15**, 1960, 2510.

Other endocrine and metabolic disturbances

BLUM, A. *et al.* 'Amyloidosis as the sole manifestation of familial Mediterranean fever. Further evidence of its genetic nature', *Ann. Int. Med.*, **57**, 1962, 795.

FORSSMAN, H. 'On heredity in diabetes insipidus' (in Swedish), *Nordisk Med.*, **16**, 1942, 3211.

— 'Heredity in diabetes insipidus', *Amer. J. Human Genet.*, **7**, 1955, 21.

WALDENSTRÖM, J. 'Recent information on porphyria diseases' (in Swedish), *Nordisk Med.*, **62**, 1959, 1443.

THE BLOOD-FORMING ORGANS, BLOOD

BANNERMAN, R. M. *Thalassemia*. New York, 1961.

VON BONSDORFF, B. 'Pernicious worm-anaemia' (in Swedish), *Nordisk Med.*, **49**, 1953, 633.

CHAREMIS, C. *et al.* 'Three inherited red-cell abnormalities in a district of Greece: Thalassemia, sickling and glucose-6-phosphatase-deshydrogenase deficiency', *Lancet*, **I**, 1963, 907.

COOLEY, T. B. *et al.* 'Anemia in children with splenomegaly and peculiar changes of the bones', *Americ. J. Dis. Child.*, **34**, 1927, 347.

ERIKSSON, A. *et al.* 'Untersuchungen über Thrombopathie (v. Willebrand-Jürgens)', *Klin. Wochenschr.*, **39**, 1961, 32.

KONDI, A. *et al.* 'Anemias of marasmus and kwashiorkor in Kenya', *Arch. Dis. Child.*, **38**, 1963, 267.

LUNDHOLM, I. *Über den Erbgang bei Anaemia hypochromica essentialis*. Thesis. Stockholm, 1937.

MEULENGRACHT, E. *Studies of chronic haemolytic icterus*. Thesis in Danish. Copenhagen, 1918.

MOORE, S. 'Bone changes in sickle cell anemia with note on similar change in skulls of ancient Mayan indians', *J. Missouri Med. Ass.*, **26**, 1929, 561.

MOSBECH, J. 'Incidence of pernicious anaemia', *Acta Med. Scand.*, **141**, 1952, 433.

MOURANT, A. E. 'Hematology, the basis of modern anthropology', *Transfusion, Paris*, **5**, 1962, 213.

REYNOLDS, J. 'An evaluation of some roentgenologic signs in sickle cell anemia and its variants', *Southern Med. J.*, **55**, 1962, 1123.

SKÖLD, E. 'On haemophilia in Sweden and its treatment with blood transfusion', *Acta Med. Scand. Suppl.*, 1944.

SUTTON, R. N. P. 'Erythrocyte glucose-6-phosphatase-deshydrogenase deficiency in Trinidad', *Lancet*, **II**, 1963, 855.

WIENER, A. S. 'Blood groups and disease. A critical review', *Lancet*, **I**, 1962, 813.

WILSON, J. G. 'Thalassemia major. Genetic basis of thalassemia', *Med. J. Austral.*, **47**, 1960, 328 and 325.

THE CIRCULATORY SYSTEM

Arteriosclerosis. History

SANDISON, A. T. 'Degenerative vascular disease in the Egyptian mummies', *Med. Hist.*, **6**, 1962, 77.

Arteriosclerosis. Geography

ANDERSON, R. S. *et al.* 'Incidence of atherosclerotic heart disease in Negro diabetic patients', *Diabetes*, **10**, 1961, 114.

BROWN, A. 'Coronary thrombosis. An environmental study', *Brit. Med. J.*, **5304**, 1962, 567.

DAVIES, J. N. P. 'Infrequency of atheromatosis and the exceeding rarity of coronary thrombosis in Africans', *Americ. Rev. Med.*, **3**, 1952, 99.

FISHBEIN, M. 'Statistics and epidemiology of atherosclerosis', *Postgrad. Med.*, **31**, 1962, 311.

LORENTIN, R. A. *et al.* 'Geographic pathology of arteriosclerosis; a study of the age of onset of significant coronary arteriosclerosis in adult Africans and New Yorkers', *Exp. Molec. Path.*, **2**, 1963, 103.

HENSCHEN, F. 'The changing panorama of diseases in Sweden during the last 50 years.' An academic lecture (in Swedish), 1946. *Verdandis Småskrifter*, 1967.

NICHAMAN, M. Z. *et al.* 'Cardiovascular mortality by race. Based on a statistical study in Charleston, S. Carolina', *Geriatrics*, **17**, 1962, 724.

SJÖVALL, J., and WIHMAN, G. 'Beobachtungen über die Arteriosklerose in Schweden', *Acta Path. Scandinav. Suppl.*, **20**, 1934.

THOMAS, W. A. 'Geographic pathology of arteriosclerosis', *New York J. Med.*, **63**, 1963, 1321.

VARTIAINEN, I., and KANERVA, K. 'Atherosclerosis and wartime', *Ann. Med. Intern. Fenn.*, **36**, 1947, 748.

WALKER, A. R., and SEFFEL, H. C. 'Coronary heart disease, strokes and diabetes in South African Indians', *Lancet*, **II**, 1962, 786.

WHO Chronicle, **14**, 1960, 228. 'Mortality from cardiovascular diseases'.

Hypertension, heart hypertrophy

ARIAS-STELLA, A., and RECAVARREN, S. 'Right ventricle hypertrophy in native children living in high altitudes', *Americ. J. Path.*, **41**, 1962, 54 and 467.

COHEN, A. M. *et al.* 'Hypertension effect of environmental change', *Lancet*, **II**, 1960, 1050.

KÖHNEN, I. *et al.* 'Grösse und Leistungsfähigkeit des Bergmanns-herzens', *Arch. Kreislauf-forsch.*, **41**, 1963, 58.

LOVE, C. R., and MCKEOWN, T. 'Arterial pressure in an industrial population; and its bearing on the problem of essential hypertension', *Lancet*, **I**, 1962, 1085.

MOSER, M. 'Epidemiology of hypertension with reference to racial susceptibility , *Ann. New York Acad. Sci.*, **84**, 1960, 989.

Endo-myocardial diseases

HIGGINSON, J. *et al.* 'The pathology of cryptogenic heart disease', *Arch. Path.*, **70**, 1960, 497.

JAFFE, R. 'Chronic myocarditis in Venezuela', *Schweiz. Zeitschr. Path.*, **18**, 1955, 942.

STEWART, K. L., and HAYES, J. A. 'A cardiac disorder of unknown aetiology in Jamaica', *Quart. Med. J.*, **32**, 1963, 99.

Thromboembolism, etc.

BARTOK, J. 'Vermehrung der Fälle von Thrombose und Lungen-embolie, und ihre Ursachen', *Virch. Arch.*, **333**, 1960, 619.

HULTQUIST, G. 'Pulmonary embolism and weather' (in Swedish), *Nordisk Med.*, **9**, 1935, 1058.

LETAC, R. *et al.* 'De la rareté de la pathologie veineuse des membres inférieurs en Afrique noire', *Schweiz. Zeitschr. Path.*, **21**, 1958, 567.

THE RESPIRATORY SYSTEM

AHLMARK, A. *et al. Silicosis and other pneumoconioses in Sweden.* Scandinav. University Books, Stockholm, 1960.

CARPENTER, R. G., and COCHRANE, A. L. 'Death rates in miners with and without pneumoconiosis', *S. Wales. Brit. J. Industr. Med.*, **13**, 1956, 102.

KURTEN, H. '"De phthisi". Ein Consilium des Memminger Stadtarztes Dr. Ulrich Ellenbog vom Jahre 1480, etc.', *Arch. Geschichte Med.*, **24**, 1931, 245.

TRAUTMANN, H. *Lunge und Berufskrankheiten.* Stuttgart, 1962.

A SELECT BIBLIOGRAPHY

THE DIGESTIVE SYSTEM

Oral cavity. Teeth

BROTHWELL, D. R. 'Teeth in earlier human populations', *Proceed. Nutr. Soc. London*, **18**, 1959, 195.
— *Digging up bones.* London, 1963.
HOLMER, U., and MAUNSBACH, A. B. 'Odontologic examination of human teeth and jaw-bones from the Nordic Stone Age' (in Swedish), *Odontol. Tidskr.*, **64**, 1956, 437.
LEIGH, R. 'Notes on the stomatology and pathology of ancient Egypt', *Americ. Archaeolog. Ethnol.*, **34**, 1934, 1.
— 'Dental morphology and pathology of pre-Spanish Peru', *Amer. J. Phys. Anthropol.*, **22**, 1937, 2.
PINDBORG, J. J. *et al.* 'Frequency of oral carcinoma, leukoplakia, leukokeratosis, leukoedema, submucous fibrosis, and lichen planus in 10,000 Indians in Lucknow, India. Preliminary report', *J. Dental Res.* (to be published).
WHO Rep. Ser., **207**, 1961, 1. 'Periodontal disease'.
WITKOP, C. J. 'Geographic and nutritional factors in dental caries', *Publ. Health Rep.*, **77**, 1962, 928.

Stomach

FALCONER, B. *Über die peptischen Läsionen. Statistisch-ätiologische Studien an einem Stockholmer Sektionsmaterial.* Jena, 1943.
HANSEN, J. L. 'Necropsy statistics on chronic gastric and duodenal ulcer in Copenhagen during forty years', *Schweiz. Zeitschr. Path.*, **21**, 1958, 441.
HURST, A. F., and STEWART, M. J. *Gastric and duodenal ulcer.* Oxford, 1929.
PULVERTAFT, C. N. 'The incidence of peptic ulceration in York and environs', *Schweiz. Zeitschr. Path.*, **21**, 1958, 220.
STRAUB, M., and SCHORNAGEL, H. E. 'General aetiology of gastro-duodenal ulcer', *Schweiz. Zeitschr. Path.*, **21**, 1958, 242.
SEGI, M. *et al.* 'Mortality for gastric and duodenal ulcer in countries, and geographical correlation to mortality for gastric and intestinal cancer', *Schweiz. Zeitschr. Path.*, **22**, 1959, 777.

Intestine

ACHESON, E. D., and NEFZGER, M. D. 'Ulcerative colitis in the US army in 1944. Epidemiology, comparisons between patients and controls', *Gastroenterol*, **44**, 1963, 7.

326

MELROSE, 'A. G. 'Geography of chronic ulcerative colitis in Great Britain', *Gastroenterol.*, **29**, 1955, 1055.

Cirrhosis of the liver

AMANO, S., and YAMAMOTO, H. 'Infectious hepatitis and cirrhosis and its sequela in Japan', *Ann. Rep. Inst. Virus. Res. Kyoto Universit.*, **3**, 1960, 185.

DAVIDSON, C. S., and POPPER, H. 'Liver-cirrhosis in alcoholics', *Americ. J. Med.*, **27**, 1959, 193.

DAVIES, J. N. P. 'Observations on the pathology of liver disease in Uganda', *Pathologia Microbiologia*, **24**, 1961, 787.

HENSCHEN, F., and BRUCE, T. *Über die Häufigkeit und Formen der Lebercirrhose in Stockholm.* Premier Conf. Soc. Internat. Path. Géographique, Geneva, 1931. Geneva, 1932.

MORRISON, L. M. *et al.* 'The relationship of viral hepatitis to cirrhosis', *Amer. J. Gastroenterol.*, **35**, 1961, 371.

SCHMIDT, W., and BRONETO, J. 'Death from liver cirrhosis and specific alcoholic beverage consumption, an ecological study', *Americ. J. Publ. Health*, **52**, 1962, 1473.

WHO Chronicle, **14**, 1960, 471. 'Cirrhosis of the liver in France'.

Gallstones

'Cholelithiasis, Statistics', *N. Carolina Med. J.*, **33**, 1962, 107.

HENSCHEN, F. 'On changes in the Swedish panorama of diseases' (academic lecture, 1946, in Swedish), *Verdandis Småskrifter*, **491**, 1947.

MÖRNER, K. T. 'A 4000-year old gallstone' (in Swedish), *Svenska Läkartidn.*, 1936.

THE URINARY SYSTEM

AURORA, A. L. *et al.* 'Endemic bladderstone disease in childhood, a problem of geographic pathology', *Acta Union. Internat. Cancr.*, **18**, 1962, 527.

JYOGETSU, M. *et al.* 'Statistical observations on urolithiasis in the urological clinic of Kobe during 10 years', *Acta Urolog. Jap.*, **8**, 1962, 458.

KARAE, I. K., and IBADOV, H. 'On endemic urolithiasis in the Andizhansk region' (in Russian), *Soviet Med.*, **26**, 1962, 120.

SHATTOCK, S. G. 'A prehistoric or predynastic Egyptian calculus', *Transact. Path. Soc. London*, **56**, 1905, 275.

A SELECT BIBLIOGRAPHY

THE REPRODUCTIVE SYSTEM

DIEKE, W. 'Die antiken Hermaphroditen', *Zentralbl. Gynäkolog.*, **78**, 1956, 889.

'Eclampsia and pre-eclampsia in pregnancy', Proc. 7 Internat. Conf. Geograph. Path. London 1960, *Pathologia Microbiologia*, **24**, 1961, 428.

MARGETTS, E. L. 'The masculine character of Hatshesup, Queen of Egypt', *Bull. Hist. Med.*, **25**, 1951, 559.

THE SKELETAL SYSTEM

General pathology

BROTHWELL, D. R. *Digging up bones.* London, 1963.

MOODIE, R. L. *Paleopathology.* Urbana, Wisc., 1923.

PALES, L. *Paléopathologie et pathologie comparative.* Paris, 1930.

STEWART, T. D. 'Pathological changes in South American Indian skeletal remains', *Handb. South Americ. Indian*, **VI**, Washington, 1950, 49.

WELLS, C. *Bones, bodies and disease.* London, 1964.

Pathology of the cranium

ADACHI, B. 'Die Porosität des Schädeldaches', *Zeitschr. Morphol. Anthropol.*, **7**, 1904, 373.

ALDRED, C., and SANDERSON, A. T. 'The Pharaoh Akhenaten. A problem in egyptology and pathology', *Bull. Hist. Med.*, **36**, 1962, 293.

COOLEY, T. B. *et al.* 'Anemia in children with splenomegaly and peculiar changes of the bones', *Americ. J. Dis. Child.*, **34**, 1927, 347.

FÜRST, C. M., and OLSSON, M. *Magnus Ladulås's and Karl Knutsson's graves in the Riddarholm Church* (in Swedish). Stockholm, 1921.

HAMPERL, H., and WEISS, P. 'Über die spongiöse Hyperostose an Schädeln in Alt-Perú', *Virch. Arch.*, **327**, 1955, 629.

HENSCHEN, F. *Morgagni's Syndrome.* Edinburgh, 1949.

— 'Cribra cranii, a skull condition said to be of racial or geographical nature', *Pathologia, Microbiologia*, **24**, 1955, 724.

HUMPHRY, G. M. 'Senile hypertrophy and senile atrophy of the skull', *J. Anat. Physiol.*, **24**, 1890, 598.

MØLLER-CHRISTENSEN, V., and SANDISON, A. T. 'Usura orbitae (Cribra orbitalia) in the collection of crania in the Anatomy Department of the University of Glasgow', *Pathologia, Microbiologia*, **26**, 1963, 175.

MOORE, S. 'Bone changes in sickle cell anemia with note on similar change in skulls of ancient Mayan Indians', *J. Missour. Med. Ass.*, **26**, 1929, 561.

Joint conditions

GEJVALL, N-G. *Westerhus: its mediaeval population and church in the light of skeletal remains.* Thesis. Lund, 1960.

ROWLING, J. T. 'Pathological changes in mummies', *Proceed. Roy. Soc. Med.*, **54**, 1961, 409.

WELLS, C. *Bones, bodies and disease.* London, 1964.

ZORAB, P. A. 'The historical and prehistorical background of ankylosing spondylitis', *Proceed. Roy. Soc. Med.*, **54**, 1961, 415.

Artificial deformities

FANG, H. S., and YU FY. 'Foot binding in Chinese women', *Canad. J. Surg.*, **3**, 1960, 195.

KINDLER, W. 'Jahrtausendalter Kult- und Modebrauch der künstlichen Schädeldeformierung und ihre gesundheitlichen Folgen, *Aesthet. Med.*, **12**, 1963, 247.

LASTRES, J. B., and CABIESES, F. *La trepanación del craneo el antiguo Peru.* Imprenta de la Universidad de Lima, 1960.

OAKLEY, K. P. *et al.* 'Contributions on trepanning or trephination in ancient and modern times', *Man*, **59**, 1959, art. 133.

VARA LOPEZ, R. *La craniectomia a través de los siglos.* Valladolid, 1949.

WOOD-JONES, F. *General pathology, fractures and dislocations, in human remains.* Archaeological survey of Nubia, Report for 1907-1908. Cairo, 1910. Vol. 2.

Malformations

DAWSON, W. R. 'Dwarfs and hunchbacks in ancient Egypt', *Ann. Med. Hist.*, **9**, 1927, 315.

GREBE, E. 'Chondrodysplasie', *Analecta Genetica*, **II**, Rome, 1956.

MØRCH, E. T. *Chondrodystrophic dwarfs in Denmark.* Thesis. Copenhagen, 1941.

RUFFER, M. A. 'On dwarfs and other deformed persons', *Bull. Soc. Archéolog. d'Alexandrie*, **13**.

THE SKIN

BJÖRNBERG, Ö. 'Total albinos among the Cuna Indians', *J. Hist. Med.*, **15**, 1960, 265.

CROCKETT, D. J. 'Colour, cancer, keloids in the Sudan', *Brit. J. Plast. Surg.*, **15**, 1962, 408.

LOMHOLT, G. *Psoriasis.* Copenhagen, 1963.

SIEGEL, M. *et al.* 'The epidemiology of systemic lupus erythematosus. Preliminary results in New York City', *J. Chron. Disease*, **15**, 1962, 131.

THE SENSORY ORGANS

Eyes

CHITNIS, V. K. 'Blindness and the prevention of blindness in India', in Holmes, *Geographic Ophthalmology.* Springfield, 1959.

HOLMES, W. J. *Geographic Ophthalmology.* Springfield, 1959.

LAULAN, R. 'Les maladies des yeux dans l'ancienne Egypte et chez le peuple d'Israel', *Presse Médicale*, **70**, 1962, 2477.

POST, R. H. 'Population differences in red and green colour vision deficiency; a review and a query on selection relaxation', *Eugen. Quart.*, **9**, 1962, 131.

SINISCALCO, M. *et al.* 'Lincage data involving G-6-P-D-deficiency, colour blindness and hemophilia', *2 Internat. Conf. Human Genet. Roma.—Excerpta Medica.*

YANG CHUN *et al.* 'Colour blindness among Chinese', *China Med. J.*, **76**, 1958, 283.

Ears

DERAEMAEKER, R. 'Recessive congenital deafness in north Belgian province', *Acta Genet. Statistic. Med.*, **10**, 1960, 295.

LIU-JUEC-HUA *et al.* '560 cases of the deaf in Peking', *China Med. J.*, **75**, 1957, 753.

NERVOUS AND MENTAL DISORDERS

Epilepsy. Hysteria

BRAIN, SIR R. 'The concept of hysteria in the time of William Harvey', *Proc. Roy. Soc. Med.*, **56**, 1963, 317.

FULTON, J. F. 'History of focal epilepsy', *Internat. J. Neurol.*, **1**, 1959, 21.

TEMKIN, O. 'The falling sickness, a history of epilepsy from the Greeks to beginning of modern neurology', *J. Hopkins Press*, **15**, 1945, 330.

Special neurology

ACHESON, E. D., and BACHRACH, C. A. 'The distribution of

multiple sclerosis in US veterans by birthplace', *Americ. J. Hyg.*, **72**, 1960, 88.

— 'MS in British Commonwealth countries in the Southern Hemisphere', *Brit. J. Prevent. Soc. Med.*, **15**, 1961, 118.

FISCHER, ANNE, and J. L. 'Aetiology of kuru', *Lancet*, **I**, 1960, 1417.

GAJDUSEK, D. C. 'Kuru', *Trans. Roy. Soc. Trop. Med. Hyg.*, **57**, 1963, 151.

GEORGI, F. *et al. Zur Problematik der MS. Geomedizinische Studien im der Schweiz und in Ostafrika.* Basel, 1961.

KIMURA, K. 'Epidemiological and geomedical studies on amyotrophic lateral sclerosis and allied diseases in Kii peninsula, Japan', *Fol. Psychiatr. Neurolog. Jap.*, **15**, 1961, 175.

KURLAND, L. T. 'Presentation of MS and other neurological studies in North America and the Western Pacific Islands', *Acta Psychiatr. Scandinav.*, **35**, suppl. 147, 1960.

LARSSON, T., and SJÖGREN, T. 'Essential tremor. A clinical and genetic population study', *Acta Psychiatr. Scandinav.*, suppl. 144, 1960.

LUNDBORG, H. *Degeneration und degenerierte Geschlechter in Schweden I. Familiäre Myoklonie.* Thesis. Stockholm, 1901.

MJÖNES, H. 'Paralysis agitans. A clinical and genetic study' (thesis, Stockholm), *Acta Psychiatr. Neurolog. Scandinav.*, suppl. 54, 1949.

RODRIGUEZ ARIAS, B., and PONS CLOTET, A. 'A large familial group and a double geographical focus of Huntington's chorea in the Spanish Levant' (in Spanish), *Res. Espan. Otoneurooftalmol.*, **20**, 1961, 154.

SJÖGREN, T. 'Die juvenile amaurotische Idiotie. Klinische und erblichkeitsmedizinische Untersuchungen' (thesis, Lund), *Hereditas*, **14**, 1931, 197.

— 'Klinische und erbbiologische Untersuchungen über Heredoataxien', *Acta Psychiatr. Neurolog.*, suppl. 27, 1943.

STEINER, G. *Multiple Sklerose.* Springer, 1962.

WELANDER, LISA. 'Late hereditary distal myopathy', *Acta Med. Scandinav.*, suppl. 265, 1951.

WHO Chronicle, **15**, 1961, 421. 'Mortality from multiple sclerosis'.

Psychiatry. Neuropathy

BERNE, E. 'Comparative psychiatry and tropical psychiatry', *Americ. J. Psychiatr.*, **113**, 1956, 193.

BLANCHLY, P. H. *et al.* 'Suicide in professional groups', *New. Engl. J. Med.*, **268**, 1963, 1278.

CAROTHERS, J. C. *The African mind in health and disease.* 1953 *WHO Monograph Series*, **17**.

DEISHER, P. W. *et al.* 'Phenylketonuric families in Washington State', *Amer. J. Diseas. Child.*, **103**, 1963, 818.

GRUENBERG, E. M. 'A review of mental health in the metropolis. The Midtown Manhattan study', *Milbank Memor. Fund Quart.*, **41**, 1963, 77.

HAGNELL, O. 'Neuroses and other nervous disturbances in a population of Southern Sweden, etc.', *Acta Psychiatr. Scandinav.*, **34**, 1959, suppl. 136, 214.

LARSSON, T., SJÖGREN, T., and JACOBSON, G. 'Senile dementia', *Acta Psychiatr. Scandinav.*, 1963, suppl. 167.

MALZBERG, B. 'The frequency of mental disease. A study of trends in New York State, *Acta Psychiatr. Scandinav.*, **39**, 1963, 19.

MARTIN, M. 'The great plague of 1665 as a study in human reactions to disaster', *Canad. Med. Ass. J.*, **88**, 1963, 420.

MURPHY, G. E. *et al.* 'Stress sickness and psychiatric disorder in a "normal" population. A study of 101 young women', *J. Nerv. Mental Disease*, **134**, 1962, 228.

OPLER, M. K. (with 22 collaborators). *Culture and mental health.* New York, 1959.

PASAMANICK, B. 'Some misconceptions concerning differences in the racial prevalence of mental disease', *Americ. J. Orthopsychiatry*, **33**, 1963, 72.

VALENTIN, MARIANNE. 'Selbstmordprobleme in Stadt und Land', *Med. Klin.*, **57**, 1962, 1305.

WHO Chronicle, **16**, 1962, 15. 'Mortality from suicide'.

— **17**, 1963, 3. 'The scope of epidemiology in psychiatry'.

YAP, P. M. 'Mental diseases peculiar to certain cultures: A survey of comparative psychiatry', *J. Mental Sc.*, **97**, 1951, 313.

TUMOURS

History

ABBOTT, K. H., and COURVILLE, C. B. 'Historical notes on meningiomas', *Bull. Los Ang. Neurol. Soc.*, **4**, 1939, 101.

BROWN, J. R., and THORNTON, J. L. 'Percival Pott and chimney sweeper's cancer', *Brit. J. Industr. Med.*, **14**, 1956, 68.

COURVILLE, C., and ABBOTT, K. H. 'Metastatic tumors of the calvarium with incidental reference to the occurrence in American aborigines', *Bull. Los Ang. Neurol. Soc.*, **10**, 1945, 12.

MØLLER, P., and MØLLER-CHRISTENSEN, V. 'A mediaeval female skull showing evidence of metastases from malignant growth', *Acta Pathol. Scandinav.*, **30**, 1952, 336.

General geography of tumours

Acta Unionis Internationalis contra Cancrum: numerous reports from recent years.

CLEMMESEN, J. 'Events in the field of geographical pathology and demography (epidemiology) of cancer', *Schweiz. Zeitschr. Path.*, **16**, 1953, 628.

CLEMMESEN, J., and SCHULTZ, G. 'Cancer incidence in Denmark 1953–1957', *Dan. Med. Bull.*, **7**, 1960, 185.

CLEMMESEN, J., and NIELSEN, A. 'Comparison of age-adjusted cancer incidence rates in Denmark and the USA', *J. Nat. Ca. Inst.*, **19**, 1957, 989.

DORN, H. F., and CUTLER, S. J. *Morbidity from cancer in the US.* Publ. Health Monograph. Washington, 1961.

EIBERGEN, R. *Cancer in Curacao.* (In Dutch.) Thesis. Groningen, 1961.

KALLNER, G. 'Cancer in Israel', *Hebrew Med. J.*, **1**, 1962, 215.

LEGON, C. D. 'Cancer in North Wales', *Brit. Med. J.*, **5352**, 1963, 265.

MANCUSO, T. F., and COULTER, E. J. 'Cancer mortality among native white, foreign-born white and non-white male residents in Ohio', *J. Nat. Ca. Inst.*, **20**, 1958, 79.

NEMEC, N. *Bösartige Geschwülste im Sektionsgut des Pathologischen Instituts Zürich.* Thesis. Zürich, 1961.

PEDERSEN, E., and MAGNUS, K. *Cancer registration in Norway. The Cancer Registry of Norway. The incidence of cancer 1953–1954.* Oslo, 1959.

POTTER, EVELYN. 'The changing cancer death rate', *Cancer Res.*, **7**, 1947, 351.

RINGERTZ, N. *et al. Cancer incidence in Sweden 1958–1960.* Stockholm, 1960–1963.

SAXEN, E. 'Report from the Finnish cancer registry', *Schweiz. Zeitschr. Path.*, **18**, 1955, 556.

SEGI, M. 'Cancer morbidity in Miyagi prefecture, Japan, and a comparison with morbidity in the United States', *J. Nat. Ca. Inst.*, **18**, 1957, 373.

Tumours of the different organs

Stomach and intestine

CLEMMESEN, J., and SÖRENSEN, J. 'Carcinomas of the digestive system in Denmark 1943–1956', *Dan. Med. Bull.*, **6**, 1959, 137.

COHART, E. M. 'Socio-economic distribution of stomach cancer in New Haven', *Cancer*, **7**, 1954, 455.

DORN, H. F., and CUTLER, S. J. *Morbidity from cancer in the United States.* Publ. Health Monograph. Washington, 1961.

DUNGAL, N. 'The special problem of stomach cancer in Iceland', *J. Amer. Med. Ass.*, **178**, 1961, 789.

HAENSZEL, W. 'Incidence of stomach cancer in USA', *Acta Un. Internat. Ca.*, **17**, 1961, 347.

HANSLUWKA, H., and KRETZ, J. 'Mortality from cancer of the digestive system in Austria', *Acta Un. Internat. Ca.*, **17**, 1961, 380.

HIGGINSON, J., and OETTLE, A. G. 'Gastro-intestinal cancer in Africa, south of the Sahara', *Acta Un. Internat. Ca.*, **17**, 1961, 333.

KUROKAWA, T. *et al.* 'Cancer of the stomach in Japan'. Report to the Congr. of Gastroenterology, 1958.

RENNAES, S. 'Statement after Torgersen's paper', *Nordisk Med.*, **57**, 1957, 515.

TORGERSEN, O., and PETERSEN, M. 'The epidemiology of gastric cancer in Oslo. Cartographic analysis etc.', *Brit. J. Cancer*, **10**, 1956, 299.

Liver

BROCK, J. F. 'Interracial studies in the south-western tip of the African continent in relation specially to cirrhosis and primary cancer of the liver', *Acta Un. Internat. Ca.*, **17**, 1961, 616.

DAVIES, J. N. P. 'Primary liver carcinoma in Uganda', *Acta Un. Internat. Ca.*, **17**, 1961, 783.

HIGGINSON, J. 'The geographical pathology of primary liver cancer', *Cancer Res.*, **23**, 1963, 1624.

MIYAKE, M. 'Primary hepatic cancer and liver cirrhosis in Japan', *Acta Un. Internat. Ca.*, **17**, 1961, 886.

Lung

BONSER, G. M., and THOMAS, G. M. 'Data relevant to the apparent rising incidence of lung cancer in Great Britain', *Schweiz. Zeitschr. Path.*, **18**, 1955, 885.

CLEMMESEN, J., NIELSEN, A., and JENSEN, E. 'The geographical and racial distribution of cancer of the lung', *Schweiz. Zeitschr. Path.*, **18**, 1955, 803.

DORMANNS, E. 'Beitrag zur Frage der Zunahme der Krebskrankheit mit besonderer Berücksichtigung des Lungenkrebses', *Schweiz. Zeitschr. Path.*, **18**, 1955, 907.

FERRARI, E. *et al.* 'Lung cancer in Venice. An epidemiological study', *Lancet*, **II**, 1961, 1347.

HAMMOND, E. C. 'Lung cancer death rates in England and Wales compared with those in USA', *Brit. Med. J.*, **5097**, 1958, 649.

KREYBERG, L., and SAXEN, E. 'A comparison of lung tumors in Finland and Norway', *Brit. J. Cancer*, **15**, 1961, 211.

Breast

MAISIN, J. H., and LANGEROCK, G. 'Racial factors in the causation of carcinoma of the breast', *Schweiz. Zeitschr. Path.*, **18**, 1955, 690.

STOCKS, P. 'Social status in relation to carcinoma of the breast', *Schweiz. Zeitschr. Path.*, **18**, 1955, 706.

Uterus, etc.

BERGGREN, C. A. G. 'Civil status and distribution in 1,822 cases of cancer of the uterine cervix', *Acta Radiolog.*, **53**, 1960, 137.

DUNHAM, LUCIA J. 'Cancer of the uterine cervix in Negro women in New York City', *Acta Un. Internat. Ca.*, **17**, 1961, 910.

EDSMYR, F. 'Carcinoma of the vulva. An analysis of 560 patients with histologically verified squamous cell carcinoma', *Acta Radiolog.*, Suppl., 1963, 217.

DAMJANOVSKI, L. *et al.* 'Circumcision and carcinoma colli uteri in Macedonia, Yugoslavia', *Brit. J. Cancer*, **17**, 1963, 406.

OBER, W. B., and REINER, L. 'Cancer of the cervix in Jewish women', *Schweiz. Zeitschr. Path.*, **18**, 1955, 774.

Urinary bladder

ABOUL NASR, A. L. *et al.* 'Epidemiology and pathology of cancer of the bladder in Egypt', *Acta Un. Internat. Ca.*, **18**, 1962, 528.

CLEMMESEN, J. 'Mortality and morbidity from bladder tumours in various countries', *Acta Un. Internat. Ca.*, **18**, 1962, 667.

PAMUKCU, A. M. 'Epidemiologic studies on urinary bladder tumors in Turkish cattle. Epizootiology of cancer in animals', *Ann. New York Acad. Sci.*, **108**, 1962, 938.

WYNDER, E. L. *et al.* 'An epidemiological investigation of cancer of the bladder', *Cancer*, **16**, 1963, 388.

Prostate

HIGGINSON, J., and SIMSON, I. 'The significance of comparative pathology in relation to prostatic cancer: with special reference to North America, Africa and Europe, etc.', *Acta Un. Internat. Ca.*, **17**, 1961, 942.

Other tumours

PINDBORG, J. J. 'Oral cancer and precancerous conditions in South East Asia', *Internat. Dental J.* (to be published).

ROTHMAN, S. 'Remarks on sex, age and racial distribution of Kaposi's sarcoma and on possible pathogenetic factors', *Acta Un. Internat. Ca.*, **18**, 1962, 326.

Leukaemia

CLEMMESEN, J. 'Distribution of leukemia in some European countries compared with USA', *Acta Un. Internat. Ca.*, **16**, 1960, 1611.

HAYHOE, F. G. *Leukemia.* London, 1960.

HEYSSEL, R. *et al.* 'Leukemia in Hiroshima atomic bomb survivors', *Blood*, **15**, 1960, 313.

The malignant lymphoma in Central Africa

BURKITT, D., and O'CONNOR, G. T. 'Malignant lymphoma in African children', *Cancer*, **14**, 1961, 258.

ROULET, F. C. (ed.). *The lymphoreticular tumours in Africa.* A symposium organised by the International Union against Cancer. Basel, 1964.

Leucosis enzootica bovis

BENDIXEN, H. J. *Leucosis enzootica bovis.* Thesis. Copenhagen, 1963.

Index

(Page numbers given in italics refer to the illustrations.)

337